Physical Agents

Theory and Practice for the Physical Therapist Assistant

Physical Agents

Theory and Practice for the Physical Therapist Assistant

Barbara J. Behrens, BS, PTA
Senior Instructor
Physical Therapist Assistant Program
Medical College of Pennsylvania and Hahnemann University
Department of Physical Therapy
Philadelphia, Pennsylvania

Susan L. Michlovitz, PhD, PT, CHT
Adjunct Associate Professor
Medical College of Pennsylvania and Hahnemann University
Department of Physical Therapy
Philadelphia, Pennsylvania
and
Physical Therapist/Hand Therapist
Temple University
Department of Orthopaedic Surgery
Philadelphia, Pennsylvania

 F. A. DAVIS COMPANY • Philadelphia

F. A. Davis Company
1915 Arch Street
Philadelphia, PA 19103

Printed in the United States of America

Last digit indicates print number: 10 9 8 7 6 5 4 3

Publisher, Health Professions: Jean-François Vilain
Developmental Editor: Crystal Spraggins
Production Editor: Glenn L. Fechner

As new scientific information becomes available through basic and clinical research, recommended treatments and drug therapies undergo changes. The authors and publisher have done everything possible to make this book accurate, up to date, and in accord with accepted standards at the time of publication. The authors, editors, and publisher are not responsible for errors or omissions or for consequences from application of the book, and make no warranty, expressed or implied, in regard to the contents of the book. Any practice described in this book should be applied by the reader in accordance with professional standards of care used in regard to the unique circumstances that may apply in each situation. The reader is advised always to check product information (package inserts) for changes and new information regarding dose and contraindications before administering any drug. Caution is especially urged when using new or infrequently ordered drugs.

Library of Congress Cataloging-in-Publication Data
Behrens, Barbara J., 1959–
    Physical agents : theory and practice for the physical therapist assistant / Barbara J. Behrens, Susan L. Michlovitz.
        p.   cm.
    Includes bibliographical references and index.
    ISBN 0-8036-0111-5
    1. Physical therapy.   2. Physical therapist assistants.
    I. Michlovitz, Susan L.   II. Title.
    RM700.B37   1996
    615.8'2—dc20   95-26022

To our parents
Marty and Bob Behrens
Mae (in memory) and Nate Michlovitz

Foreword

For many years, thermal, mechanical, and electrical modalities have been applied in facilities ranging from physician's offices to university-based medical centers. All too often these agents have been administered without regard to the distinct physiological effects they can produce or the specific therapeutic goals intended. In addition, the education given to those who apply these modalities has been lacking, as evidenced by my own observations and experience, as well as those of the authors.

The authors are to be commended for simplifying and logically presenting the material and, challenging the reader. Every important aspect is considered, discussed, and questioned to aid in clinical decision making. The principles and physiological actions relative to each modality, as well as precautions and contraindications, form the foundation and also direct the reader into further research.

The major technological advances of recent years and the increasing number and variety of devices and their different mechanisms of delivery have led to an even greater need for education, training, and thought. This excellent text thus discusses the concept that these modalities are adjunctive to one or more of the therapeutic goals that must be individualized by the clinician. A modality by itself should not constitute the entire treatment, but it can be a valuable adjunct when properly sequenced into a comprehensive treatment paradigm. In addition, proper selection of a specific thermal agent, mechanical device, or electrical parameter is needed to selectively obtain the desired physiological effect relative to an acute, subacute, or chronic condition.

Health care is presently in a state of transformation that is creating increased use of clinicians such as physical and occupational therapist assistants. Cross-training among professions is becoming an issue, as well. In addition, occupational therapists are increasingly involved in the rehabilitation of patients with acute injuries to the hand or upper extremity, necessitating an intimate knowledge of adjunctive modalities to assist in the reduction of inflammation, edema, pain, and reflex muscle guarding. Indications for one or more adjunctive modalities at this stage is, however, different from that in the subacute or chronic stage, in which it is distinctly presented as a clinical decision-making challenge. This text presents numerous other situations that challenge the reader to think about the integrative modality of choice with specific parameters for administration.

Both authors and their contributors have a wealth of knowledge and clinical experience dealing with the logical and properly sequenced administration of adjunctive modalities. They have thus collaborated to produce an extremely comprehensive text that will be widely used by many in the field of physical rehabilitation.

Jeffrey S. Mannheimer MA, PT
Clinical Assistant Professor
University of Medicine and Dentistry of New Jersey
Newark, New Jersey
President
Delaware Valley Physical Therapy Associates,
Lawrenceville, New Jersey

Preface: For The Student

Physical agents include the use of heat, cold, water, electricity, light, and mechanical devices for the rehabilitation of physical dysfunction and movement disorders. This text is targeted toward students preparing to work in the field of rehabilitation and clinicians who use these agents as an adjunct to their practice. The book is written at a level for undergraduate education and for the student who has not had a thorough foundation in general physics or physiology. The book has sections devoted to principles for practice, to application of physical agents, and to decision-making paradigm. We are fortunate to have talented and well-experienced authors for each chapter. These authors are involved in the education of physical therapists, physical therapist assistants, and occupational therapists. Many have research interests in the topics about which they have written.

Each chapter begins with objectives and concludes with study questions and an extensive reference list. The body of each chapter reflects practice concepts based on theoretical and scientific evidence for the use of physical agents. The underpinnings of the use of physical agents are based on empiric observations and scientific principles tested in laboratory and clinical research. Students are often given a summary of that research during their course work. Important information can be gained from the research literature but must be put into perspective as it relates to clinical practice. The authors have attempted to do this by integrating information gained from the basic research. The research that has been performed with physical agents has included that from laboratory animal models, from normal subjects, and from clinical settings. The result of each has provided valuable insight for clinical practice, allowing for the establishment of guidelines for the safe and effective selection of physical agents. Examples can be used to illustrate these points. We know that the use of therapeutic doses of ultrasound on patients with malignancies is not safe because tumor growth can be accelerated. This information was learned from studies on laboratory animals. Electrical stimulation promotes circulation to tissues and has been used to heal wounds. We gained this knowledge from studies with animal models and in clinical studies. Each physical agent has similar research paradigms by which we have gained knowledge for clinical practice. This is important for you to appreciate as you study physical agents and then later apply these agents in clinical practice. The "machines" are not just "bells and whistles" to be used randomly and without thought.

We, the editors felt that a text like this has been needed for many years. There have not been any other texts written that have addressed Physical Agents comprehensively with an emphasis on patient outcome. Clinicians and students preparing to work in the field of rehabilitation need to be able to take research data and understand its potential application. They also need to be able to understand the information well enough to be able to communicate it with their patients and determine whether or not it worked.

We, the editors, hope to have been successful in presenting a text that emphasizes the safe, efficacious, and effective use of physical agents. We look forward to feedback from you, the reader.

Barbara J. Behrens and Susan L. Michlovitz, editors

Acknowledgments

We thank the following for their assistance with this book:

—all the authors

—the students and clinicians we have instructed for the last decade plus. . . .

—Ellen Price, MEd, PT and Margaret Snell, EdD, RN, who B.J.B. has studied under

—Carol Morgan, a superb cartoonist.

—Joseph Thoder, MD for giving B.J.B. back the use of her right hand

—Maureen McBeth for photographs in the chapters on ultrasound and TENS

—Crystal McNichol, a gem of a developmental editor . . .

—Sam and Casey, who were there underfoot when we needed warm fuzzies

Barbara J. Behrens and Susan L. Michlovitz, editors

Contributors

Joyce L. Adcock, MA, PT
Chief Physical Therapist
Temple University Hospital
Philadelphia, Pennsylvania

Robert W. Babb, PT
Vice President of Rehabilitation
The Center for Aquatic Rehabilitation
Philadelphia, Pennsylvania

Barbara J. Behrens, BS, PTA
Senior Instructor
Physical Therapist Assistant Program
Medical College of Pennsylvania and
Hahnemann University
Department of Physical Therapy
Philadelphia, Pennsylvania

Jane Brighton Cedar, MS, PT
Instructor
Physical Therapist Assistant Program
Mt. Hood Community College
Gresham, Oregon

Joy C. Cohn, PT
Chestnut Hill Rehabilitation Hospital
Wyndmoor, Pennsylvania

Mary-Ann Dalzell, BScpht, MSc(A)
Faculty Lecturer
McGill University
School of Physical and Occupational
  Therapy
Executive Director
L'Esprit Sport Orthopaedic and
  Sports Medicine Center
Montreal, Quebec, Canada

Elizabeth R. Gardner, MS, PT, NCS
Assistant Professor
Department of Otolaryngology—
Head and Neck Surgery
The Johns Hopkins Hospital
Baltimore, Maryland

Cheryl A. Gillespie, MA, PT
Associate Professor
Physical Therapist Assistant Program
Suffolk Community College
Selden, New York

Burke Gurney, MA, PT
Formerly
Director and Instructor
Physical Therapist Assistant Program
San Juan College
Farmington, NM
Currently
Instructor
Division of Physical Therapy
School of Medicine
University of New Mexico
Albuquerque, New Mexico
and
Physical Therapist
Horizon Specialty Hospital
Albuquerque, New Mexico

Thomas J. Harrer, BA, BSPT
Instructor
Physical Therapist Assistant Program
Kapiolani Community College
University of Hawaii
Honolulu, Hawaii

Kathleen M. Kenna, PT MEd, ATC
PTA Program Director
College of Health Sciences
Physical Therapist Assistant Program
Roanoke, Virginia

Gisele Larose, OTR, CHT
Contract Hand Therapy Services
Larose Ltd., A Consulting Firm
Philadelphia, Pennsylvania

Susan L. Michlovitz, PhD, PT, CHT
Adjunct Associate Professor
Allegheny University of the
    Health Sciences
Department of Physical Therapy
Philadelphia, Pennsylvania
and
Physical Therapist/Hand Therapist
Temple University
Department of Orthopaedic Surgery
Philadelphia, Pennsylvania

Cecilia Mullin, PTA
Research Associate
Shriners Hospitals—Philadelphia
    Unit
Research Department
Philadelphia, Pennsylvania

Elaine Muntzer, PT, CHT
Partner
Hand and Orthopedic Rehabilitation
    Services
Levittown, Pennsylvania

Ethne L. Nussbaum, MEd, PT
Assistant Professor
Department of Physical Therapy
Faculty of Medicine
University of Toronto
Toronto, Ontario, Canada
and
Clinical Associate in Physiotherapy
Department of Rehabilitation Medi-
    cine
Mount Sinai Hospital
Toronto, Ontario, Canada

Wayne Smith, MEd, PT, ATC, SCS
Chief
Assistant Professor and
Academic Clinical Coordinator
Program in Physical Therapy
Kirksville Osteopathic Medical
    College, Southwest Center
Phoenix, Arizona
Trainer
USA Rugby Association

Kristin von Nieda, MEd, PT
Assistant Professor
Department of Physical Therapy
Medical College of Pennsylvania and
Hahnemann University
Philadelphia, Pennsylvania

Contents

Section II. Thermal and Mechanical Agents 49

Chapter 3. Heat and Cold Modalities 51
Kristin von Nieda, MEd, PT, Barbara J. Behrens, BS, PTA, and
Thomas Harrer, BA, BSPT

Chapter 4. Therapeutic Ultrasound 81
Ethne L. Nussbaum, MEd, BSc, PT

Chapter 7. Passive Motion Devices for Soft Tissue Management: Traction

Burke Gurney, MA, PT

Chapter 8. Passive Motion Devices for Soft Tissue Management: Continuous Passive Motion

Gisele Larose, OTR, CHT

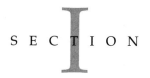

SECTION

I

The Concept of Adjunctive Therapies

C H A 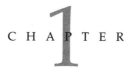 T E R

From Injury to Repair: Pain and Inflammation

Jane Cedar, MS, PT

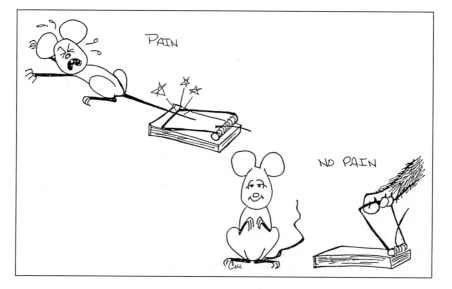

CHAPTER OBJECTIVES

- Define pain.
- Describe the factors that affect an individual's perception of pain.
- Define acute and chronic pain.
- Explain the gate control theory of pain; give examples of the use of physical agents based on this theory.
- Define endogenous opiates; list events that can trigger the release of these substances.
- Describe therapy for a patient in acute pain, including methods of encouraging active patient participation in the recovery process.
- Describe the team approach to the treatment of patients with chronic pain.
- Describe key events that occur in the three stages of wound healing.
- Identify precautions for handling a wound in each of the three stages.
- Describe appropriate therapy for a wound in each of the three stages.

CHAPTER OUTLINE

Pain is one of the most common problems facing patients referred for rehabilitation. It is a symptom of physical, physiologic, or psychologic dysfunction.[1] Pain is often thought of as the body's warning system,[2] the body's way of letting the individual know that something is wrong. Without the sensation of pain, additional tissue damage or injury may occur. Pain may, however, have numerous adverse effects, resulting in symptoms such as muscle spasm and weakness, decreased range of a motion, fatigue, insomnia, increased irritability, anxiety, depression, decreased appetite, sexual dysfunction, and emotional distress.[3–6]

DEFINITIONS

Pain is defined as "an unpleasant sensory and emotional experience associated with actual or potential tissue damage, or described in terms of such damage."[7] This definition avoids tying pain to just a physical stimulus and instead emphasizes that our willingness to call something painful can be influenced by other factors. These factors include our focus of attention, level of anxiety, degree of suggestibility, level of arousal, degree of fatigue, previous emotional and psychologic experience and cultural mores.[3,4,8] In other words, while a sensation may start as a physical stimulus to a nociceptor (pain receptor), our willingness to call the sensation painful is variable depending on past learning and current circumstances, and is purely subjective.

The body's response to trauma is a complex interaction of sensory, motivational, and cognitive processes that determine a sequence of behavior that characterizes pain[1,6] (Fig. 1–1). On a systemic level, the sympathetic component of the autonomic nervous system responds to the perceived threat by a "fight-or-flight"

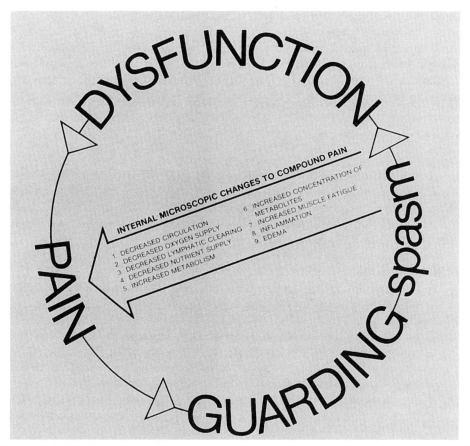

Figure 1–1. Primary pain cycle and associated internal changes. (*From Mannheimer and Lampe,[1] p 10, with permission.*)

reaction. This reaction involves numerous body systems and typically includes increased heart rate and sweating, expansion of the bronchioles (small airways), dilation of the pupils, shunting of blood from the skin and digestive tract to the muscles and brain, decreased peristalsis, and contraction of the sphincters.[9] On a local level, the body will react in three primary ways through (1) muscle spasm, (2) edema, and (3) release of endogenous pain chemical mediators. Initially, when experiencing pain resulting from trauma, the body will try to withdraw from the stimulus. Then a reflex occurs in an attempt to immobilize the injured area through muscle splinting or spasm. This response may occur as the body's built-in way to prevent further damage. This reaction of the muscles requires a high level of metabolic activity at the same time as it compresses the blood vessels. The compromised circulation is often inadequate to supply metabolic needs, leading to ischemia, a new source of pain.

Edema also commonly results from injury because of a disruption of the capillaries and lymphatics by trauma or secondary to compression from muscle spasm. This further compounds the problems of nutrient supply and waste removal and also frequently causes more pain. Finally, endogenous pain-producing substances such as potassium, serotonin (5-HT), bradykinin, histamine, prostaglandins, leukotrines, and substance P are commonly released into the injured area.[6,10] These substances can directly activate nociceptors, or may act alone or in combination to sensitize nociceptors to other agents. For example, histamine excites polymodal nociceptors, bradykinin increases the synthesis and release of prostaglandins from nearby cells, and prostaglandin E produces hyperalgesia and sensitizes nociceptors.[6]

ACUTE AND CHRONIC PAIN

Pain is classified as acute or chronic.[6,11–13] Acute pain is the result of infection, injury, or internal disease. If the cause is diagnosed and treated or removed, the pain is eliminated relatively quickly.[14] Chronic pain may or may not relate to an actual physical injury, and often persists despite treatment.[5,15] The longer the pain persists, the more likely it is to be referred away from the site of the lesion.[11] The reasons for this are not completely understood.

Various mechanisms have been proposed to account for chronic pain. The most commonly described mechanisms follow:[6,10,13,16–18]

1. Mechanical: Clinical examples of mechanical irritation include entrapment syndromes such as carpal tunnel syndrome.
2. Chemical: Chemical irritation in the injured area occurs as the body releases various substances in reaction to trauma, inflammation, or ischemia. These substances increase the sensitivity of the nociceptor,[6] enhance each other's action, and facilitate the release of prostaglandin E. A positive-feedback loop of pain causing inflammation causing more pain results.
3. Regeneration: As nerves are regenerating following surgery or trauma, there can be a period of marked increase in discharges from the peripheral nerve fibers that transmit pain signals (A-delta and C fibers[6,13,19]).
4. Reflexes: Motor reflexes that normally act to protect tissue from acute pain can persist and produce changes associated with chronic pain such as muscle spasm. This can result in ischemia and nerve compression. Overactivity of sympathetic reflexes can result in vasoconstriction, ischemia, and trophic changes.
5. Inhibitory failure: Inhibitory failure involves a breakdown in the usual response of the central nervous systems (CNS).[6,20–22] In response to significant pain, the CNS normally releases chemicals called *endogenous opiates*. These chemicals exert control at the first relay of incoming injury signals in the dorsal horn of the spinal cord and decrease or block the transmission of further pain signals. Some examples of this inhibitory failure are thalamic pain, pain associated with brain or spinal cord injury, and pain associated with demyelinating diseases such as multiple sclerosis.

The transition from acute to chronic pain has not been well defined. If pain meets the following three criteria, however, it is usually termed chronic pain: (1) the cause is uncertain or not correctable, (2) medical treatments have been ineffective, and (3) it has persisted for 1 month beyond the usual course of acute disease or a reasonable time to heal.[6]

Chronic pain is often treated by a team approach with a heavy emphasis on psychologic support and guidance.[11,16–18,20,23,24] The team can include a coordinating physician and/or nurse practitioner, a psychologist, a physical therapist, an occupational therapist, a social worker, and a vocational rehabilitation counselor.

Recreational therapists, dieticians, biofeedback technicians, and other health professionals may also play roles on some teams. The team attempts to empower the patient and his or her family through education. Physical therapy emphasizes active management of the pain[6,22,25] through the proper use of activity alternating with rest, body mechanics, posture, stretching, strengthening, cardiovascular conditioning, relaxation techniques, work hardening, and home use of modalities such as heat, ice, and transcutaneous electrical nerve stimulation (TENS). Manual techniques and modality treatments are kept to a minimum but may include mobilization, manipulation, myofascial release, ultrasound, and electrical stimulation. Other members of the team deal with drug dependency, stress management, assertiveness training, behavioral modification, family therapy, and vocational counseling as needed.

Psychologic Implications

On a psychologic level, the individual reacts to the ongoing misery of chronic pain, the failure of the medical system to provide relief, changes in role and social status, and financial hardship. Many people suffer from depression in the face of these problems. They may also engage in pain behavior and pain games as maladaptive behavioral responses to their situation.[5,6,16,17]

REFERRED PAIN

Pain arising from deep body structures but felt at another distant site is called *referred pain*.[19,26–28] It is considered an error in the localization of pain.[27,28] Mechanisms that cause the referral of pain are based on the convergence of cutaneous (skin) and visceral (internal organ) afferent nerve fibers within the spinal cord and dermatomes, sclerotomes, and myotomes. Referred pain may be an indicator of the spinal segment in which there is a problem.[27] Pain in the L5 dermatome (buttock, leg, and foot) could arise from the irritation around the L5 nerve root, the L5 disk, any facet involvement of L4 to L5, any muscle supplied by the L5 nerve root or any visceral structure having L5 innervation.[27] Another common example of referred pain is the pain associated with angina (ischemia of the heart) and with myocardial infarction (heart attack). An individual experiencing these conditions may feel pain radiating down the arm in the T1 and T2 dermatomes.[22] Pain is felt here because the pain fibers innervating the heart arise from the T1 to T5 nerve roots.

It is important to be aware of common referral patterns in order to identify the anatomic source of pain correctly and treat it appropriately.[29] Also, since pain that is perceived by the patient appears to arise from the area of referral and not the deeper, more distant structures, it is important to be able to explain to the patient why you may not be treating them "where it hurts," but rather that you are treating the source of the pain.

PAIN ASSESSMENT

Pain is a subjective experience and as such it is difficult to measure. It is essential, however, to have some means of monitoring an individual's perception of pain at any given time in order to monitor response to treatment and activity. The McGill pain questionnaire[30–32] and visual analog scales[33] are some pain assessment tools commonly used in physical therapy.

MCGILL PAIN QUESTIONNAIRE

The McGill pain questionnaire is made up of several parts and attempts to measure the patient's perception of pain. Body diagrams for pain location and word descriptors for pain quality are included. The patient's description of pain intensity and the pattern of pain related to activity compose the remainder of the questionnaire. The benefits of using the McGill pain questionnaire include collecting quantitative information regarding pain and providing information on the effects of different treatments and activities on pain perception.

VISUAL ANALOG SCALES

The visual analog scale is another quick and accurate means by which patients can rate their pain[6,33] (see Fig. 2–1). The patient is given a piece of paper marked with a line 10 cm long. At one end is written "the worst pain I ever felt" and at the other "no pain at all." The patient is asked to mark the line at the point corresponding to the intensity of pain felt at that moment. Records can be kept by measuring the position of the marks on the scale from treatment to treatment. Verbal reporting of pain is a variation of the visual analog scale. The patient is asked to rate his or her pain "on a scale of 1 to 10, 10 being the worst pain imaginable, 1 being no pain." This information is then recorded in the patient's chart. Further descriptors of pain assessment are detailed in Chapter 2.

PAIN PERCEPTION

The mechanisms of pain perception are not completely understood,[6] although some pieces of the puzzle are better identified and understood than others. "Pain signals" must be picked up by sensory receptors in the periphery and the signals must be transmitted to the brain for us to perceive pain (Fig. 1–2). This is not a simple stimulus-response situation.[6,10] Many factors modify the signal before and after it reaches the brain.[6,34–38] The following is a brief review of the neural mechanisms of pain perception.

PAIN RECEPTORS

Specialized receptors called *nociceptors* signal actual or potential tissue damage.[2,6,29] The receptors in the skin are understood better than the receptors found in the viscera and cardiac and skeletal muscle.[6] The nociceptors are actually three distinct types of free nerve endings that respond to different stimulus modalities (Table 1–1). The nociceptors do not normally respond to sensory stimuli in nondamaging ranges. For example, high-threshold mechanoreceptors (HTM) do not usually respond to light touch. The sensitivity of HTM receptors increases following mild injury, however, causing the surrounding tissue to become more sensitive to pressure. Polymodal nociceptors become increasingly sensitive following repeated heat or chemical activation,[6,29,34] possibly accounting for the hyperalgia experienced in injured skin.

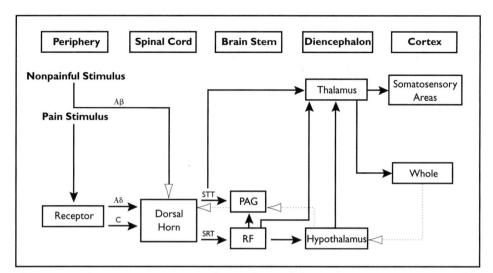

Figure 1–2. Schematic representation of ascending and descending connections responsible for pain sensation. Ascending pathways are represented by solid lines. Pain stimulus triggers a response in the peripheral sensory receptors. Stimulus is sent to spinal cord via the A-delta (Aδ) and C fibers, then to the brain stem (PAG = periaqueductal gray matter and RF = reticular formation) via two tracts (STT = spinothalamic tract and SRT = spinoreticulothalamic pathway). Information is relayed to the thalamus and hypothalamus, then on to the somatosensory areas and other areas of the cortex. Descending, inhibitory pathways are represented by dashed lines. Descending modulation of pain perception is thought to block pain signal transmission in the dorsal horn of the spinal cord. Nonpainful sensory stimulus [transmitted via A-beta (Aβ)] is also thought to block pain signal transmission in the dorsal horn.[10,21]

PERIPHERAL FIBERS

Each type of nociceptor is attached to one of two distinct types of primary afferent (sensory) neurons: small myelinated A-delta fibers and small unmyelinated C fibers (see Table 1–1). The A-delta fibers conduct impulses at a rate faster than the C fibers. Stimulation of A-delta fibers evokes a sharp and pricking pain sensation that is well-localized and of short duration (sometimes referred to as "first pain"[36]). Stimulation of C fibers produces a longer lasting burning sensation, which is dull and poorly localized (sometimes referred to as "second pain"[36]).

DORSAL ROOT GANGLIA

The cell bodies of the A-delta and C fibers, together with those of the larger sensory fibers (A-beta), are found in the dorsal root ganglia at the various levels of the spinal cord. Primary afferent (sensory) signals are transmitted from these ganglia by axonal processes to specific areas of the spinal cord.

DORSAL HORN OF THE SPINAL CORD

A-delta and C fibers carrying pain signals travel through the lateral division of the dorsal root. They may then travel several spinal segments before entering the spinal gray matter. "The dorsal horn of the spinal cord acts like a computer that

Table 1–1   **Types of Nociceptors**

Type	Responds to	Fiber Connection	Sensation	Speed of Conduction
High-threshold mechanoreceptor	Strong mechanical stimulation	A-delta	Sharp "Pricking" Well localized	Fast
Mechanothermal nociceptor	Strong mechanical stimulation Noxious heat	A-delta	Sharp "Pricking" Well localized	Fast
Polymodal nociceptor	Strong mechanical stimulation Noxious heat Irritant chemicals	C	Dull Aching Burning Poorly localized	Slow

processes the incoming sensory signals, rearranging and modulating them before sending them on to the next higher level."[39] Many factors influence which signals are emphasized and which are ignored.

Within the dorsal horn, A-delta and C fibers communicate with several different types of neurons in different layers of the gray matter[6,10,37]. These include nociceptive-specific neurons that receive input only from A-delta and C fibers (pain fibers) and wide-dynamic-range neurons that receive input from A-beta mechanoreceptive (nonpainful) fibers as well as from A-delta and C fibers (see Table 1–1). Nociceptive-specific neurons assist in discrimination of the specific type of pain, that is, thermal, mechanical, or chemical, but do not localize the pain sensation well. The wide-dynamic-range cells contribute to the localization of burning or pricking pain as well as the discrimination between touch and noxious pinching. These cells receive input from the viscera as well as the skin. It is thought that this convergence of noxious stimuli may be the basis for referred pain, because the brain may be unable to discriminate between a visceral or cutaneous source of stimuli.[6] Wide-dynamic-range cells are also called T (transmission) cells and form the basis for the gate control theory[35,37,38,40,41] (see below).

PAIN PATHWAYS

Ascending

In order for an individual to be aware of pain, the noxious input to the dorsal horn of the spinal cord must travel to the brain (see Fig. 1–2). Several ascending tracts are responsible for the transmission of pain signals.[6,10,42] The axons of most of the transmission cells cross over and ascend via the spinothalamic tract. This tract transmits the pain signal to the thalamus. The thalamus acts as a general relay station for sensory information and has precise projections to the portion of the brain called the *somatosensory cortex*.[6,29] Once the signal reaches the cortex it is perceived as a sharp, discriminative, and relatively localized sensation.[6] The second pathway is called the *spinoreticulothalamic pathway*. As the name implies, signals travel from the spine to the reticular formation of the brainstem and to the thalamus. Signals are also thought to connect to nuclei in the periaqueductal gray area of the midbrain and to areas of the limbic system. The information that this pathway conveys is perceived as diffuse, poorly localized somatic and visceral pain.[6]

Descending

The descending control system for modulation of pain is not completely understood. There is evidence that naturally occurring substances called endogenous opiates exist that inhibit the perception of pain.[6,10] Examples include methionine enkephalin (met-enkephalin), beta-endorphin (β-endorphin), serotonin, and dopamine. They work by various mechanisms and are effective for different lengths of time (see below). Release of endogenous opiates is stimulated by systemic pain, intense exercise, laughter, relaxation, meditation, acupuncture, and electrical stimulation.[6]

PAIN THEORIES

A number of theories have been proposed to explain the nature of pain and how it is perceived.[6] Currently, the gate control theory is considered the most complete model of pain.[6] The reader should be aware, however, that knowledge of the nature of pain and the mechanisms of its perception continue to expand.

GATE CONTROL THEORY

The gate control theory was proposed in 1965 by Melzack and Wall[35] and was modified in 1978[43] and 1982[44] (Fig. 1–3). They stated that sensory mechanisms alone failed to account for the fact that nerve lesions do not always cause pain. Instead, they proposed a more complex interaction of peripheral and central mechanisms. Injury activates small-diameter myelinated afferent nerve fibers (A-delta fibers) and small-diameter unmyelinated afferent fibers (C fibers). These nerve impulses excite central transmission cells (T cells) that were proposed to be in the substantia gelatinosa of the dorsal horn of the spinal cord. These T cells receive a convergence of excitatory and inhibitory influences, some from nociceptors and some from other sensory nerve endings. Whether or not further transmission occurs and the pain signal is sent on to higher centers to be perceived by the individual depends on the summation of inhibitory and excitatory influences. In addition, Melzack and Wall proposed that descending control from the brainstem and cortex also strongly influenced the excitability of the transmission cells. They stated that "psychological factors such as past experience, attention, and emotion influence pain response and perception by acting on the gate control system."[45]

ENDOGENOUS OPIATES

In the years since 1965 much has been learned about pain control mechanisms. The accuracy of the original statement by Melzack and Wall that facilitation and inhibition occur and influence the perception of pain is clear; where and how this facilitation and inhibition occur is not clear. A new class of neurotransmitters called *endogenous opiates*[6,10] has been discovered. These naturally occurring "pain killers," including enkephalins, endorphins, serotonin, and dopamine, operate in

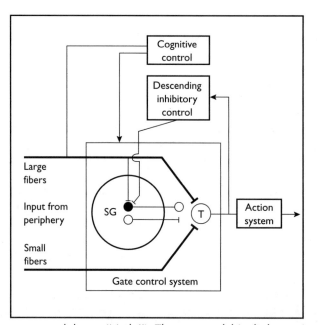

Figure 1–3. The gate control theory (Mark II). The new model includes excitatory (white circle) and inhibitory (black circle) links from the substantia gelatinosa (SG) to the transmission (T) cells as well as descending inhibitory control from brain stem systems. The round knob at the end of the inhibitory link implies that its actions may be presynaptic, postsynaptic, or both. All connections are excitatory, except the inhibitory link for the SG to T cell. (*From Bonica,[6] p 10, with permission.*)

different parts of the nervous system and are effective for varying lengths of time. They may partially account for the "descending control mechanisms" referred to by Melzack and Wall. Enkephalins, short-acting endogenous opiates that operate at the spinal cord level, are now thought to "block the gate" by interfering with A-delta and C fiber signal transmission to T cells. They have a very short half-life, meaning that they are effective while actually present in the tissue and for only a short time afterward. Nonpainful sensory stimulus is effective in triggering the release of enkephalins.

Endorphins are another class of endogenous opiates. They act in several different areas of the nervous system (including the dorsal horn) to inhibit pain signal transmission or to decrease the amount of chemical irritants present in the system.[6,10] The half-life of these neurotransmitters is 4 hours. The release of endorphins is stimulated by a variety of factors including intense pain, intense exercise, acupuncture, laughter, meditation, and relaxation.

Serotonin (5-hydroxytryptamine or 5-HT) and dopamine are also capable of influencing pain perception; however, the mechanisms of their actions are not well understood. Serotonin is released from platelets and activates the primary afferent pain fibers,[6,46] which would seem to increase the number of pain signals. However, serotonin is also involved in the descending (brain to spinal cord) system that inhibits signals from peripheral nociceptors.[47,48] Whether or not serotonin is a necessary link in the analgesic system is not known at this time.[48] Dopamine, a neurotransmitter well known for its role in influencing movement through basal ganglion functioning, may also be used by the body to synthesize morphine and codeine.[49] More continues to be learned all the time regarding these substances and the roles they play in the human body.

CLINICAL VERSUS EXPERIMENTAL PAIN

Experimental pain is pain that is induced in order to study physiologic, psychologic, emotional, and behavioral responses to stimuli. Subjects are often healthy volunteers who are aware of the controlled nature of the study or patients with pain who are submitting to induced pain in order to measure their responses or pain tolerance. Although experiments with pain have greatly expanded our knowledge of the responses to such stimuli, the controlled nature of the stimulus and the situation may very well bias subjects' responses. Care should be taken in extrapolating experimental results to clinical situations. As Wall stated, "in the real world outside the laboratory, the variation in the relationship between pain and injury occupies all portions between injury with no pain and pain with no injury."[44]

PAIN RELIEF

PAIN AS A SYMPTOM OF DYSFUNCTION

Rehabilitation typically focuses on pain which is caused by physical dysfunction or that is the result of disease. Pain is usually a symptom of dysfunction. The underlying dysfunction or problem as well as the symptom of pain should be treated. A complete approach to working with a patient who presents in pain should include:[50]

1. Gathering background information, including mechanism of injury (if applicable), prior medical problems, work background, recreational activity, health habits, and sleep patterns
2. Pain assessment forms, including various pain rating scales
3. Physical examination, including range-of-motion measurements, volume and girth assessments (if applicable), strength assessments, postural evaluation, joint alignment and mobility, soft tissue evaluation, and functional ability

The treatment plan that results from this evaluation should prioritize, then address all pertinent problems. Effective initial treatment of the pain with pain-relieving modalities or medications prescribed by a physician is important to minimize the pain-dysfunction-guarding-spasm cycle (see Fig. 1–1) and is critical to the success of the plan; however, limiting the treatment of pain to medication or physical modalities such as ice massage, hot packs, ultrasound, and light massage is seldom effective in addressing the underlying causes of pain.

Frequently, poor posture and body mechanics, decreased flexibility, and an overall decline in fitness will be contributing factors to the pain problem.[50] Common examples include the patient with a severe forward head and rounded shoulders who complains of neck pain or supraspinatus tendinitis, or the truck driver with shortened hamstring muscles who complains of low back pain. If these patients are only treated symptomatically with pain-relieving modalities and the larger issues are not addressed, there is a high likelihood that they will either achieve poor control of their pain or become "revolving door patients" who return on a frequent basis with the same or related pain complaints.

It is also important that the psychologic and emotional aspects of the patient's pain problem not be ignored. Positive reinforcement of pain behavior may increase the likelihood of an acute pain problem becoming a chronic pain problem.[14,16] Involvement in decision-making and treatment activities by the patient is important to foster a sense of personal responsibility over dependency. If properly administered, even the physical modalities may include education and active involvement on the part of the patient. For example, instruction in proper body mechanics, positions of rest, the appropriate use of moist heat, and relaxation techniques including deep breathing and visualization can all be part of a treatment of "hot packs and massage" and create a sound base for an effective home program.

THERAPEUTIC INTERVENTION—CLINICAL DECISION MAKING

The form that treatment takes, the timing with which it is administered, and the attitude of the health care professional toward the patient and his or her problem are all critical to the successful treatment of pain. The importance of correcting dysfunction as a means of treating pain was discussed above. The various tools that can be used in physical therapy to provide analgesia will be briefly reviewed below. They will be discussed in greater depth in subsequent chapters of this text.

THERMAL MODALITIES

Thermal modalities include: (1) superficial heating agents such as hot packs, paraffin, Fluidotherapy, infrared lamps, and warm whirlpool baths (above 96°F),[51] (2) deep heating agents such as ultrasound and shortwave diathermy and (3) cold agents such as cold packs, ice massage, ice towels, and cold baths. The decision of which thermal modality to use should include consideration of several factors (Table 1–2), most notably, goal of treatment, stage of healing of the injury, depth of the target tissue, patient tolerance and preference, and ease of application (especially for home use).

ELECTRICAL MODALITIES

Transcutaneous electrical nerve stimulation (TENS) is an application of electrotherapy specifically designed for the treatment of pain.[42] TENS units are small, portable, battery-powered pulsatile stimulators. The stimulus parameters used with these devices are based on the theories of pain perception. Two of the more commonly used protocols are sensory-level (conventional or high-rate) TENS, which is set at 75 to 100 pulses per second (pps), a short pulse duration, and sensory paresthesia level of intensity[52] in order to "block the gate," and low-rate TENS, which is set at a low rate (1 to 4 pps), a moderate duration, and a motor threshold level of intensity in order to stimulate the release of endorphins.[52]

Biofeedback is another electrical modality that is frequently used in the management of pain. Biofeedback is used to monitor various functions in the body, including muscle activity, skin temperature, skin conductance, heart rate, respiratory rate, blood pressure, and brain waves. The information picked up by the

Table 1–2   **Treatment Choices: Heat versus Cold**

HEAT			COLD	
Advantages	Disadvantages	Potential Depth of Effect	Advantages	Disadvantages
↓ Pain	May cause ↑ swelling	Superficial: approx. 0.5 cm	↓ Pain May prevent further swelling	↑ Stiffness
↑ Tissue extensibility				↓ Tissue extensibility
		Deep: approx. 4–6 cm		
↓ Stiffness				

Source: Adapted from Michlovitz, SL: Thermal Agents in Rehabilitation, ed 3. FA Davis, Philadelphia, 1996.

biofeedback unit in the form of electrical potentials is then translated into an audio and/or visual signal that the patient can then relate to activity of the body. The idea is to bring physiologic functioning that normally occurs below our level of awareness to our conscious attention so that we can learn to control various body systems. A common application in physical therapy is the monitoring of muscle function[53] to enhance muscle activity in a weak muscle or to promote relaxation in a tense muscle.

TISSUE REPAIR

The body will experience a predictable sequence of reactions from injury through the completion of healing. There are both physical and psychologic factors that may influence the phases of this sequence. Estimates of the length of each phase vary,[54,55] but it is generally agreed that they overlap.[56,57] Certainly factors such as the size of the wound; the general health of the individual, including cardiovascular and pulmonary systems; the presence of underlying disease processes or infection; and the administration of immunosuppressant drugs will influence the course of recovery.

The goals of this next section are to (1) describe the normal response to tissue trauma, (2) discuss factors that affect wound healing, and (3) introduce ways in which physical agents and electrotherapy can be used to influence tissue healing.

TISSUE RESPONSE TO TRAUMA: INFLAMMATION AND REPAIR

The body responds to injury of vascularized tissue with a series of events, collectively called inflammation and repair.[54] Vascular, cellular, hormonal, and immune system responses occur in order to minimize tissue damage and restore function. Skin, muscle, peripheral nerves, and bone can regenerate to a certain extent following cell death; other human tissue, such as the brain and spinal cord cannot. Scar tissue replaces damaged tissue that cannot regenerate. While scar tissue may restore a certain structural integrity to the tissue, it is not as strong as the original tissue (maximal tensile strength of scar tissue is between 70% and 80% of normal tissue[57,58]), is poorly vascularized, may disrupt organ functioning, may restrict movement (especially if it occurs near a joint), and may be disfiguring.

Inflammation (Days 1 to 10)

The initial phase of healing is described as the inflammatory or "self-defense" response.[59] This normal process, which is a prerequisite to healing, does have uncomfortable and sometimes distressing symptoms, including the "cardinal signs of inflammation": redness, heat, swelling, and pain. In addition there is typically a loss of function.[54] These signs are the result of complex interactions of the vascular, hemostatic, cellular, and immune systems.

Immediately following injury, changes in severed vessels occur as the body attempts to wall off the wound from the external environment.[58] Platelets aggregate, blood coagulation is initiated, severed lymph channels are sealed off, and arterioles constrict. These brief but important compensatory mechanisms serve to protect the individual from excessive blood loss and increased exposure to bacterial contamination.

Within a few minutes of injury vasodilation of the injured vessels occurs, resulting in increased blood flow, redness, and heat. Noninjured vessels dilate in response to chemicals such as histamine and prostaglandins released from injured tissues.[55] An increase in the hydrostatic pressure also occurs within the vessels. At the same time, the capillaries and venules become more permeable (because of chemicals called bradykinins and histamine), allowing the release of cells, macromolecules, and fluid from the vascular system into the interstitial spaces. Lymph vessels that normally clear osmotically active particles from this area are unable to keep up with the demand. Edema occurs as fluid moves in to the interstitium to restore the balance of osmotic pressures.

The make-up of the edema fluid changes as the stages of inflammation progress and with the magnitude of injury. Initially the fluid is a clear, watery substance called *transudate*. As more cells and plasma proteins enter the interstitial space, the edema fluid becomes viscous and cloudy and is called *exudate*. If the exudate contains large numbers of leukocytes (white blood cells), it is called *pus*.[54]

For healing to commence, the wound must be decontaminated (by phagocytosis) and a new blood supply must be established (revascularization).[55] Phagocytosis is carried out first by polymorphonuclear leukocytes. In a few days another type of phagocyte called a *macrophage* appears. These cells will remain in the wound until all signs of inflammation are gone. Macrophages attack and engulf bacteria and dispose of necrotic tissue in the wound. They have been called the "director cells" of repair because, by emitting certain chemical signals, macrophages recruit fibroblasts to form scar tissue. The number of fibroblasts relates to the amount of scar tissue. If there are not enough macrophages or they cannot function well enough because of a lack of oxygen, there will be no signal to stimulate the fibroblasts. A chronic wound will result.

As this phase comes to a close, chemicals are released from blood vessels to dissolve clots. The lymphatic channels open to assist in reducing wound edema.[55]

Proliferative Phase (Days 3 to 20)

Revascularization and rebuilding of the tissue occur in the proliferative phase. Revascularization is thought to be triggered by the macrophages[55] ("director cells" of the inflammation phase). Intact blood vessels at the edges of the wound develop small buds and sprouts that grow into the wound area (Fig. 1–4). These outgrowths eventually come in contact with and join other arteriolar or venular buds and form a functioning capillary loop. These loops are what create the bright pink color seen throughout healing wounds. They are extremely fragile when first formed and can be easily disrupted. Immobilization or protected movement is important to prevent bleeding. Vigorous heating at this time may also cause increased bleeding and is contraindicated.[60]

Rebuilding of the structure of the wound occurs by resurfacing with epithelial tissue and restrengthening with connective tissue. This phase is extremely active and is highly dependent on the oxygenation of the tissue. Hypoxic wounds will build friable, poor quality scars. Fibroblasts, which form scar tissue, respond to changes in the electrical potential at the wound (chemotactic influence) and migrate into the inflamed area along fibrin strands.

Three processes occur simultaneously to close the wound (Table 1–3). The process of wound contraction deserves special mention. The purpose of this process is to decrease the open area that the skin must ultimately cover.[61] It occurs by action of the myofibroblasts located at the edge of the wound. This is a normal part of the healing process, starting around day 4 postinjury and continuing to days 14 through 21. Depending on the location of the wound, the results of this contraction process may or may not restrict movement. For example, the contraction of a large scar in the hand may cause functional problems, while the contraction of a large scar on the buttocks may not. Wound contraction is one of many different forces that may lead to a contracture.

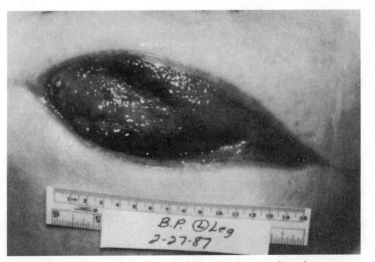

Figure 1–4. Wound bed filled with well-vascularized tissue. Beefy-red appearance indicates good endothelial growth and capillary perfusion. (*From Feedar and Kloth,[63] p 142, with permission.*)

Table 1–3 **Three Stages of the Proliferation Phase of Healing**

Stages of Proliferation Phase	Changes Within the Wound
Epithelization (granulation)	Wound is filled in with granulating tissue, from the edges in and from structures like hair shafts and sweat glands out Epithelial cells seek out a moist, oxygen-rich environment Epithelial cells can only cover 2 cm of open wound
Wound contraction	Myofibroblasts pull the entire wound together Occurs from 4 to 14–21 days
Collagen production	Wound tensile strength is dependent on crosslinking Weak electrostatic forces hold edges together

Remodeling or Maturation Phase (Day 9 Onward)

The long-term goal of wound healing is the return of function.[55] During the final phase of healing, remodeling occurs. There is a balance between continued formation of new collagen and the breakdown of old collagen. As long as the scar looks "rosier" than normal, remodeling is under way;[55] this process may continue for years. Abnormal scars may form when more collagen is produced than reabsorbed. Overproduction of collagen can result in a heterotropic scar or keloid scar (Fig. 1–5).

During remodeling, randomly oriented collagen fibers are replaced with fibers that are oriented both linearly and laterally. By processes not fully under-

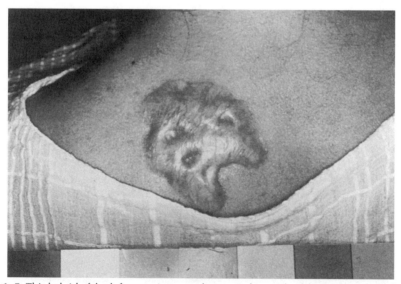

Figure 1–5. This keloid of the left posterior scapula area is the result of thermal injury to the back. This thermal injury occurred as the result of carbon dioxide laser treatment of a decorative tattoo. (*Courtesy of David B. Afelberg, MD, Palo Alto, CA, as shown in Reed and Zarro,[54] p 11.*)

stood, the scar takes on some of the characteristics of the structure it is replacing: repaired ligamentous tissue will ultimately have a different structure than the repaired joint capsule only millimeters away. Two theories have been proposed to explain how collagen realigns appropriately.[55] The induction theory hypothesizes that scar tissue tries to mimic the characteristics of the tissue it is healing. The tension theory hypothesizes that the collagen fibers that lay down during remodeling respond to internal and external stresses that are placed on the wound, and align accordingly. The application of dynamic splints, serial casting, constant passive motion (CPM) machines, neuromuscular electrical stimulation (NMES), and positional stretching techniques to wounds or scars in order to increase flexibility and range of motion is based on this theory. CPMs and NMES are detailed in Chapters 8 and 15.

DELAYS IN WOUND HEALING

Delayed closure of a wound simply means that a wound is taking longer than expected to heal.[62] There are two types of delayed closure. The first is intentionally created by the medical staff when a choice is made not to suture a wound closed (healing by first intention), but rather to leave it open to granulate and re-epithelialize on its own (healing by second intention). Reasons for promoting healing by second intention include dirt in the wound, infection, and excessive drainage. The second type of delayed closure is not deliberate and involves many factors affecting the conservative treatment of a wound. It is important to consider whether the delay is caused by (1) a factor related to the patient's general physical or mental condition, or (2) iatrogenic factors, such as the way the wound is physically managed and treatments including drugs and therapies.[62,63] Factors that can be changed should be addressed (Table 1–4).

An important area beyond the scope of this chapter is wound dressing. The traditional concept of promoting wound healing by "airing" the wound has given way to an understanding of the importance of maintaining a moist environment at the wound bed. Semiocclusive or occlusive dressings are now used to promote re-epithelization, avoid the formation of a crust (scab or eschar), decrease bacterial exposure, and decrease the secondary trauma of frequent dressing changes.[63–67]

Chronic wounds are wounds that are not healing despite conservative or surgical treatment[62] (Fig. 1–6). This does not mean that healing is impossible but that intervention will be needed to improve the chances of successful wound closure. Factors that increase the likelihood of a wound becoming chronic include: (1) medications such as certain nonsteroidal anti-inflammatory drugs, steroids, and immunosuppressive drugs used for transplant patients; (2) acquired immune deficiency syndrome (AIDS): (3) cellular toxicity of commonly used antimicrobial agents such as povidone iodine (e.g., Betadine; Benton-Dickinson Acute Care, Franklin Lakes, NJ), hydrogen peroxide and acetic acid; (4) radiation therapy; and (5) chemotherapy.[62]

FACTORS THAT INFLUENCE WOUND HEALING

Balance is critical to the success of the healing process. If there is no inflammatory response, there is no healing. If there is too little inflammatory response, healing is slow. If there is too much inflammatory response, healing is prolonged and ex-

Table 1–4   **Effect of Local Factors on the Promotion or Impairment of Wound Healing**

Local Factors	Promotion of Wound Healing	Impairment of Wound Healing
Surgical technique	Close approximation of wound edges	Excessive tension Devitalized tissue
Blood supply	Patent	Atherosclerosis Venous stasis Tissue ischemia
Infection	None	Bacteria Mycobacteria Fungi or yeast
Medications	Some topical antibiotics (e.g., mupirocin-Bactroban)	Topical steroids Many systemic and topical antibiotics Antineoplastic drugs Hemostatic agents (aluminum chloride or Monsel's solution)
Trauma	None	Chronic trauma Foreign body Factitial trauma
Microenvironment	Occlusive dressings	Dry dressings Photo-aged skin Radiation injury
Ulcer type	—	Decubitus ulcers Tumor (Marjolin's ulcer) Neuropathic ulcers (mal perforans ulcers)

Source: From Daly,[57] p 41, with permission.

cessive scar tissue forms.[55] Some of the factors that can impair the effectiveness of the inflammatory response include the virulence of the bacteria, the presence of foreign objects, the presence of necrotic tissue, poor oxygen supply, dehydration, certain vitamin deficiencies, lack of protein, radiated tissues, and immunosuppression (see Tables 1–4 and 1–5).

Age is also a factor in wound healing. The neonate may have a modified response because of the immaturity of organ system functioning. Children have a greater capacity for tissue repair than adults but lack the reserves necessary to counteract any significant trauma. This is shown by "an easily upset electrolyte balance, sudden elevation or lowering of body temperature, and rapid spread of infection."[68] Older adults undergo the same healing process as young adults, but more slowly. They are, however, "more susceptible to wound healing problems due to the interactions of body systems, environmental stresses, and disease with an aging process that takes place over many years."[69] Aging leads to decreased efficiency in many body systems, including the cardiovascular, pulmonary, immune, and integumentary.[68,71] This decrease in efficiency affects healing

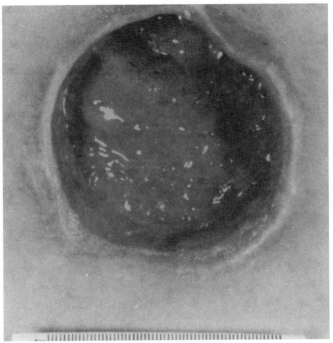

Figure 1–6. Wound edema that contains necrotic debris and bacterial toxins that contribute to chronic inflammation. (*From Feedar and Kloth,[63] p 139.*)

Table 1–5   **Effect of Systemic Factors on the Promotion or Impairment of Wound Healing**

Systemic Factors	Promotion of Wound Healing	Impairment of Wound Healing
Nutrition	No deficiencies	Deficiency of protein, calories, vitamins (especially A and C), trace metals (especially zinc and copper)
Age	Young	Advanced chronic illness (hepatic, renal, hematopoietic, cardiovascular, autoimmune, carcinoma)
Illness	None	
		Endocrine disease (e.g., diabetes mellitus, Cushing's disease)
		Systemic vascular disorders (periarteritis nodosa, vasculitis, granulomatosis, atherosclerosis)
		Connective tissue disease (e.g., Ehlers-Danlos syndrome)
Systemic medications		Corticosteroids, aspiring, heparin, coumadin, penicillamine, nicotine, phenylbutazone, and other nonsteroidal anti-inflammatory drugs; antineoplastic agents

Source: From Daly,[57] p 41, with permission.

(Table 1–6). It is important to remember, however, that there is more variability in the older population than in any other age group: what may be true for a fragile, debilitated 60-year old with diabetes mellitus may not be true for a healthy, robust 80-year-old.

PHYSICAL THERAPY AND WOUND HEALING

Although the medical and nursing staff are primarily responsible for injury management and wound repair, physical therapy may be involved with many aspects of trauma management. Individuals with soft tissue injuries, including sprains and strains, are often referred to physical therapy. Management to avoid an excessive inflammatory reaction includes rest, ice, compression, and elevation (RICE) of the affected part. As healing progresses, other physical agents can be applied, including ultrasound, hot packs, whirlpool, shortwave diathermy, and electrical stimulation.[70,73] Range-of-motion exercises, strengthening exercises, and functional activities may complete the program.

If the trauma includes an open wound, therapy may be involved in treatments including:

1. Hydrotherapy to cleanse and debride the wound
2. Electrical stimulation to promote wound healing[64,72–75]
3. Ultrasound to promote wound healing during the proliferative and remodeling phases[76,77]
4. Hyperbaric oxygen chambers[78] to promote healing of chronic wounds
5. CPM machines to promote organized scar formation and assist in the avoidance of contractures
6. Early controlled mobilization of the injured part, including management of bracing with adjustable locks and exercise to prevent contractures and minimize muscle atrophy

Table 1–6   **The Effects of Aging on the Healing Response[53,56]**

Phases of Healing	Effects of Aging
Inflammatory, "self-defense" phase	↓ 'd and disrupted vascular supplies → ↓'d clearance of metabolites, bacteria, and foreign materials
and	↓'d supply of nutrients ↓'d inflammatory response → ↑'d likelihood of "chronic wounds" ↓'d rate of wound capillary growth
Proliferation phase	↓'d metabolic response ↓'d migration and proliferation of cells Delayed maturation of cells Delayed wound contraction
Remodeling phase	Delayed collagen remodeling ↑'d tertiary cross-linking of collagen → less flexible and weaker scars

7. Positioning programs to protect healing tissue and avoid the development of pressure sores or contractures
8. The design of seating systems (if applicable) to prevent the development of pressure sores and provide optimal mobility
9. Advising staff, patients, or family members in the selection of pressure-relieving devices (specialty beds, mattresses, and seat cushions)
10. Patient and family education in appropriate home activities

SUMMARY

This chapter has dealt with the topics of pain and wound healing. It is important to be aware that knowledge of pain perception and control mechanisms and wound healing continues to expand rapidly. In order to provide the most effective treatment for patients, health care providers must be ready to modify treatment choices as new information and modalities become available.

Pain is a frequent concern for patients involved in rehabilitation. Skillful management of the physical, physiologic, and psychologic aspects of the patient with pain is a responsibility of all members of the rehabilitation team. An understanding of pain mechanisms will lead to appropriate choices of treatment areas and approaches.

Wound healing progresses through a series of predictable stages, each of which may require different handling. Wound closure may be intentionally delayed if there is dirt in the wound, infection, or excessive drainage. Errors in wound management, as well as factors relating to the patient's underlying physical and mental condition, may lead to the development of chronic wounds. The rehabilitation team may be involved in numerous aspects of wound care ranging from debridement to the prevention of secondary complications to optimization of mobility during the patient's recovery.

DISCUSSION QUESTIONS

1. If a patient asked you to explain the nature of pain, how would you explain why some people seem to feel more pain than others? What terminology would you use to ensure that your explanation is easily understood by the patient?

2. How would the psychologic implications of pain perception influence your approach to a patient with chronic pain? Would this approach change in any way if this were an acute pain syndrome rather than a chronic pain syndrome?

3. If the patient asked you why he or she were feeling pain in an amputated limb or pain that travels down an arm or leg, how would you explain it? Be careful to use terminology that a patient would understand.

4. How would you explain the inflammation and tissue repair process to a patient? Be careful to use terminology that the patient would understand.

Your explanation should address the significance and necessity of the process.

5. Prepare an explanation for a patient that would discuss the importance of proper nutrition and wound care to promote tissue healing. Your explanation should include the rationale for keeping the wound moist as opposed to the patient's expressed desire to "let the wound dry."

REFERENCES

1. Mannheimer, JS and Lampe, GN: Clinical Transcutaneous Electrical Nerve Stimulation. FA Davis, Philadelphia, 1984.

2. Sherrington, CS: The Integrative Action of the Nervous System. Scribner, New York, 1906.

3. Tyrer, SR (ed): Psychology, Psychiatry and Chronic Pain. Butterworth and Heinemann, Oxford, 1992.

4. Sternbach, R: Psychology of Pain, ed 2. Raven Press, New York, 1986.

5. France, RD and Krishnan, KRR: Chronic Pain. American Psychiatric Press, Washington, 1988.

6. Bonica, JJ: The Management of Pain, Vols I and II, ed 2. Lea & Febiger, Malvern, PA, 1990.

7. Merskey, H and Able-Fessard, DG: Pain terms: A list with definitions and notes on usage. Pain 6:249, 1979.

8. Kwako, J and Shealy, CN: Psychological consideration in the management of pain. In Mannheimer, JS and Lampe, GN: Clinical Transcutaneous Electrical Nerve Stimulation. FA Davis, Philadelphia, 1984, p 29.

9. Cunningham, DJ: Cunningham's Textbook of Anatomy. Oxford University Press, London, 1981.

10. Kandel, ER, Schwartz, JH and Jessell, TM: Principles of Neural Science, ed 3. Elsevier, New York, 1991.

11. Sternbach, RA: Acute versus chronic pain. In Wall PD and Melzack, R (eds): Textbook of Pain. Churchill Livingstone, New York, 1994, p 173.

12. Bowsher, D: Acute and chronic pain and assessment. In Wells, PE, Frampton, V, and Bosher, D (eds): Pain Management in Physical Therapy. Appleton and Lange, Norwalk, CT, 1988, p 11.

13. Wall, PD: Mechanisms of acute and chronic pain. In Kruger, L and Liebeskind, JC (eds): Advances in Pain Research and Therapy, Vol 6. Raven Press, New York, 1984, p 95.

14. Milnes, S: The Conquest of Pain. Grossett & Dunlap, New York, 1974.

15. Mannheimer, JS and Lampe, GN: Pain and TENS in pain management. In Mannheimer, JS and Lampe, GN: Clinical Transcutaneous Electrical Nerve Stimulation. FA Davis, Philadelphia, 1984, p 7.

16. Miller, TW: Chronic Pain, Vol I and II. International Universities Press, Madison, 1990.

17. Aronoff, GM: Evaluation and Treatment of Chronic Pain. Williams & Wilkins, Baltimore, 1992.

18. Watt-Watson, JH and Donovon, MI: Pain Management. CV Mosby, St Louis, 1992.

19.   Fields, HL: Pain. McGraw-Hill, New York, 1987.

20.   Tollison, CD (ed): Handbook of Pain Management, ed 2. Williams & Wilkins, Baltimore, 1994.

21.   Bowsher, D: Central pain mechanisms. In Wells, PE, Frampton, V, and Bowsher, D (eds): Pain Management in Physical Therapy. Appleton and Lange, Norwarlk, CT, 1988, p 22.

22.   Newton, RA: Contemporary views on pain and the role played by thermal agents in managing pain symptoms. In Michlovitz, SL: Thermal Agents in Rehabilitation, ed 2. FA Davis, Philadelphia, 1990, p 18.

23.   Raj, PP: Practical Management of Pain, ed 2. CV Mosby, St. Louis, 1992.

24.   Ramamurthy, S and Rogers, JN: Decision Making in Pain Management. CV Mosby, St. Louis, 1993.

25.   Wasserman, JB: Physical therapy in the treatment of chronic pain. Clin Manag 6:6, 1986.

26.   Cyriax, J: Textbook of Orthopedic Medicine, Vol I: Diagnosis of Soft Tissue Injuries. Tindell, London, 1975.

27.   Magee, DJ: Orthopedic Physical Assessment, ed 2. WB Saunders, Philadelphia, 1992.

28.   Travell, JG and Simmons, DG: Myofascial Pain and Dysfunction: The Trigger Point Manual. Williams & Wilkins, Baltimore, 1983.

29.   Hanegan, JL: Principles of nociception. In Gersh, MR: Electrotherapy in Rehabiliation. FA Davis, Philadelphia, 1992, p 26.

30.   Melzack, R and Torgerson, WS: On the language of pain. Anesthesiology 34:50, 1971.

31.   Melzack, R: The McGill pain questionnaire: Major properties and scoring methods. Pain 1:277, 1975.

32.   Melzack, R: A short form of the McGill pain questionnaire. Pain 30:91, 1987.

33.   Bond, MR and Pilowsky, I: The subjective assessment of pain and its relationship to the administration of analgesics in patients with advanced cancer. J Psychosomat Res 10:203, 1966.

34.   Perl, ER: Characteristics of nociceptors and their activation of neurons in the superficial dorsal horn: First steps for the sensation of pain. In Kruger, L and Liebeskind, JC (eds): Advances in Pain Research and Therapy, Vol 6. Raven Press, New York, 1984, p 23.

35.   Melzack, R and Wall, PD: Pain mechanisms: A new theory. Science 150:971, 1965.

36.   Bowsher, D: A note on the distinction between first and second pain. In Mathews, B and Hill, RG (eds): Anatomical and Physiological Aspects of Trigeminal Pain. Excerpta Medica, Amsterdam, 1982.

37.   Wall, PD: Modulation of pain by painful and nonpainful events. In Bonica, JJ and Able-Fessard, D (eds): Advances in Pain Research and Therapy, Vol 1. Raven Press, New York, 1976, p 1.

38.   Wall, PD: The gate control theory of pain mechanism: An examination and restatement. Brain 101:1, 1978.

39.   Travell, JG and Simmons, DG: Myofascial Pain and Dysfunction: The Trigger Point Manual. Williams & Wilkins, Baltimore, 1983, p 30.

40.   Wall, PD: On the relation of injury to pain. Pain 6:253, 1979.

41.   Wall, PD: The role of substantia gelatinosa as a gate control. In Bonica, JJ (ed): Pain. Raven Press, New York, 1980, p 205.

42. Mannheimer, JS and Lampe, GN: Differential evaluation for the determination of TENS effectiveness in specific pain syndromes. In Mannheimer, JS and Lampe, GN: Clinical Transcutaneous Electrical Nerve Stimulation. FA Davis, Philadelphia, 1984, p 63.

43. Wall, PD: The gate control theory of pain mechanism: An examination and restatement. Brain 101:1, 1978, p 2.

44. Melzack, R and Wall, PD: The Challenge of Pain. Basic Books, 1983.

45. Melzack, R and Wall, PD: Pain mechanisms: A new theory. Science 150:971, 1965, p 976.

46. Jensen, K, et al: Pain, wheal and flare in human forearm skin induced by bradykinin and 5-hydroxytryptamine. Peptides 11:1133, 1990.

47. Loomis, CW, et al: Monomaine and opioid interactions in spinal analgesia and tolerance. Pharmacol Biochem Behav 26:445, 1987.

48. Roberts, MH: Involvement of serotonin in nociceptive pathways. Drug Des Deliv 4:77, 1989.

49. Matsubara, K, et al: Increased urinary morphine, codeine and tetrahydropapaveroline in parkinsonian patient undergoing L3, 4-dihydroxyphenylalanine therapy: A possible biosynthetic pathway of morphine from L-3, 4 dihydroxyphenylalanine in humans. J Pharmacol Exp Ther 260:974, 1992.

50. Saunders, HD: Orthopedic Physical Therapy: Evaluation, Treatment, and Prevention of Musculoskeletal Disorders. Educational Opportunities, Edina, MN, 1985.

51. Walsh, MT: Hydrotherapy: The use of water as a therapeutic agent. In Michlovitz, SL: Thermal Agents in Rehabilitation, ed 2. FA Davis, Philadelphia, 1990, p 109.

52. Gersh, MR: Transcutaneous electrical nerve stimulation (TENS) for management of pain and sensory pathology. In Gersh, MR: Electrotherapy in Rehabilitation. FA Davis, Philadelphia, 1992, p 149.

53. LeCraw, DE and Wolf, SL: Electromyographic biofeedback (EMGBF) for neuromuscular relaxation and re-education. In Gersh, MR: Electrotherapy in Rehabilitation. FA Davis, Philadelphia, 1992, p 291.

54. Reed, B and Zarro, V: Inflammation and repair and the use of thermal agents. In Michlovitz, SL: Thermal Agents in Rehabilitation, ed 2. FA Davis, Philadelphia, 1990, p 3.

55. Hardy, MA: The biology of scar formation. Phys Ther 69:1014, 1989.

56. Kloth, LC and McCulloch, JM: The inflammatory response to wounding. In McCulloch, JM, Kloth, LC, and Feedar, JA: Wound Healing: Alternatives in Management, ed 2. FA Davis, Philadelphia, 1995, p 3.

57. Daly, TJ: The repair phase of wound healing: Re-epithelialization and contraction. In McCulloch, JM, Kloth, LC, and Feedar, JA: Wound Healing: Alternatives in Management, FA Davis, Philadelphia, 1990, p 14.

58. Cooper, DM: Optimizing wound healing. Nurs Clin of North Am 25:165, 1990.

59. Jones, PL, and Millman, A: Wound healing and the aged patient. Nurs Clin of North Am 25:263, 1990.

60. Paletta, FX, Shedi, SI, and Mudd, JG: Hypothermia and tourniquet ischemia. Plast Reconstr Surg 29:531, 1962.

61. Messer, MS: Wound care. Crit Care Nurs Q 11:17, 1989.

62. Mulder, GD: Factors complicating wound repair. In McCulloch, JM, Kloth, LC, and Feedar, JA: Wound Healing: Alternatives in Management, ed 2. FA Davis, Philadelphia, 1995, p 47.

63.   Feedar, JA and Kloth, LC: Conservative management of chronic wounds. In McCulloch, JM, Kloth, LC, and Feedar, JA: Wound Healing: Alternatives in Management, ed 2. FA Davis, Philadelphia, 1995, p 143.

64.   Feedar, JA, Kloth, LC, and Gentzkow, GD: Chronic dermal ulcer healing enhanced with monophasic pulsed electrical stimulation. Phys Ther 71:639, 1991.

65.   Hollinworth, H: Wound care: Pathway to success. Nursing Times 88:66, 1992.

66.   Bayley, EW: Wound healing in the patient with burns. Nurs Clin North Am 25:205, 1990.

67.   Krasner, D: The 12 commandments of wound care. Nursing 12:34, 1992.

68.   Garvin, G: Wound healing in pediatrics. Nurs Clin North Am 25:181, 1990.

69.   Jones, PL, and Millman, A: Wound healing and the aged patient. Nurs Clin of North Am 25:263–273, 1990.

70.   Rosenburg, CS: Wound healing in the patient with diabetes mellitus. Nurs Clin North Am 25:247, 1990.

71.   Hotter, AN: Wound healing and immunocompromise. Nurs Clin North Am 25:193, 1990.

72.   Kloth, LC: Electrical stimulation in tissue repair. In McCulloch, JM, Kloth, LC, and Feedar, JA: Wound Healing: Alternatives in Management, ed 2. FA Davis, Philadelphia, 1995, p 275.

73.   Nelson, RM and Currier, DP (eds): Clinical Electrotherapy, ed 2. Appleton and Lange, Norwalk, CT, 1991.

74.   Charman, RA: Part 3: Bioelectric potentials and tissue currents. Physiotherapy 76:643, 1990.

75.   Mulder, GD: Treatment of open-skin wounds with electric stimulation. Arch Phys Med Rehabil 72:375, 1991.

76.   Ziskin, MC, McDiarmid, T, and Michlovitz, SL: Therapeutic ultrasound. In Michlovitz, SL (ed): Thermal Agents in Rehabilitation, ed 2. FA Davis, Philadelphia, 1990, p 134.

77.   Dyson, M: The role of ultrasound in wound healing. In McCulloch, JM, Kloth, LC, and Feedar, JA: Wound Healing: Alternatives in Management, ed 2. FA Davis, Philadelphia, 1995, p 318.

78.   McWhorter, JW: Hyperbaric oxygen in wound healing. In McCulloch, JM, Kloth, LC, and Feedar, JA: Wound Healing: Alternatives in Management, ed 2. FA Davis, Philadelphia, 1995, p 405.

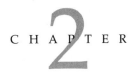

Integration of Physical Agents into Therapeutic Treatment Approaches: Observable Responses

Barbara J. Behrens, BS, PTA

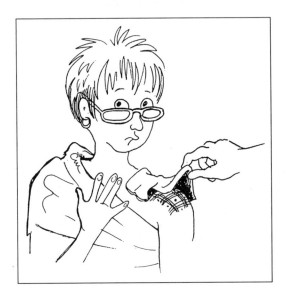

CHAPTER OBJECTIVES

- Discuss the differences in treatment approaches based on experience.
- Outline the treatment goals for physical agents.
- Describe the observable responses to therapeutic treatment interventions.
- Outline patient assessment techniques for pain, edema, muscle spasm, and muscle strength.

CHAPTER OUTLINE

Therapeutic interventions for the treatment of soft tissue injuries may involve the use of some form of a physical agent—whether it be heat, light, sound, compression, vibration, or traction—to accomplish a positive goal for a patient. The selection of the individual modality or physical agent is based on several differing factors such as (1) the diagnosis of the patient, (2) the medical stability of the patient, (3) the identified goals for treatment, (4) the experience of the clinician, (5) the choices available to the clinician, and (6) the cognitive ability of the patient. The influence of each of these factors will vary from individual to individual. Patient safety and appropriate patient selection must remain foremost in this aspect of the decision-making process.

APPROACHES

There are several different approaches to treatment that will result in favorable results for the patient. The clinician should be a good observer and know what to look for when performing any therapeutic intervention. Several approaches to the treatment process will be discussed, including the dogmatic approach, the psychologic approach, and the experimental approach (Table 2–1).

THE DOGMATIC APPROACH

"Dogmatic" refers to the practice of a technique based on the published research, or commonly held beliefs and opinions regarding the validity of a given technique.[1] Experienced clinicians will draw on their past experience in making ob-

Table 2–1 **Treatment Approaches**

Dogmatic approach	Based on published research, commonly held beliefs and opinions (new graduate)
Psychologic approach	How to approach the patient in addition to knowing what to use based on a review of the literature
Experimental approach	Based on clinical experience, the clinician makes treatment selections on the current reports in the literature, previous patient responses to the technique, and the concept of "what if I try....?" (seasoned practitioner)

Source: From Rothstein[2], with permission.

servations of treatment outcomes. New practitioners will use their ability to read scientific literature, consult with peers, and perform accepted treatment techniques to establish their own "bag of tricks" to draw from. Because of their proven reliability, dogmatic approaches lend credibility to both the recent graduate and to the seasoned practitioner. These approaches represent recipes for success or a common ground for all clinicians.[2]

THE PSYCHOLOGIC APPROACH

The psychologic approach involves more than just a knowledge of treatment interventions for a given condition or knowledge of a particular patient diagnosis; it involves just how to approach the patient. A significant portion of the favorable responses seen with any form of therapeutic intervention centers around the patient's ability to comprehend what and why techniques are being done. A patient's understanding of the rationale for a particular treatment, or the mere fact that a rationale was presented, may "make or break" the outcome of the treatment.[3–5] One must be cognizant of the realities of human nature and understand that the treatment techniques are for tissue healing for the benefit of the *patient* with the torn cartilage, not just for tissue healing of the torn cartilage. This simple concept is often overlooked.

Once a patient has had someone take the time to explain what is happening, it can be easier to accept the potential outcome. The explanations need not be technical, unless the patient responds best to technical explanations. They should be phrased in simple terms so that the patient will be able to understand enough to ask a question or report inappropriate sensations during the treatment.

THE EXPERIMENTAL APPROACH

The experimental approach to therapeutic intervention often involves an element of "hit or miss" that is heavily biased toward clinical experience. This is the area where once the dogmatic, accepted techniques have been explored and the literature has been read, the clinician starts to question things by saying "what if. . . ?" Typically this is the world of the seasoned practitioner with years of clinical experience who has observed many patients and their individual responses to a wide variety of both explanations and combinations of treatments. This is the arena for efficacy in treatment approaches. Efficacy refers to the ability to produce results from a set of actions.[6] This becomes the measurement for the success or failure of both the technique and the clinician. Successful clinicians become skillfull in collecting a body of case studies to help justify not only the technique, but how they chose to implement it.

Experimentation with combining and sequencing individual treatment techniques is the mark of the confident and successful practitioner. New ground is broken when clinicians start to look at their rationales, question them, and test their assumptions. This form of experimentation produces both positive and potentially negative or null results in terms of patient progress; however, it allows the establishment of new dogmas or new recipes.[2]

These potentially unsubstantiated approaches or sequences of approaches are performed with one central theme that does not change: the safety of the patient. With any new idea for treatment, the first and foremost concern must be the safety of the patient. Experimental approaches must never cross the boundary of placing the patient at risk. The use of therapeutic modalities, especially electrical or thermal modalities presents many potential dangers to the patient if used incorrectly. These modalities also present many potential benefits for the patient if used correctly and at the appropriate period of recovery. Imprecise usage of a modality can result in a waste of time for both the clinician and the patient, as well as wasting the reimbursement dollar.

The approaches described represent three different components of a successful intervention with a patient. Experience, professional interests, continuing education, and the specific characteristics of the patient population in the particular clinic or treatment setting will greatly influence an individuals' approach to the patient (see Table 2–1).

THERAPEUTIC TREATMENT GOALS: IS A PHYSICAL AGENT MODALITY APPROPRIATE?

The physical agent modalities that this text will address are typically utilized in the management of soft tissue injuries. Soft tissue injuries can produce pain, altered sensation, edema, muscle guarding, muscle weakness, or lack of muscle function. Each of these can be managed by the use of one or several physical agents. These signs and symptoms can also be addressed through the use of "manual techniques," therapeutic exercise, pharmacologic intervention, and rest. However, the modality approaches can also be used in combination with any or all of the other approaches to help facilitate recovery for the patient. The ultimate question for all clinicians will remain the same: "Am I doing all that I can do to improve the condition of the patient safely and expediently?"

The overzealous or inexperienced clinician may use the "shotgun" approach. This involves the use of multiple techniques both manual and mechanical to accomplish a goal. Unfortunately, the patient may report a negative treatment outcome that then could not be traced back to any individual source, since all of the pieces given alone had not produced the effect. For example, suppose a patient is referred for treatment with a primary complaint of pain, which upon evaluation is thought to be caused by protective muscle spasm throughout the cervical spine, limiting movement and guarding the injured site from further trauma. The treatment approach includes hot packs, traction, electrical stimulation, ultrasound, massage, joint mobilization, and therapeutic exercises. Several of the chosen treatment techniques would address the primary complaint of pain, and several of the techniques might be capable of relieving the cause of the underlying pain or muscle spasm. The combination of treatment techniques may or may not relieve the symptoms. The patient's symptoms may increase if any one of the techniques used is not appropriate for this patient.

Clinicians also can get lost in the multitude of symptoms that a patient may offer. Prudent practitioners will identify primary goals, address them with a given technique or modality, and observe and record patient responses. If there are remaining symptoms, another modality or approach might be indicated. Reduction of the patient's "chief complaint" may reflexively reduce his or her other symptoms, but this will only be evident to the observant clinician. If, for example, pain is worsened by the underlying muscle spasm, reduction of the spasm should reduce the pain. It may or may not be true that relieving the pain will reduce the muscle spasm.[8] A patient may not respond well to the specific modality chosen.

Traction, for example, may increase the anxiety level of a patient, therefore exacerbating their muscle guarding, and increasing their perception of pain. If, however, the traction was applied with or following superficial heat, and followed by deep heat and soft tissue mobilization or massage, the patient's initial increase in guarding may be relieved by the deep heat or the soft tissue mobilization rather than the traction. The potential exists that the therapeutic application of deep heat and soft tissue mobilization may decrease the reported symptoms more efficiently than the traction for this patient, but other patients may respond better to the traction. The focus of this discussion, and any therapeutic intervention with physical agents must be *the individuality of the patient*, and his or her responses, both positive and negative.

OBSERVABLE RESPONSES TO THERAPEUTIC PHYSICAL INTERVENTIONS

Several references have been made to the importance of careful observation by the clinician. These observations need to encompass the condition of the soft tissue being treated locally, distally, and proximally. Skin condition can be identified in terms of its color which refers to the amount of melanin, or pigmentation in the skin. Skin condition also refers to the overall tone of the skin and whether or not there are palpable changes in the underlying muscle tone. Skin temperature and surface moisture content are additionally easily palpated and observed, respectively.

SKIN COLOR

It is important to initially observe and document the condition and color of the patient's skin prior to the application of any therapeutic modality. This observation should provide descriptive information such as fair, olive, or dark skin appearance rather than "normal," which gives no substantive information. It should also address the general skin condition for the area being treated and whether or not there are any visible scars in the treatment tissue. Skin coloring gives an indication of the local circulation for the area and the potential sensitivity of the skin to thermal agents. Thermal agents are commonly applied to promote an increase in circulation to help enhance the nutrient base for tissue healing. Fair skin appears "pinker" when local circulation is enhanced by heat. Immature scar tissue is well vascularized and may turn bright red in response to the application of superficial heat. Mature scar tissue may not be as well vascularized as noninjured or repaired tissue; subsequently, mature scar tissue may not take on the same appearance as uninvolved tissue when heated or cooled. For this reason, the presence of a scar in the treatment area is important to note and watch during the application of any thermal agent.[11]

Human skin color is pigmented by a biochemical compound known as *melanin*. The presence of melanin darkens the color of skin.[9,10] Darker-skinned individuals, who may have "olive" or "black" skin tones have more melanin present in the skin than fairer-skinned individuals. Melanin presence will alter the visual responses to local increases in subcutaneous circulation. Typically the skin of "fair-skinned" patients will appear "pink" or "red" after prolonged exposure to the sun. It is readily visible because of the lack of melanin. Darker-skinned patients also respond to prolonged exposure to the sun; however, the changes in skin color with changes in local circulation will be less apparent to the unobservant eye. Patients who have continually experienced severe weather conditions, and have marked "weathering" of their skin, will also respond less noticeably to changes in local circulation.

Circulatory Irregularities and Skin Blanching

Since circulatory changes can be noted to some degree by appearance, it is important for the clinician to observe and identify various skin types and their responses to local changes in circulation. One simple test for circulatory changes is known as "blanching," or the action of capillary refill. Blanching of the skin is the term used to describe the response to applied pressure on the surface of the skin following an increase in local circulation. Fair skin will temporarily lose color when pressure is applied, and as the capillary beds refill with blood, the color returns. Mature scar tissue, when depressed, may not respond by blanching; it may remain unchanged, indicating that the underlying tissue has impaired circulatory function. It also may indicate that the patient will have an increased sensitivity to heat or cold. This simple exercise will also indicate the ability of the capillary beds and arterioles in response to stimuli.[12]

Mottling of the Skin

Mottling of the skin following the application of superficial heat would be manifested by spotting patches of erythema. This may be an indication of overheating of the skin, but it also may be indicative of an individual who has had repeated or prolonged use of superficial heat. Mottling should be considered a warning sign of potential overheating.

To summarize, changes in blood flow to the skin may alter "coloring" of the skin. Scar tissue may alter the ability of a patient to describe sensation in a large treatment area accurately. The patient is thus unable to report overheating. Therefore both the color and the scar tissue of the skin should be examined prior to any thermal modality application.

PALPABLE OBSERVATIONS

Muscle Guarding and Spasm

Muscle guarding is an indication of the degree of motor unit firing present to protect the area whereby a muscle responds to trauma by contracting. This form of contraction helps to prevent any movement from occurring in the injured area, so that damaged or injured structures will not be placed at any further risk. It may be voluntary or subconscious contraction. Prolonged increases in muscle guarding can result in a shortening of the underlying tissue and a feeling of "hardening" so that the spasm now feels harder than the surrounding tissue. The actual number of sarcomeres in the muscle may decrease because of immobility if the resting length is that of a shortened position of the muscle.[13]

Patients will report that they "feel a muscle spasm"; there is still a degree of controversy regarding the nature of the physical existence of the phenomenon the patient describes. Some thermal agents are utilized to help reduce or eliminate these reported spasms or perceived increases in guarding, and it is important to palpate the area before and after applying a modality to it to determine whether or not the treatment technique produced any changes for the clinician and the patient. Palpation before and after treatment is also a way to validate the outcome of the chosen approach. If the clinician assesses the area via palpation prior to the initiation of treatment and fails to reassess the area after the application of a modality, it is difficult to determine the result of the approach. Palpation also assists clinicians in setting up their own library of experiences to draw from in the future. If they routinely notice that muscle guarding appears to reduce following the application of a particular modality, then the next time they treat a patient who reports similar complaints, they will have a potential tool to utilize.

Skin Surface Temperature

Surface skin temperature should change in response to environmental influences. The application of heat will typically cause an increase in the skin surface temperature, accompanied by erythema and possibly perspiration. The application of cold will typically cause a decrease in the surface skin temperature accompanied by a reflex vasodilation erythema. Human skin responds to the application of superficial heat by local vasodilation, which should be observable visually and palpably by a skin surface temperature change.

Skin temperature, color, and overall tone can provide the clinician with valuable information regarding the response or the potential response to the application to a thermal agent by indicating vascular status of the treated tissue. Clinical observation skills will improve with experience and can form the foundation for choices in therapeutic treatment modalities in the future.

ASSESSMENT OF THE PATIENT

Following a thorough evaluation,[14] several treatment goals may emerge, each with its own set of assessment or evaluative criteria. The most commonly treated signs and symptoms using physical agents include pain, edema, muscle spasm, muscle weakness, and the failure of muscle to respond by voluntarily contracting or relaxing.

PAIN ASSESSMENT

Pain represents the most difficult complaint to quantify and document objectively. Pain assessment may encompass a wide variety of approaches to measure the impact of pain on the performance of the patient experiencing the pain. There may be a strong psychologic component to the expression of pain, and the intensity of the experience can only be described by the patient. Because of its complexities, many researchers and clinicians have attempted to compile an objective set of baseline measures to reflect the pain experience.

Analog scales have been utilized in an attempt to quickly measure the level or quantity of discomfort a patient is experiencing. These scales may be visual or verbal and involve the patient assigning a number to his or her expression of discomfort on a scale from 0 (no pain) to 10 (severe pain).

Visual and Numerical Analog Pain Scales

Visual and analog scales involve the use of a 10-cm line drawn on a piece of paper, with a beginning and an end identified by word descriptors "no pain" and "pain as bad as it can be," respectively (Fig. 2–1). Patients are asked to place a mark on the line indicating their level of discomfort[15] (Fig. 2–2). The clinician then measures the distance in centimeters from the start of the line and records the measurement. Following treatment, the patient is given a new, unmarked 10-cm line and asked to reassess their level of discomfort and mark the line again. The clinician then measures the distance to the new mark and once again records the length of the line in centimeters. The patient is given a clean new line to indicate their level of discomfort so that their past responses may not easily be remembered or altered. If the results of the analog line measurements are recorded regularly, then it will be possible for the clinician to actually chart the patient's progress. This may assist in determining if modalities are effective in relieving the patient's pain, according to the patient's reported responses. A similar assessment may be done with numbers from 0 to 10 marked along a 10-cm line, and thus a numerical scale[16].

Pain Ratings

Utilization of either of the analog scale measures for pain involves assessment of the level of discomfort before and after treatment for accuracy. The type of questions asked of the patient are important, and clinicians should be careful not to encourage the patient to respond to the presence of pain, but rather the presence of whatever sensation or symptom is the greatest. Optimally, a clinician would ask the patient to rate their discomfort, and following treatment, let the clinician know just what they are feeling. The questions should not reinforce the perception of pain by using the word in the question.[17] Rather than asking a patient "do you still hurt?", ask "what are you feeling now?" to find out what the primary complaint is.

Patients who are not motivated to recover may skew their responses and invalidate the subjective results of treatment. The patient may also attempt to control the "recovery time" by assigning an arbitrary number to their "acceptable" level of pain in order for them to be able to return to work. They may decide that they are unwilling to discontinue with therapy until their pain, as they

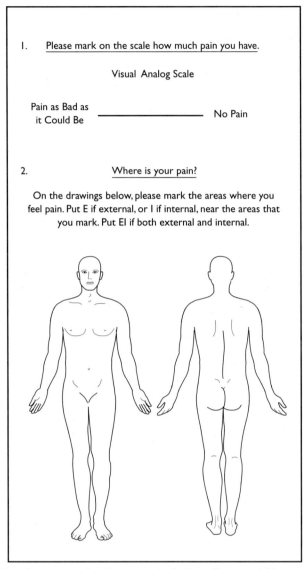

Figure 2–1. (1) Visual analog scale. The unmarked 10-cm line would be given to patients for them to indicate what level of pain they are experiencing. The distance from the start point of the line would be measured and recorded for future assessment comparisons. (2) Anatomical pain drawings. (*Adapted from Parts 1, 2, and 3 of the McGill Pain questionnaire.*)

report it, returns to a level of 3. If utilizing the unmarked line, they may arbitrarily decide that their assessment of their pain must be one third of the distance from the starting point before *they* will be satisfied that they can return to work. This is another reason why pain ratings are just one factor in pain assessment. Analog scales are simple, quick, subjective measures for a complaint. They are not flawless, however, and should not be used as the sole source of pain assessment.

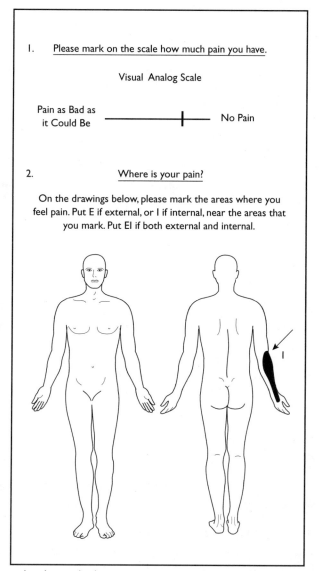

1. <u>Please mark on the scale how much pain you have.</u>

Visual Analog Scale

Pain as Bad as
it Could Be ———————|——— No Pain

2. <u>Where is your pain?</u>

On the drawings below, please mark the areas where you
feel pain. Put E if external, or I if internal, near the areas that
you mark. Put EI if both external and internal.

Figure 2–2. A sample of a marked pain assessment scale. Use of this scale would mean that the distance from the start of the line would not have to be measured to establish a baseline pain assessment. (*Adapted from Parts 1, 2, and 3 of the McGill Pain questionnaire.*)

Pain Inventories as Assessment Tools

Inventories for pain assessment represent another tool for quantifying and documenting the subjective complaints of pain. The McGill-Melzack pain questionnaire was formulated in an attempt to be universally applicable for many cultures, diagnoses, and multiple levels of cognitive understanding. Patients in pain were surveyed to describe their pain with whatever words they could use to capture their experience adequately. The responses were categorized in terms of affective, emotional, and behavioral responses. Participants in the survey were then asked to rank order the phrases or words that were offered in terms of least annoying to the worst experience. Many translations took place so that the information could be utilized with virtually any culture. A standardized version of the test was formulated and a methodology for grading or interpreting it was formulated. Individual categories of descriptors are graded according to their ranking within the category. Thus if there are four words in a category, the first word listed is ranked as the least bothersome, and the fourth word as the most annoying and potentially serious.

Some of the descriptors include words such as "sharp" or "dull," which will assist the clinician in assessing the ease of localization of the discomfort. As discussed in Chapter 1, pain receptors can be A-delta fibers, transmitting fast "pain of injury," or they may be C fibers, which are responsible for the transmission of the "pain of suffering" or a difficult-to-identify aching sensation.

The McGill-Melzack pain questionnaire records information about sensory, affective, and evaluate components of the patient's pain experience and is quite comprehensive[29,30](Fig. 2–3).

Anatomic Pain Drawings

Anatomic line drawings allow the patient to locate just where he or she is experiencing discomfort. This drawing guides the clinician to the primary area(s) of discomfort. This type of information can be extremely important if radiating pain is present, since it may indicate the original source. It also acts as a road map for patients who are experiencing multiple areas of involvement, since they may "color in" the worst area first. Caution should be observed when interpreting these drawings if the clinician is unable to solicit responses directly from the patient, since some patients may have difficulty recognizing a particular part of the body on the line drawing. This would be another reason that the drawing should be completed in the presence of a clinician who is available to answer questions as they arise. Technology has introduced computer animation to pain drawings and pain drawing analysis, which may lead to further refinement of the data obtained.[31-35]

Inventories should be filled out by patients while they are comfortably positioned and relaxed, possibly while waiting to be seen by the clinician. The anatomic pain drawing, however, should be completed in the presence of a clinician so that any sequencing can be noted.[18] Although the information obtained in these inventories is useful, it is by no means complete and should be accompanied by other performance-related assessments.

Facial Expression of Pain

Facial expression can be another way of assessing a patient's subjective complaints of pain. Facial musculature, particularly in the forehead and around the eyes, will contract in response to pain perception. A patient may not verbally express discomfort because of his or her cultural background, but may "look like" he or she is in pain.[19] Following treatment the patient appears more comfortable, despite responses indicating no change in level of discomfort (Fig. 2–4).

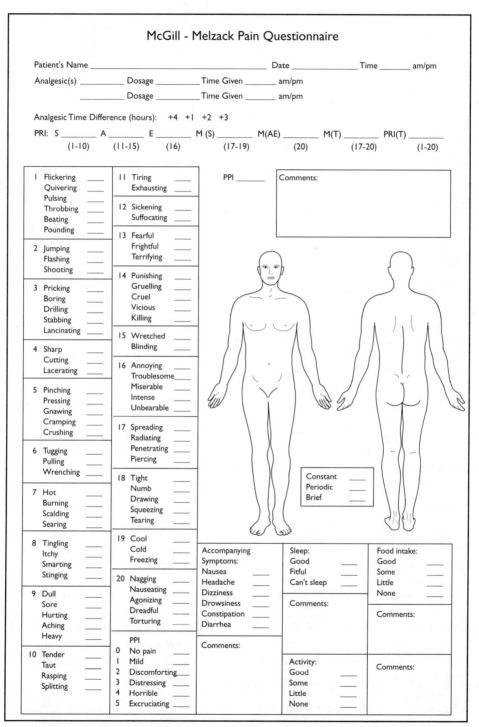

Figure 2–3. The McGill-Melzack pain questionnaire. (*Courtesy of R. Melzack.*)

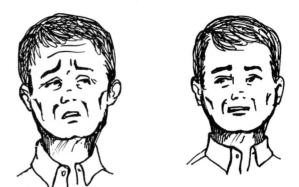

Figure 2–4. Facial expression can indicate whether or not an individual is experiencing pain.

Mobility and Function

Mobility and function are objective assessment tools for the patient complaining of pain. Range-of-motion (ROM) measurements can document the pain-free movement of an extremity. If following treatment a patient is able to increase the available range of motion, then we may assume pain has diminished.

Since pain can only be quantified by the person experiencing it, the importance of multiple avenues to assess it are critical. It is also important to remember that not all patients who seek assistance in the management of pain have legitimate complaints. Secondary gain, or the potential of a legal battle, may influence a patient's responses to treatment, so that the patient does not report any decrease in discomfort until monetary settlement has been made. Working with patients who are influenced by outside sources to prolong the course of treatment may be particularly frustrating for the new graduate or inexperienced clinician[20] but can be difficult for the seasoned clinician as well.

Documentation of as many indicators of pain as are feasible and appropriate for the situation should be recorded. Both time and experience are required to become comfortable and knowledgeable in assessing treatment effectiveness.

EDEMA ASSESSMENT

Edema, or swelling, is an abnormal increase in the amount of interstitial fluid. It may be diffuse throughout the area or localized to the injury site.[21] Edema in small quantities is a normal response to trauma, and it is necessary for repair. Prolonged and or massive edema can interrupt repair by impeding diffusion of nutrients to cells or perhaps by leading to tissue fibrosis. To assess the degree of edema present in an area accurately, there are several options, depending on the location of the edema. The options include circumferential joint measurements, volumetric water displacement, joint mobility, and the performance of an activity that may have been limited by edema. (Refer to Chapter 9 for an in-depth explanation of the physiology of edema.)

Circumferential Joint Measurement

Using a tape measure can be one of the quickest, easiest, and most accurate ways to assess the presence of edema. For consistency of measurement, the following factors must be adhered to:

1. Use of a tape measure that does not stretch
2. Measurement with the same tape each time
3. Measurement by the same individual
4. Measurement at the same time of day
5. Measurement using the same bony landmarks
6. Measurement using the same technique
7. Measurement using the same unit of measure (inches or centimeters)

If these factors are adhered to, then there will be a reasonable degree of accuracy of the measurements. Further details regarding circumferential measurement can be found in Chapter 9.

Volumetric Water Displacement

When edema is confined to distal extremities, volumetric measures are practical and accurate. A volumeter is a device that measures water displacement to record the volume that an extremity submerged in water occupies. If an edematous extremity is placed in a known volume of water, and the volume of water is measured again while the extremity is immersed, then the volume of that part of the extremity can be calculated. Subsequent measurements will reveal the status of the edema and whether the volume displaced will increase, decrease, or remain stationary. Some critical factors for accuracy of this form of measurement include the following:

1. The time of day of the measurement should be the same
2. The temperature of the water should be the same
3. The depth of the immersion of the extremity must be the same
4. The unit of measure of water displacement must be the same, whether ounces or milliliters.

There are commercially available Plexiglas hand and foot volumeters (Volumetrics Limited, Idyllwild, CA) whose accuracy is known (Fig. 2–5). There can be several disadvantages to volumetric measurements as the sole source of assessment of edema. This form of assessment looks at total volume of the part immersed, but does not account for individual areas of excessive edema relative to the diffuse edema. It does not enable the clinician to document precisely where the edema is located, simply that there is swelling. It is not as practical to use for the assessment of an entire extremity as circumferential joint measurements would be. Despite these disadvantages, it can be a useful and time-efficient form of edema assessment for foot and ankle, wrist or hand.[22]

Joint Mobility or Ease of Movement

The presence of edema can impede joint movement. It would not be uncommon for joint ROM to be restricted because of edema. Measurements of available joint ROM with a goniometer can provide additional objective baselines with which to compare following therapeutic intervention.[23]

Performance of an Activity Limited by Edema

A patient's ability to perform activities of daily living (ADLs) may be impaired by the presence of edema.[24] The limitation of movement caused by an increase in edema may inhibit the patient's ability to don a garment, such as difficulty putting on socks or stockings because of the edema in a foot or ankle.

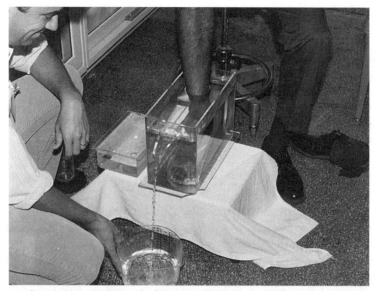

Figure 2–5. Volumetric assessment of edema can be performed utilizing a volumeter and water displacement. (*From Watkins, MP: Clinical evaluation of thermal agents. In Michlovitz, S [ed]: Thermal Agents in Rehabilitation, ed 2. FA Davis, Philadelphia, 1990, p 236, with permission.*)

What Should Be Monitored for Edema Management?

Assessment of edema will take into account all of the elements that apply to the individual patient. If the possibility of volumetric and circumferential joint measurements is feasible, then both should be monitored. To be considered valid, the form of assessment should be kept consistent for a given patient. If a patient has an acute ankle sprain, and the initial evaluation utilized volumetric measurements for edema, then any reassessment of the edema should also employ volumetric measurements. If, however, the initial evaluation utilized circumferential joint measurements, then the subsequent assessments of edema should utilize circumferential joint measurements.

Since there are several methods that can be used, it is not incorrect to use whatever will give the most comprehensive picture of the patient's condition and therapeutic results. If the initial evaluation utilized a volumetric measure, reassessment would employ the same technique; however, it would not be inappropriate to monitor circumferential joint measurements, ROM, and independence in the performance of ADLs as well.

MUSCLE SPASM ASSESSMENT

Muscle spasm or muscle guarding may severely inhibit a patient's recovery. The assessment of muscle spasm may also take several forms, muscle tone assessment, postural assessment, tissue compliance, and the ease of movement or ROM. Each of these assessments may be utilized as part of the total picture of the patient's condition.

MUSCLE TONE AND TISSUE COMPLIANCE

Muscle tone refers to the resistance of the muscle to passive stretch or elongation, or how "tight" it feels. When a muscle guards, it assumes a shortened state to help protect the area from further injury. Its tone may therefore be increased protectively, and it feels harder than uninvolved tissue when palpated.[25] The ease of reaching the determination that a muscle is guarding comes with experience in palpating a multitude of soft tissue injuries on a wide variety of patients. Muscle tightness and its cause are difficult to assess objectively without an external source of measurement such as a surface electromyographic (EMG) reading of the electrical activity taking place within the muscle.

Tissue tone or tissue compliance assessments rely heavily on the experience of the clinician monitoring them. In many acute pain conditions, the patient will experience some degree of tenderness in the injured soft tissue. Tissue tone changes may or may not be one of the first palpable signs of injury. If muscle guarding is present, then it will typically occur in both the agonist and antagonistic muscle groups crossing or surrounding the injured area. Palpation comparisons of the involved and uninvolved side will provide further insight as to the level of discomfort that the patient is experiencing. This is another subjective assessment that can be employed.

Objective tools have been developed to help determine tissue compliance in the form of strain gauges; however, their use clinically is not yet widespread. Most of the determinations that are made are based on the clinical experience of the practitioner. Strain gauges are calibrated to detect the amount of applied pressure administered to a patient. They then can objectively quantify just how much force was exerted on the surface of the skin before the patient complained of discomfort. These devices are referred to as dolorimeters or algometers.[27,28,36–38]

This section has dealt with the concept of tissue compliance and its impact on the condition of the patient as well as on the progress of the patient. Since most of the aforementioned tools rely heavily on the clinical experience of the practitioner, the emergence of tools to measure and document clinical observations objectively was logical.

POSTURAL ASSESSMENT

If the patient is experiencing muscle guarding with an increase in muscle tone, and the injured area involves postural muscles, this may be reflected in the patient's sitting or standing posture. Patients who have injured the cervical spine or who have had a "whiplash" or cervical strain will have different sitting postures than individuals who have not experienced this type of trauma. In many patients with cervical strains, the cervical muscles guard in both anterior and posterior regions supporting the head, and limiting the mobility of the head. They may visually look as if they have a "forward head posture," where the head is displaced anteriorly on the cervical spine because of the increased anterior cervical musculature tone or guarding, and the increased posterior guarding increasing the posterior lordosis of the cervical spine[39,40] (Fig. 2–6).

Lumbar musculature may respond in a similar manner to the cervical musculature. Postural assessment of the lumbar region may reveal that there is a unilateral shift away from the site of injury or toward the site of injury. In most cases,

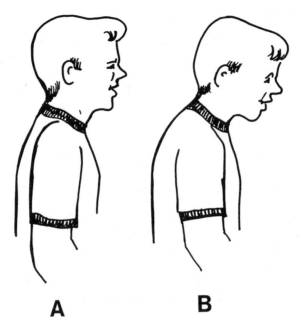

A   **B**

Figure 2–6. Illustration depicts (A) normal cervical posture and (B) "forward head posture."

there will be some palpable or observable change in the normal symmetry of the patient.[26]

RANGE OF MOBILITY

As with other forms of assessment, the measurement of joint ROM can give an objective measure of the available movement of a joint. In the case of muscle spasm, an agonist muscle spasm may limit the antagonistic direction of joint ROM. This simple assessment tool should be a part of every peripheral joint assessment to determine whether or not progress has been made with a particular procedure.

MUSCLE STRENGTH ASSESSMENTS

Muscle strength assessment can be accomplished either manually or with the use of sophisticated equipment to record force or torque production. A manual test of the strength of a muscle is known as a *manual muscle test* (MMT). MMTs assess specific muscle contractions or gross muscle actions and can provide the clinician with insight into the strength of response. MMTs are performed when the area to be tested is stabilized and the active and passive ROM have been assessed. Resistance is then applied. The patient is given verbal instructions to resist the movement or force being applied to the area. If a patient fails to complete the full ROM or fails to elicit a muscle contraction, there are "grades" given to the response.

More reproducible testing of muscle performance may involve the use of a commercially manufactured dynamometer such as those by CYBEX isokinetic dynamometer (Ronkonkoma, NY) to apply force to the limb being tested. This equipment also provides for proximal stabilization for the patient when resistance is applied to the distal extent of the tested extremity. There is a force reading or torque output recorded by the equipment during the test. Subsequent tests should reveal increases in torque output if a patient is progressing and all testing factors are kept constant, such as position, speed, stabilization, and test position.

PUTTING IT ALL TOGETHER

A physical agent is applied to effect a positive change in the condition of the patient. Observation of the initial condition and then reassessment of the patient following any therapeutic intervention will justify either the continuation of care, with or without modification, or the termination of treatment. Without a carefully constructed process for these assessments, it is difficult to ascertain whether or not progress is being made. If a patient is beginning to regain his or her strength, has experienced a decrease in the level of discomfort, has less edema, and has less muscle spasm limiting function, then he or she can start to become more independent. Patient independence is the cornerstone of therapeutic intervention: management of the dysfunction and encouragement to perform as much as can safely be performed.

DISCUSSION QUESTIONS

1. What are the differences among the approaches that can be taken in any therapeutic intervention approach?

2. Where does clinical experience influence the approach that is taken in determining a therapeutic intervention to enhance patient recovery?

3. Of what significance is the cognitive ability of the patient in response to a therapeutic intervention approach?

4. What are the components of pain assessment?

5. What are the components of edema assessment?

6. Which assessment tool(s) would provide data for the determination of several individual symptoms, for example, edema and muscle spasm, and how?

REFERENCES

1. Webster's 9th New Collegiate Dictionary. Merriam-Webster, Springfield, MA, 1987, p 373.

2. Rothstein, JM: Cookbooks and aphorisms (editor's note). Phys Ther 74:6, 1994.

3. Clark, WC and Yang, JC: Applications of sensory decision theory to problems in laboratory and clinical pain. In Melzack, R (ed): Pain Measurement and Assessment. Raven Press, New York, 1983, pp 15–19.

4. Melzak, R and Wall, PD: The Challenge of Pain. Basic Books, New York, 1983, pp 332–333.

5. Cousins, N: Anatomy of an Illness. Bantam Books, New York, 1979, pp 49–69.

6. Webster's 9th New Collegiate Dictionary. Merriam-Webster, Springfield, MA, 1987, p 397.

7. Melzack, R: Seminar notes. Pain Management Seminar, New York, NY, October, 1982.

8. Dwarakanath, GK: Pathophysiology of pain. In Warfield, CA (ed): Manual of Pain Management. JB Lippincott, Philadelphia, 1991, p 3.

9. Miller, MA, Drakontides, AB, and Leavell, LC: Kimber-Gray-Stackpole's Anatomy and Physiology, ed 17. Macmillan, New York, 1977, p 317.

10. Scanlon, VC and Sanders, T: Essentials of Anatomy and Physiology, ed 2. FA Davis, Philadelphia, 1995, pp 88–89.

11. Lehmann, JF and DeLateur, BJ: Therapeutic heat. In Lehmann, JF (ed): Therapeutic Heat and Cold, ed 3d. Williams & Wilkins, Baltimore, 1982, p 424.

12. McCulloch, JM: Evaluation of patients with open wounds. In McCulloch, JM, Kloth, LC, and Feedar, J: Wound Healing: Alternatives in Management, ed 2. FA Davis, Philadelphia, 1995, p 125.

13. Soderberg, GL: Skeletal muscle function. In Currier, DP and Nelson, RM: Dynamics of Human Biologic Tissues. FA Davis, Philadelphia, 1992, pp 92–93.

14. Rothstein, JM: Task force on standards for measurement of physical therapy. Phys Ther 71:595, 1991.

15. Melzack, R: Pain Measurement and Assessment. Raven Press, New York, 1983, p 33.

16. Warfield, CA (ed): Manual of Pain Management. JB Lippincott, Philadelphia, 1991, pp 20–23.

17. Melzack, R: The Challenge of Pain. Basic Books, New York, 1983, pp 37–47, 173–179.

18. Melzack, R: The Challenge of Pain. Basic Books, New York, 1983, pp 41–47.

19. Melzack, R: The Challenge of Pain. Basic Books, New York, 1983, pp 173–179.

20. Warfield, CA (ed): Manual of Pain Management: JB Lippincott, Philadelphia, 1991, pp 16–19.

21. Scanlon, VC and Sanders, T: Essentials of Anatomy and Physiology, ed 2. FA Davis, Philadelphia, 1995, p 439.

22. McCulloch, JM: Evaluation of patients with open wounds. In McCulloch, JM, Kloth, LC, and Feedar, J: Wound Healing: Alternatives in Management, ed 2. FA Davis, Philadelphia, 1995, p 123.

23. Krusen, FH, Kotke, FJ, and Ellwood PM: Handbook of Physical Medicine and Rehabilitation. WB Saunders, Philadelphia, 1971, pp 709–711.

24. Kessler, RM and Hertling, D: Management of Common Musculoskeletal Disorders. Harper and Row Publishers, Philadelphia, 1983, pp 44–46.

25. Saunders, HD: Evaluation and Treatment of Musculoskeletal Disorders. H Duane Saunders, Minneapolis, 1982, p 11.

26. Saunders, HD: Evaluation and Treatment of Musculoskeletal Disorders. H Duane Saunders, Minneapolis, 1982, pp 20–22.

27. Fischer, AA: Clinical use of tissue compliance meter for documentation of soft tissue pathology. Clin J Pain 3:23, 1987.

28. Fischer, AA: Pressure threshold measurement for diagnosis of myofacial pain and evaluation of treatment results. Clin J Pain 2:207, 1987.

29. Lowe, NK, Walker, SN, and MacCallum, RC: Confirming the theoretical structure of the McGill Pain Questionnaire in acute clinical pain. Pain 46:52, 1991.

30. Holroyd, KA, et al: A multi-center evaluation of the McGill Pain Questionnaire: Results from more than 1700 chronic pain patients. Pain 48:301, 1992.

31. Swanston, M, et al: Pain assessment with interactive computer animation. Pain 53:347, 1993.

32. Chan, CW, et al: The pain drawing and Waddell's nonorganic physical signs in chronic low-back pain. Spine 18:1717, 1993.

33. North, RB, et al: Automated "pain drawing" analysis by computer-controlled, patient-interactive neurological stimulation system. Pain 50:51, 1992.

34. Toomey, TC, et al: Relationship of pain drawing scores to ratings of pain description and function. Clin J Pain 7:269, 1993.

35. Mann, HN, et al: Initial-impression diagnosis using low-back pain patient pain drawings. Spine 18: 41, 1993.

36. Atkins, CJ, et al: An electronic method for measuring joint tenderness in rheumatoid arthritis. Arthritis Rheum 35:407, 1992.

37. Bryan, AS, Klenerman, L, and Bowsher, D: The diagnosis of reflex sympathetic dystrophy using an algometer. Bone Joint Surg (Br), 73:644, 1991.

38. Cott, A, et al: Interrater reliability of the tender point criterion for fibromyalgia, Rheumatology 19:1955, 1992.

39. Cailliet, R: Neck and Arm Pain, ed 3. FA Davis, Philadelphia, 1991, pp 74–75.

40. Saunders, HD: Evaluation and Treatment of Musculoskeletal Disorders. H Duane Saunders, Minneapolis, 1982, p 66.

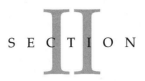

S E C T I O N

Thermal and Mechanical Agents

Heat and Cold Modalities

Kristin von Nieda, MEd, PT
Barbara J. Behrens, BS, PTA
Thomas Harrer, PT

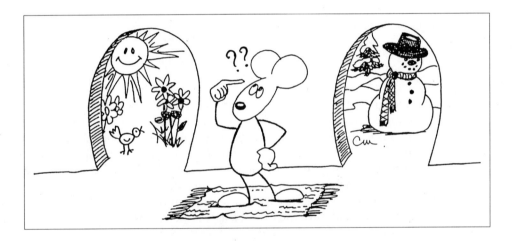

CHAPTER OBJECTIVES

- Describe the different types of heat modalities.
- Discuss the application techniques for heat modalities.
- Differentiate between the possible choices of heat modalities.
- Describe the different types of cold modalities.
- Discuss the application techniques of cold modalities.
- Differentiate between the possible choices of cold modalities.
- Discuss the clinical decision making involved in utilizing heat or cold modalities.

CHAPTER OUTLINE

Hippocrates recognized the benefits of using hot rocks and thermal baths to relieve joint stiffness and to promote relaxation, as well as the use of snow for relief of soft tissue injuries. Since that time, the methods of applying thermal agents have progressed, but many of Hippocrates' application principles remain viable. This chapter provides a review of the literature and the necessary background for developing critical thinking processes and problem-solving skills for appropriate clinical application of heat and cold modalities. Knowledge of the body's physiologic responses to heat and cold provides the basis for decisions regarding the use, method of application, and treatment duration of thermal agents.

TEMPERATURE REGULATION

Temperature regulation in the presence of temperature fluctuations occurs to maintain homeostasis through the interaction of local and central neural mechanisms. Sensory receptors in the skin, muscles, and joints respond to changes in temperature. Sufficient intensity of and exposure to the stimulus are needed for activation of the temperature-regulating center in the hypothalamus. Upon reaching the hypothalamus, the information is integrated and interpreted, resulting in the activation of temperature-regulating mechanisms, such as circulatory changes, shivering, or sweating.[1] Knowledge of basic neuroanatomy and neural transmission is necessary to understand temperature regulation in the body. Neural transmission is a function of first-, second-, and third-order afferent and efferent neurons or nerve fibers. Afferent neurons conduct sensory information from the periphery to the brain. Efferent neurons conduct motor information from the brain to the periphery. First-order neurons transmit information from thermal receptors or free nerve endings and terminate in the dorsal horn of the spinal cord. Second-order neurons transmit information along ascending or descending tracts of the white matter of the spinal cord and terminate in the thalamus. Third-order neurons transmit ascending sensory and descending motor information between the thalamus and the cerebral cortex. For example, the *affect* of stepping on a nail has the *effect* of withdrawing from a nail. The sensory afferent input to the cerebral cortex stimulates an efferent response resulting in a motor effect (Figs. 3–1, 3–2). Chapter 1 of this text provides detailed information.

PHYSICAL MECHANISMS OF HEAT EXCHANGE

The means by which therapeutic heat or cold is delivered to the target tissue is attributed to the following physical mechanisms: conduction, convection, radiation, conversion, or evaporation. The extent of temperature change results from several of the following factors:

1. Temperature difference between the thermal agent and the treatment tissue
2. Time of exposure to the thermal agent.
3. Thermal conductivity of the treatment tissue.
4. Intensity of the thermal agent.

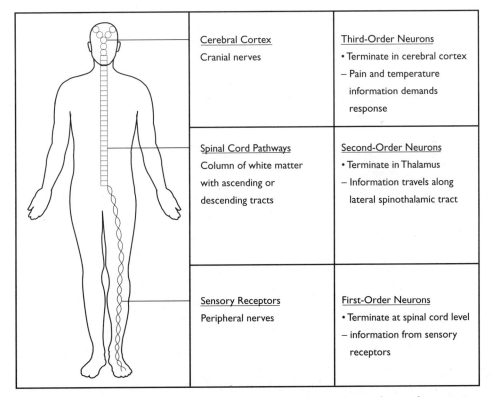

Figure 3–1. The first-, second-, and third-order neuron transmission pathways for sensation perception.

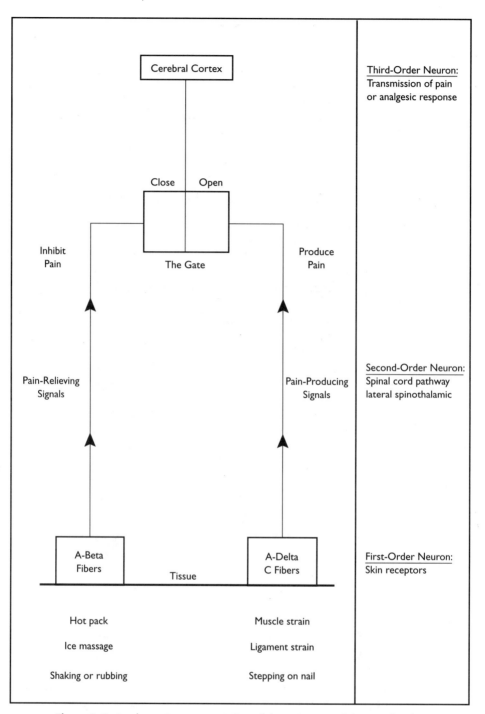

Figure 3–2. A schematic representation of the gate control theory of pain.

Adipose tissue, skeletal muscle, bone, and blood have different levels of conductivity to heat or cold. Adipose tissue acts as insulation to underlying tissues, thus limiting the degree of temperature change in deeper tissues. Blood and muscle, which contain a relatively high water content, readily absorb and conduct heat.

CONDUCTION

Heat loss or gain through direct contact between materials with different temperatures is called *conduction*. Heat absorbed by the body when using a heating pad is an example of heat exchange by conduction.

CONVECTION

Convection is defined as the transference of heat to a body by the movement of air, matter, or liquid around or past the body. An example of convective heat is a hot-air furnace. A furnace circulates warmed air around a room, and the temperature of the contents changes. A clinical example is a warm or cool whirlpool, in which movement of the water around a body part results in a temperature change.

RADIATION

Radiation or radiant energy transfers heat (usually through air) from a warmer source to a cooler source. Examples of radiant heat include the glowing coals of an open fire or the heating element on an electric stove. A therapeutic example is an infrared heat lamp. The infrared element in the lamp does not come in contact with the tissue. When radiant heat is generated from the lamp, only those body areas in the immediate vicinity of the lamp receive direct heating effects.

CONVERSION

Conversion refers to the temperature change that results when energy is transformed from one form to another, such as the conversion from mechanical or electrical energy to thermal energy. A clinical example is therapeutic ultrasound, in which sound waves (mechanical energy) are transformed to heat (thermal energy) as they pass through tissue.

EVAPORATION

Evaporation is defined as the transformation from a liquid state to a gas state. This transformation requires an energy exchange. Heat is given off when liquids transform to gases. Sweating results from heat production within the body. Cooling occurs as the perspiration evaporates from the surface of the skin.

THERAPEUTIC HEAT

Several thermal agents are available for heat application to tissues. Generally two categories are described: superficial and deep heating agents. Superficial heating agents, such as hot packs, warm whirlpool, and paraffin, primarily increase the temperature of the skin, with little or no effect on deeper structures. Deep heating agents, such as ultrasound and diathermies, can increase the temperature of tissues at depths of 3 to 5 cm. Diathermy is discussed later in this chapter. Ultrasound is addressed in Chapter 4.

PHYSIOLOGIC EFFECTS OF HEAT

Physiologic changes in response to heat application vary according to the intensity of the agent, the duration of application, and the area being treated. Therapeutic levels of heating are categorized as mild and vigorous. Heating is considered mild when tissue temperatures are less than 40°C, and vigorous heating occurs when tissue temperature reaches 40° to 45°C.[2] At these temperatures hyperemia or redness is noted, which indicates an increase in blood flow. Temperature increases greater than 45°C may potentially result in thermal pain and irreversible tissue damage.[3,4]

Elevating the tissue temperature results in an increase in blood flow to the area, attributable in part to the vasodilatory response in surface blood vessels.[5] The increase in blood flow removes heat from the area, while blood that is relatively cooler flows into the area, thus preventing excessive heat accumulation. Conversely, therapeutic heating levels may not be reached because the increased blood flow may not allow for adequate heat buildup in the area. Heat accumulation is affected by the intensity and duration of the stimulus, as well as the rate of heat absorption by the tissue. If therapeutic heating levels are reached with local application, reflex heating in other areas of the body may also occur. Local heat application has both direct and indirect heating effects. For example, when heat was applied to the low back area, an increase in subcutaneous blood flow and vasodilation to the distal extremities was reported.[1,5,6] When milder or less vigorous heating is desired, it may be reasonable to apply the principles of reflex heating to achieve the therapeutic goals. Patients with peripheral vascular disease may not be able to accommodate the vascular changes associated with vigorous heating. If the treatment plan includes the use of heat, indirect or reflex heating may be preferable. To provide a therapeutic level of heat to the distal leg of a patient with compromised circulation, heat may be applied over the anterior aspect of the ipsilateral thigh.

The application of superficial heating agents generally does not allow for increases in muscle temperatures, unless those structures are themselves superficial. Increased temperature in the muscles and tendons of the hand and foot may occur with the use of superficial heating agents, because insulation from adipose tissue is not prevalent in these areas.

Changes in metabolic rate in association with changes in tissue temperature have been reported. An increase is tissue temperature correlates with an increase in metabolic rate.[7]

Heat may have a beneficial role in wound healing based on the increase in blood flow, which decreases susceptibility to infection. The increase in blood flow also improves perfusion of the wound and periwound tissue. Improved perfusion results in an increase in oxygen tension of the wound, and the increase in oxygen allows for greater clearing of bacteria from the wound site.[8]

TREATMENT GOALS

Based on the physiologic effects of therapeutic heat, treatment goals are easy to identify. Therapeutic heating agents are used as adjunctive treatment techniques for achieving functional goals. Heat contributes to the alleviation of pain and to pain management, which may allow increased work productivity or improved range of motion. The increase in motion may in turn lead to improvement in activities of daily living. When heat is used for reduction of muscle guarding or spasm, it may lead to pain reduction and further improvement in mobility. By affecting the viscoelastic properties of tendon and muscle with the use of heat, tissue extensibility is enhanced, potentially allowing for return to normal function.

Each of the therapeutic goals, pain reduction and management, reduction of muscle guarding and spasm, and increased tissue extensibility, are addressed in relationship to the specific thermal agent. It is important to recognize the connection between these therapeutic goals and the overall functional goals.

Pain Reduction

The use of superficial heat for the alleviation or management of pain is well recognized, but the mechanism by which heat produces analgesia is not fully understood. Several mechanisms have been proposed to explain pain relief in response to therapeutic heat.

Melzack and Wall[9] proposed the gate control theory of pain, in which a spinal "gating" mechanism was responsible for pain mediation. Small A-delta fibers and C fibers are primary afferents that transmit pain impulses from free nerve endings or nociceptors to the spinal cord. When therapeutic heat is used, the thermal stimuli provide input to the spinal gating mechanism, that in effect override the painful stimuli. When there is greater nonnoxious input (heat) than noxious input (pain), the "gate" is in a relatively closed position, thus inhibiting transmission of pain to second-order neurons or ascending tracts.

Gammon[10] postulated that thermal stimuli (heat or cold) produced counterirritation. Pain was not as readily perceived because the thermal input "countered" painful stimuli. This may explain why a common response to initial injury is rubbing or pressure, both of which could be considered counterirritants.

Heat has also been shown to elevate pain threshold[10,11] and increase nerve conduction velocity.[12] An elevated pain threshold may delay the onset and perception of pain. Clinical relevance associated with the change in nerve conduction velocity has not been demonstrated.

Reduction of Muscle Guarding or Spasm

Muscle guarding or spasm may occur in response to: (1) trauma, as a protective mechanism to guard against the potential pain and further injury or pain associated with joint movement, or (2) a painful stimulus that activates or perpetuates the pain-spasm-pain cycle.[13] Heat has been used to relieve muscle guarding and spasm.[14,15] When muscle temperature is sufficiently elevated, as can be seen with the use of deep heating agents, the firing rate of the muscle spindle afferents (type II) is decreased, while that of the Golgi tendon organs (type Ib) is increased.[16] The resultant decrease in alpha motor neuron activity leads to a decrease in tonic muscle activity. In other words there is a decrease in muscle guarding resulting from decreased stimuli to the muscle.

The reduction in muscle guarding and spasm as the direct result of elevated muscle temperature does not explain the reduction seen with the use of superficial heating agents. This muscle relaxation may be explained by an indirect reduction in muscle spindle firing as a direct result of elevating skin temperature. The increase in skin temperature causes a decrease in gamma efferent activity, thus altering stretch on the muscle spindle and producing a decrease in the firing rate and an overall decrease in alpha motor neuron activity.[7]

Heat application has a direct affect on pain and muscle spasm such that the pain-spasm-pain cycle[13] can be interrupted by influencing pain as well as the muscle spasm. A reduction in pain can lead to a reduction in spasm, thus further reducing pain.

Tissue Extensibility

Shortening of connective tissue may result from injury or immobilization. The viscoelastic properties of muscle, tendon, and ligament are also affected.[18] The use of heat has been shown to decrease viscosity and increase the elastic properties of connective tissue, specifically muscle, tendon, and joint capsule.[2] However, a sufficient load must also be applied to produce residual elongation of the tissue over a long time.[17] The temperature range needed for residual length changes is 40° to 45°C.[2] If stretching is performed without heat application, the resultant elongation may only be temporary, and it is likely that the tissue will revert to its original length after the stretch is removed. Furthermore, the potential for irritation and tissue damage is lessened when heat is applied during the stretching procedure.

Residual elongation of connective tissue is dependent on a sufficient increase in tissue temperature, the timing of the application, and the type of stretch applied. The stretch is best applied during heat application, if possible, or immediately after removal of the heat source. A low-load prolonged stretch was reported as preferable to a high-load brief stretch because it resulted in less tissue damage and greater increases in range of motion.[18–21]

Patients with arthritis who have pain and limited motion associated with joint stiffness may benefit from the use of therapeutic heat. The direct effect of heat is an increase in the elastic properties of the joint capsule,[22] and the reduction of associated pain may also contribute to the resultant increased range of motion.

HEAT AND EXERCISE

A greater increase in blood flow is reported with heat and exercise than with either heat or exercise alone.[23] An initial decrease in isometric muscle strength was seen during the first 30 minutes after deep heat application and subsequent increase in strength was measured during the next 2.5 hours.[24] Endurance was shown to decrease after heat applications.[25,26] These findings are of particular interest because muscle performance may be altered in response to heat. The clinical implications of the relationship between the use of heat and exercise are important considerations for planning and implementing exercise programs and for evaluating patient performance. To assess progress or limitations in strength and endurance accurately, measurements should be taken consistently either before or after exercise. If an initial measurement is taken prior to exercise and a subsequent measurement is taken after exercise, comparison of the results may lead to erroneous conclusions about the patient's performance and the efficacy of the treatment.

METHODS OF HEAT APPLICATION

SUPERFICIAL HEATING AGENTS

Heat from superficial heating agents generally penetrates to depths of less than 1 cm from the surface of the skin. Subcutaneous tissue that is well vascularized reaches its maximum temperature increase within 6 to 8 minutes of application.[27-29] Skin and subcutaneous tissue temperatures increase 5° to 6°C after 6 minutes and are maintained up to 30 minutes after application. A treatment duration of 15 to 30 minutes is necessary for an increase in muscle temperature of 1°C at depths up to 3 cm.[27,28,30] Temperature of a joint capsule in the foot increased 9°C in response to 20 minutes of heat exposure at 47.8°C.[31] It is therefore possible to heat joint structures using superficial heating agents when these structures are closer to the skin surface.

Hydrocollator Packs

The commercial hydrocollator pack or hot pack is one of the most common ways to deliver superficial moist heat. Generally, hot packs contain a hydrophilic substance, such as silica gel or betonite, encased in channeled canvas covers. They are stored in thermostatically controlled units that are filled with water at a temperature range of 71° to 79°C.[2] Frequent use, low water levels, and faulty thermostats can affect the temperature of the hot packs, so it is important to check the water level and temperature to assure optimal heat delivery so therapeutic heat levels are achieved. The hot packs should be checked for ruptures in the canvas or mold formation, which can weaken the canvas and allow leakage.

The temperature of the hot pack itself is regulated by the length of time it is stored and the temperature of the water in which it is stored. After a hot pack has been used, 20 to 30 minutes is needed for the hot pack to reach the temperature of the water in the storage unit. This is an important consideration if hot packs are frequently used in a clinic.

Prior to application to the patient, the hot pack is covered with six to eight layers of toweling that insulate the hot pack from heat loss and protect the patient from potential burn. Commercial terrycloth covers are also available and are equivalent to two to four layers of toweling (Fig. 3–3).

Thermal energy is conducted from hot packs to the skin surface, and heat is absorbed superficially. The resultant change in temperature depends on the thermal conductivity and the size of the area being treated, the temperature of the hot pack, the size of the hot pack, and the duration of the application.

Hot packs are manufactured in several sizes and shapes to better match the body part to which they are applied. The standard size of 10 × 12 inches is suitable for treating medium-sized flat surface areas. The oversize pack is approximately twice the size of the standard pack and is suited for larger flat surface areas. Cervical packs are designed to fit the contours of the neck and are also appropriate for use around peripheral joints (Fig. 3–4). Size and shape are important because the mechanism of heat transfer is conduction, so optimal contact with the skin surface assures optimal heat absorption. The weight of the hot packs also helps to maintain contact with the body surface. Weight of the pack increases with the size and is a consideration when deciding to use this form of superficial heat. Patients may not tolerate the weight of the pack during treatment.

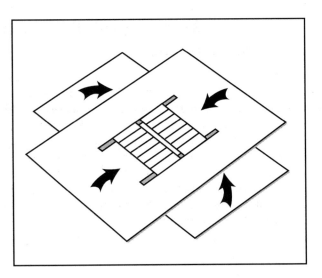

Figure 3–3. Hot pack that has been placed on two towels, folded in half to provide eight layers of toweling.

Preparing the patient for treatment includes proper positioning and draping of the patient, visual inspection of the area to be treated, and assessment of the patient's ability to report sensory changes. The area to be treated should be clear of clothing and jewelry to assure even heating. Select and prepare the hot pack with the appropriate layers of toweling. Apply the hot pack and make sure the patient

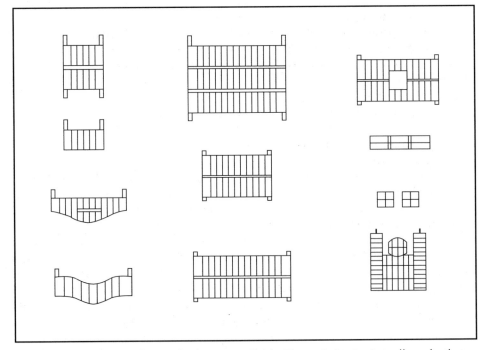

Figure 3–4. The variety of hot packs that are available. The variation in sizes allows for the selection of the appropriate size pack to fit the treatment area. Left column *(top to bottom):* standard size, half size, cervical packs. Middle column *(top to bottom):* oversize, "spinal" sizes. Right column *(top to bottom):* "knee or shoulder pack," obstetric size, others.

is in a comfortable position, considering the weight of the hot pack. Instruct the patients in what they should expect to experience from the treatment, and ask them to report any abnormal or unusual sensations. Monitor the initial response to treatment during the first 5 to 10 minutes by asking the patient for feedback and by visually inspecting the skin. If necessary, adjust the layers of toweling. Maximum skin temperature change is achieved within the first 10 minutes of hot pack application and maintained for approximately an additional 10 minutes. Therefore treatment time is typically 20 minutes. Observe the skin again after the hot pack is removed and assess the patient's response to the treatment.

Commercial hot packs are also available for home use. In addition to hydrocollator packs, there are reusable, microwavable products that deliver heat in a similar manner to hydrocollator packs. Detailed instruction to patients and care providers regarding safe and appropriate use is essential, and return demonstration is recommended. Use of superficial heating agents at home as part of an established home program may be beneficial to the patient in maintaining range of motion, managing pain, and alleviating joint stiffness.

Paraffin

Paraffin is another superficial heating agent in which conduction is the method of heat transfer. Paraffin baths contain a mixture of paraffin wax and mineral oil, which combine to lower the melting point and the specific heat in comparison to water.[2] Paraffin is stored in double-walled, thermostatically controlled, stainless steel tanks, and temperatures are maintained in the range of 47.0° to 54.4°C. The low specific heat of paraffin allows patients to tolerate the higher temperatures.

Paraffin is best suited for distal extremity joints, such as the wrist, hand, and foot, because of the primary methods of application: "dip and wrap" and "dip and immerse." The dip-and-wrap method involves dipping and removing the body part from the paraffin bath for 8 to 10 repetitions. A solid glove is formed that serves to insulate the body part against heat loss. It is common to place a plastic bag over the glove and to wrap a towel around the extremity to further assist in heat retention. The wrapped extremity is then positioned in elevation to minimize edema formation. Treatment duration is 15 to 20 minutes, after which time the glove is removed, and the wax is discarded or returned to the unit to be reused (Figs. 3–5, 3–6).

The dip-and-immerse method is similar to the above method in that the patient is asked to dip and reimmerse the body part allowing the glove to form. Rather than wrapping the hand or foot, the part is reimmersed and left in the paraffin bath for the duration of the treatment. This method is more effective in raising tissue temperature, but places the patient at greater risk for burn. This method also does not allow for elevation of the body part being treated and an increase in edema may result. As with any therapeutic heat application, careful monitoring of the patient during and after treatment is essential to safe and ethical practice.

Prior to treatment, the patient should be instructed to remove clothing and jewelry from the area and to thoroughly wash and dry the area to be treated. The skin should be visually inspected and sensation and heat tolerance assessed. The patient should be instructed in what to expect during the treatment and to report any abnormal sensations. Care should be taken by the patient to avoid touching the sides or bottom of the unit to prevent burns.

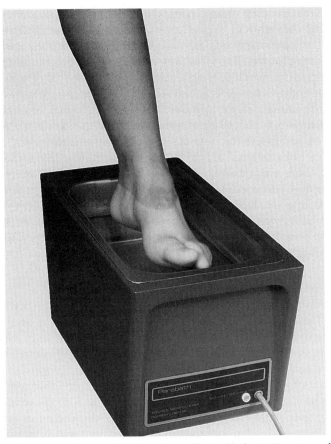

Figure 3–5. Paraffin unit with an application of paraffin to the foot. (*Courtesy of Talcott Laboratories, Houston, TX.*)

Paraffin has advantages over hydrocollator packs in that it conforms to the body part and may provide more evenly distributed and intense heat. However, the higher temperatures may not be as easily tolerated, and there is no way of adjusting the level of heat delivery to the patient, as is the case with hot packs. Home units are available but more expensive than commercial hot packs. Paraffin also poses environmental concerns regarding its disposal.

Fluidotherapy

Fluidotherapy allows stimulation of both thermoreceptors and mechanoreceptors. Fluidotherapy units contain particles of natural cellulose enclosed in a cabinet, through which dry, warm air is circulated. The method of heat exchange, which oc-

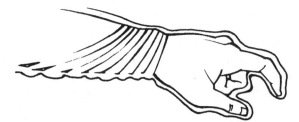

Figure 3–6. A hand that has had paraffin applied in eight layers via a "dip method."

curs with Fluidotherapy, is convection. The units are thermostatically controlled, and specific temperatures can be selected. The turbulence level has a separate control. The moving suspended particles create a medium similar to that of a liquid, and stretching and exercise can be performed during the heat application.

Fluidotherapy units have been manufactured to accommodate the upper extremity (Fig. 3–7), the lower extremity (Fig. 3–8), and the back. Fluidotherapy is used for pain relief, tissue healing, and for increasing range of motion. It is also indicated to promote desensitization of hypersensitive tissues. The effects of Fluidotherapy are the result of the combination of heat and the movement of the natural cellulose particles.

Unlike paraffin and hydrocollator packs, there is no loss of heat over time. The temperature is selected and maintained for the duration of the treatment when using Fluidotherapy. The constant temperature may result in greater heating, and elevated temperatures in joint capsules of the hand and foot have been reported.[32] Unlike paraffin and hot packs, Fluidotherapy allows movement during its use.

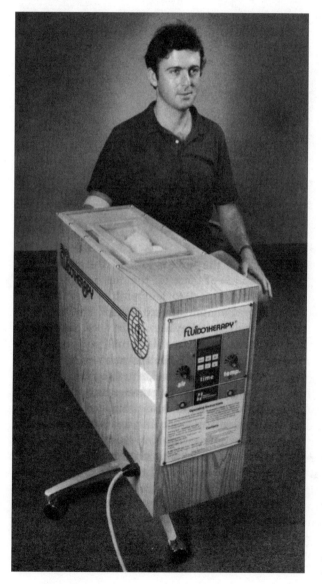

Figure 3–7. Fluidotherapy unit for the upper extremity. (*From Michlovitz, SL: Biophysical principles of heating and superficial heat agents. In Michlovitz, SL (ed): Thermal Agents in Rehabilitation, ed 2. FA Davis, Philadelphia, 1990, p 98, with permission.*)

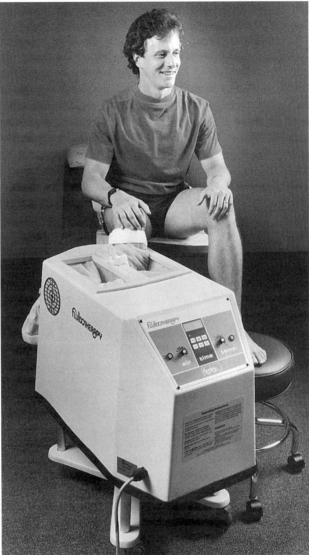

Figure 3–8. Fluidotherapy for the foot and ankle. (*From Michlovitz, SL: Biophysical principles of heating and superficial heat agents. In Michlovitz, SL (ed): Thermal Agents in Rehabilitation, ed 2. FA Davis, Philadelphia, 1990, p 99, with permission.*)

Preparation for Fluidotherapy treatments is similar to that of paraffin. The area to be treated should be thoroughly washed and dried, and jewelry and clothing should be removed from the area. Sensation and heat tolerance should be assessed, and the skin carefully inspected. Open lesions should be covered with a plastic barrier prior to treatment to prevent the cellulose particles from entering the wound. The plastic barrier contributes to a moist wound environment.

Fluidotherapy has been reported to be safe when used in the presence of splints, bandages, tape, metal implants, plastic joint replacements, and artificial tendons.[32] Splints that are designed to apply a stretch to joints can be applied prior to treatment in the Fluidotherapy unit, such that the stretch can be applied during the heat application to the joint. Exercise equipment, such as small balls, can also be used by patients during treatment.

Fluidotherapy units are available for home use on a rental or a purchase basis. The home units are designed to sit on a tabletop and are practical to heat a hand and wrist.

Diathermy

Diathermy is a deep heating agent and causes increases in tissue temperature at depths of 3 to 5 cm,[33] without overheating the skin and subcutaneous tissues. The literal meaning of *diathermy* is "to heat through." Electromagnetic radiation in a nonionizing form is within the range of radiofrequency waves. As the high-frequency waves pass into the body, the internal kinetic energy of the tissue is increased. Heat is generated from the conversion of electromagnetic energy to mechanical energy.

The benefits of diathermy are the same as those associated with superficial heating agents, namely increased blood flow, decreased pain, and increased tissue extensibility. The primary difference lies in the depth of penetration, thus allowing for heating of deeper tissues. Selected tissues may be targeted depending on the method of energy transfer associated with the type of diathermy used.[2,33]

Two types of diathermy are described: microwave (MWD) and shortwave (SWD). Both use electromagnetic energy that falls within the radiofrequency portion of the electromagnetic spectrum. The Federal Communications Commission has assigned specific frequencies for shortwave and microwave diathermies. The most widely used frequency associated with SWD is 27.12 MHz, and 2450 MHz is the most widely used frequency for MWD.

There are two methods of application for SWD: capacitance and inductance. Electrical fields (capacitance) and magnetic fields (inductance) are generated by the SWD unit. The body part being treated is placed between two electrodes and essentially becomes part of the circuit. As energy passes through the tissue, more heat is generated in tissues of low conductivity or high resistance, such as fat, ligaments, tendons, and cartilage. The ratio of the electrical field to the magnetic field is higher for capacitance SWD.

Inductance SWD primarily utilizes the magnetic field. The body part is not part of the circuit, and heat is generated as eddy currents generated by the magnetic field pass into the tissue (Fig. 3–9). Tissues with high conductivity, such as blood, muscle, and sweat, are most affected because they allow greater current flow.

Selection of the method of SWD depends on the tissue characteristics of the area being treated. If the goal of treatment is to increase tissue extensibility and the limitation is primarily to capsular tightness, then capacitance SWD is the more appropriate choice. If the treatment goal is to increase blood flow to aid healing of a muscle injury, then inductance diathermy should be chosen.

Shortwave diathermy is not commonly used in clinical practice, in part because of the variety and portability of other therapeutic heating agents. The amount of heat generated in the tissues is not easily quantified, and there are more contraindications associated with diathermy than with other thermal agents. Microwave diathermy is even less common in the United States and will not be discussed further in this chapter.

TREATMENT CONSIDERATIONS

The selection of the appropriate thermal agent is based on the size and location of the area to be treated, the depth of tissue targeted for treatment, the treatment

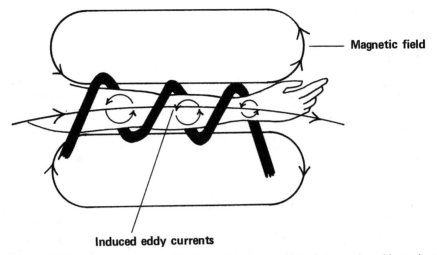

Induced eddy currents

Figure 3–9. Eddy currents are induced in tissues by the magnetic field produced by inductive applicators. (*From Kloth, LC, and Ziskin, MC: Diathermy and pulsed electromagnetic fields. In Michlovitz, SL (ed): Thermal Agents in Rehabilitation, ed 2. FA Davis, Philadelphia, 1990, p 179, with permission.*)

goals, and the contraindications and precautions associated with the treatment and the thermal agent. Table 3–1 lists the contraindications and precautions for superficial heating agents and diathermy. For example, use of a hot pack is appropriate for treatment of a patient with low back pain if the goals of the treatment are to decrease pain and muscle spasm. Diathermy may also be appropriate, especially if deeper muscles are to be heated. However, diathermy would not be considered appropriate if the patient had low back pain after a surgical procedure for the spine, in which a metal rod was used as a fixation device.

Treatment and the response to treatment should be carefully monitored, regardless of the thermal agent used. Prior to treatment the area should be carefully inspected; the patient's sensation, heat tolerance, cognitive status, and ability to communicate should also be determined, because deficits in any of these areas require more careful monitoring during treatment.

CRYOTHERAPY

Cryo means "cold" or "freezing," and cryotherapy refers to the practice of using cold to achieve therapeutic goals. Cooling agents, such as cold packs, cool whirlpool, and ice massage, are used in the management of pain and edema and are effective in decreasing muscle guarding and spasm. The primary methods of heat transfer, or in this case heat abstraction or cooling, are conduction and convection.

PHYSIOLOGIC EFFECTS OF COLD

When cold is applied to the surface of the skin, the initial response is vasoconstriction of superficial blood vessels. If skin temperature is sufficiently lowered, the cooler temperature stimulates free nerve endings, which in turn causes reflex vasoconstriction. Local blood flow is also decreased. However, when a sufficient

Table 3–1   Contraindications to and Precautions for the Use of Superficial Heating Agents and Diathermy

General Contraindications for Heating Agents	Rationale
Acute inflammation	Local heat application may exacerbate the inflammatory response.
Existing fever	Heat application may further elevate body temperature.
Malignancies	The increased blood flow that results from localized heat application may promote a metastasis.
Acute hemorrage	Hemorrhage may be prolonged if heat is applied after an acute injury.
Peripheral vascular disease	Heat increases metabolic demands and a patient with peripheral vascular disease has a diminished capacity to meet the increase in metabolic demands of heated tissue.
Radiation (x-ray therapy)	Tissue that is devitalized by x-ray therapy should not be heated.

Specific Contraindications for Diathermy*	
Metal implants or any metal within the treatment area (snaps, zippers, hair pins)	Metal will alter the flow of electromagnetic energy and may result in a burn.
Cardiac pacemakers	Pacemaker function may be altered.

Precautions to the Use of Heat	
During menses	May have an increase in blood flow if heat is applied to the low back.
In the presence of sensory deficit	There is an increased potential for a burn; need to be monitored closely.
During pregnancy	The effect on the fetus has not been established; heat application to peripheral joints may be given with caution.

*Diathermy equipment should not be operated within close proximity to cardiac pacemakers or other equipment that may be adversely affected by electromagnetic radiation (traction, electrical stimulation equipment).

amount of cooled blood flows through the general circulation, the hypothalamus may be stimulated, resulting in further reflex vasoconstriction. The vasoconstriction and the resultant reduction in blood flow are a means for the body to retain heat by restricting the volume of cooled blood in systemic circulation. Shivering is also a heat-retaining mechanism and may result if a large area of the body is exposed to cooler temperatures.

Vasodilation has been reported to occur in response to extended exposure to cold.[34,35] Lewis[34] postulated that cycles of vasodilation followed periods of vasoconstriction to increase the flow of relatively warmer blood to the body areas affected by cold. He termed this phenomenon the "hunting response," and proposed that it occurred as a result of an axon reflex. Cold vasodilation was also reported to occur without the cycling component and was attributed to local responses in deeper tissues.[36] Responses have included the following: (1) skin vessels were shown to maximally constrict at 15 °C followed by vasodilation at temperatures below 15 °C, reaching maximal vasodilation at 0 °C.[36] Other studies have also reported cold-induced vascular responses, to which the prevention of local tissue injury is ascribed.[34,37,38] The hunting response is described as cycles of vasoconstriction-vasodilatoin lasting approximately 12 to 30 minutes during cold exposure.[39–47] Vasodilation occurs prior to the vasoconstrictive phase of the hunting response, and changes in sensation accompany the cycles. Cold vasodilation was also reported to occur without the cycling component and was attributed to local responses in deeper tissues.[37]

Tissue temperature changes in response to cold applications have been reported at depths of 1 to 4 cm,[48] depending on the temperature gradient and the duration of the exposure. More intense cold and longer durations result in greater decreases in tissue temperature. The presence of adipose tissue also affects the depth of cold penetration because it acts as insulation. It may not be possible to lower temperatures of deeper structures if the intensity of the cooling agent and the duration of the application are not adequate, and if the area of the body being treated has low conductivity. However, cooling of muscles and joints is possible when these structures are located more superficially without the presence of excessive adipose tissue. For tissue temperature changes at greater depths to be noted, longer application times are needed.

Decreases in tissue temperature to 10 °C or below may result in thermal damage to tissues.[48] Thermal damage may trigger an inflammatory response and result in an increase in edema. This may account, in part, for somewhat conflicting results in animal studies of the effect of cryotherapy on posttraumatic edema.[49–52]

The viscoelastic properties of tissue are also affected by cold application. Just as heat increases elasticity and decreases viscosity, cold has the opposite effect. Tissues that are cooled may not respond as favorably to length changes, and range of motion measures after cold application may not be accurate.

Therapeutic cold reduces the metabolic rate and slows the production of metabolites, resulting in less metabolically generated heat production. The reduction in the metabolic rate also decreases the oxygen demand for tissues, such that tissues can accommodate the decreased blood flow.

TREATMENT GOALS

Knowledge of the physiologic effects of cold helps to identify the benefits of the use of therapeutic cold as an adjunctive treatment in physical therapy. The rationale for using cold is similar to that of the use of therapeutic heat. Addressing impairments, such as edema, pain, muscle guarding and spasm, and abnormal muscle tone, helps in attaining meaningful therapeutic goals related to mobility and function (Table 3–2).

Table 3–2   **Treatment Goals for Therapeutic Cold**

Indication	Rationale
Pain reduction	A-beta and C fiber stimulation
Muscle spasm reduction	Decreased muscle spindle activity
Inflammation reduction	Decreased vascular responses
Edema reduction	Vasoconstriction
Hemorrhage containment	Decreased by minimizing effects of active bleeding

Edema Reduction

Cold is commonly used in the management of acute inflammation and edema. Vascular responses to cold affect cell wall permeability, thus inhibiting fluid accumulation in the interstitium. In a recent study of microcirculatory changes in response to cold, Smith and colleagues[53] suggested that the amount of interstitial fluid is controlled by an increase in the reabsorption rate. They reported that there was an increase in the diameter of venules, but no change in arteriolar diameter in response to cold.

The decrease in blood flow associated with vasoconstriction and the decrease in metabolic rate with cold application may result in less accumulation of metabolites and chemical irritants in the injured area. The presence of chemical irritants may themselves trigger an inflammatory and pain response. By minimizing the presence of these irritants, a decrease in the rate of the inflammatory response may be possible, resulting in less edema formation.

Cold applications in combination with compression have been reported to be more effective than compression alone for the management of edema. Basur and associates[54] compared the use of cold and compression to the use of compression alone in the management of acute ankle sprains. They reported that edema was better controlled when using combined cold and compression rather than compression alone. Levy and Marmar[55] reported similar findings in their study of the postoperative management of patients with total knee arthroplasties. In addition to improved edema control with cold and compression, they also reported less pain and a greater increase in range of motion. Healy and associates[56] found no difference in the amount of postoperative swelling in knees when comparing the use of a commercial cold compressive device to the use of ice packs and Ace wraps.

The intensity and duration of cold application appear to influence the effect on edema. More intense cold applied for longer durations may have an adverse effect. Therefore, less intense cold applied for durations of 20 to 30 minutes are recommended. To maximize edema reduction concomitant compression is also advised.

Pain Reduction

Cryotherapy is commonly used to decrease pain. The proposed mechanisms by which cold influences pain are similar to those for heat. Cooling agents applied to the skin surface may elevate the pain threshold. Cold is also a counterirritant and may lessen pain sensation by stimulating thermal receptors.

Pain associated with edema and inflammation is both directly and indirectly mediated with cryotherapy. Analgesia is a direct effect of therapeutic cold. Further pain reduction may result from the decrease in chemical irritant response to the decrease in metabolic rate. There may be a decrease in stimulation of mechanoreceptors in the area of injury as swelling is reduced.

Reduction of Muscle Spasm

Muscle guarding or spasm is a local reaction to injury, in which a tonic contraction is sustained in an attempt to "guard" or protect the tissue from further injury. It is also a component of the pain-spasm-pain cycle, and as such may be reflexively affected by a decrease in pain. Muscle tightness may be reduced following cryotherapy if sufficient analgesia is induced to allow stretch of the muscle.

Reduction of Muscle Spasticity

Spasticity is differentiated from muscle spasm in that it is associated with increased resistance to passive stretch, an increase in deep tendon reflexes (DTRs), and clonus. Clonus is defined as the spasmodic alteration of contractions between antagonistic muscle groups because of a hyperactive stretch reflex from an upper motor neuron lesion. Several studies indicate that spasticity can be reduced by cryotherapy.[57–62] Cold application temporarily decreases the amplitude of DTRs. The reduction may be a result of direct cooling of the muscle and can be attributed to stimulation of skin receptors.

Miglietta[59] investigated the effects of cold on sustained ankle clonus and reported that clonus was either decreased or eliminated after cold whirlpool at 18.3°C for 15 minutes. The changes were maintained for several hours.

The decrease in spasticity associated with cryotherapy may have a positive effect on mobility and may allow an increased level of participation in a therapy program. Because the reduction in spasticity can be sustained for several hours, the exercise or activity should be initiated within that time frame. This becomes especially important when establishing a home program and instructing the patient, family members, and other care providers in carrying out the program.

METHODS OF COLD APPLICATION

Ice Massage

Ice massage is the application of ice directly onto the skin surface. Because it is an intense cold application, it is usually applied to small areas, such as a muscle belly or trigger point. To cover an area 10 cm by 15 cm, 5 to 10 minutes is needed.[63] Treatment time for ice massage can also be determined by the amount of time needed to numb the area. Before numbness or analgesia occurs, a patient experiences stages of cold, burning, and aching. It is important for the patient to understand that these sensations are normal responses so that the patient may better tolerate the treatment. The ability to produce numbness depends on the size of the area treated. Smaller areas are recommended because the intensity and localization of the cold application does not allow for effective local temperature regulation, and tissue cooling is achieved.

Paper or Styrofoam cups are filled with water and placed in a freezer. The use of paper or Styrofoam cups provides insulation to the therapist handling the ice cup. The skin surface to be treated should be exposed and the surrounding area draped with a towel to absorb the water as the ice melts.

Cold Packs

Cold packs are a simple and effective method for cooling tissue. There are commercially available cold packs, as well as cold packs that can easily be made a means of delivering very cold temperatures to the treatment area and are considered a good choice for cold treatments. Commercial cold packs are contain a semi-gelled substance, covered in durable plastic. They are manufactured in sizes similar to those of hydrocollator packs. The cold packs are stored in freezer units and remain cold for up to 10 minutes after removal from the cooling unit. They may be applied either directly to the skin or can be used with a wet or dry interface, depending on the desired intensity of the cold application. These cold packs conform to irregular surface areas, but maintaining a constant cold temperature is problematic. Commercial cold packs are reusable and self-contained.

Ice packs can be made using a plastic bag or towel and crushed ice or ice cubes. The use of crushed ice allows for better conformity when applying the ice pack to the body part. The pack can be applied directly to the surface of the skin or it may be applied using a wet or dry towel as an interface. An Ace wrap or second towel may be used to secure the cold or ice pack and to absorb water as the ice melts. Ice packs can be easily made at home and are inexpensive.

The patients should be positioned comfortably and draped appropriately for the duration of the ice application. Average treatment time for a cold or ice pack application is 10 to 15 minutes.

Cold or Ice Baths

Immersion in water that contains partially melted ice cubes is primarily used for distal extremities or larger body parts. Immersion of the body part allows complete conformity of the cooling agent to the skin. Therapeutic temperature ranges for cold baths are between 13° and 18°C, and lower temperatures within this range are tolerated for shorter durations. This method of cryotherapy is easily applied in the home setting.

TREATMENT GUIDELINES

Patient preparation and proper positioning are primary considerations for any method of cold application. The treatment should be explained prior to its initiation. Encourage the patient to ask questions, and stress the importance of verbalizing the response to treatment. Patients should be positioned for comfort, and the area to be treated should be clear of clothing and jewelry. Proper body mechanics for both patient and clinicians are also important considerations in treatment preparation and patient positioning.

Visual inspection includes an assessment of skin integrity and appearance and tissue response prior to, during, and after cryotherapy treatments. In addition to visual inspection, the patient's subjective response should be checked periodically throughout the duration of the treatment.

SAFETY CONSIDERATIONS WITH THE APPLICATION OF COLD TREATMENT

Precautions

Cryotherapy should be used with caution on patients with thermoregulatory problems, sensory deficits, hypersensitivity to cold, and impaired circulation. If cryotherapy is to be used, careful monitoring is essential. Appropriate adjustments of the treatment parameters may be necessary to decrease stress to body systems. For example, if a patient reports an abnormal level of discomfort in response to ice massage, perhaps a method involving less intense cold could be substituted. Cold should not be applied directly over an area of compromised circulation.

Cold applications can cause a transient increase in blood pressure.[64,65] Careful monitoring of blood pressure should be performed prior to, during, and after cold application if the patient is hypertensive. Treatment should be discontinued if an excessive elevation in blood pressure occurs.

Contraindications

Cryotherapy is contraindicated for patients with particular cold sensitivities. Cold urticaria may include both local and systemic reactions. The local response is characterized by wheals or raised, reddened areas that appear in direct response to a local cold application.[66,67] The systemic response may include facial flushing, a drop in blood pressure, an increase in heart rate and syncope.[68]

Patients with cryoglobulinemia are at risk for developing ischemia or gangrene because of an abnormal blood protein. This protein forms a gel when exposed to cold. This condition is seen in patients with multiple myeloma, chronic liver disease, and several rheumatic diseases.[69]

Patients with Raynaud's disease exhibit cycles of pallor, cyanosis, rubor, and normal color in the hands and feet in response to cold. Numbness, tingling, or burning may also occur. These sensations are similar to the normal stages of sensation experienced with cold, so it is important to pay attention to visual cues as well as subjective responses from the patient.

Paroxysmal cold hemoglobinuria is characterized by the presence of blood in the urine. It can result from either local or systemic exposure to cold. It may not be possible to observe this response in the clinic, but a complete and thorough patient history will help in identifying those individuals at risk.

CLINICAL DECISION MAKING: HEAT OR COLD?

Responses to both therapeutic heat application and cryotherapy may be similar. Both heat and cold are effective pain management techniques and both are beneficial in reducing muscle guarding or spasm. Some guidelines apply when making recommendations for the use of heat or cold. The benefits of cold in the management of acute injuries are well documented. For painful conditions associated with acute injuries, cryotherapy is the treatment of choice. Neither heat nor cold provide lasting benefit in the management of chronic pain,[70] but heat may aid in promoting relaxation and could be recommended for home use. Either heat or cold could be used for relief of joint stiffness. Heat enhances the viscoelastic properties of connective tissue and may result in increased motion and decreased pain. Although cold has the opposite effect on connective tissue, it may provide greater pain relief for a given patient. An increase in motion may result, because pain no longer limits the motion.

For pain associated with muscle guarding, either heat or cold may be effective. If a patient has received heat treatments, and there is no documented change in the pain level or in range of motion, then a trial of therapeutic cold may be indicated.

Acute injuries are treated with cold because the rate of the inflammation and edema formation are reduced. Heat is contraindicated for acute injuries because it may exacerbate the inflammatory process. However, an increase in blood flow may promote the reabsorption of exudates and may be appropriate in the management of chronic edema and inflammation.

Precautions and contraindications may guide the treatment choice when the treatment goal could be achieved with either heat or cold. Patient tolerance of the thermal agent should not be discounted. If either heat or cold produces discomfort, and if the treatment goal can be achieved with either heat or cold, then patient preference may be the primary determinant. Table 3–3 summarizes the use of thermal agents in the clinical setting and treatment goals.

DOCUMENTATION

The goals of documentation are to provide an accurate and complete description of the treatment and the patient's response to treatment. Documentation should include all the necessary parameters and components, such that the treatment could be easily reproduced by another clinician. Documentation of the use of any thermal agent should include a description of the type of agent used, the method of application, the area treated, and the position of the patient. For example, report that a "cervical" hot pack was applied to a patient's shoulder using eight layers of toweling. Also report the position of the patient and the involved extremity if it was supported in a particular position.

Documentation of the patient's response to treatment is important, because it provides a means for evaluating the effectiveness of the treatment and the patient's readiness to progress in the treatment plan. Both subjective and objective responses should be documented. Subjective statements by the patient regarding pain and activity levels are indications of how effective the use of thermal agents are for pain management. Pain levels can be better quantified by using a visual analog scale or verbal rating scale. Objective measures are essential in determining treatment efficacy. Girth and volume measures should be reported to reflect changes in edema and can be used to determine whether changes have been maintained over time. The same is true for goniometric measurements, which are useful in assessing changes in range of motion in response to treatment. Improvement in function is the ultimate therapeutic goal. Although the use of heat or cold may not have a direct effect on function, the functional status of the patient reflects the overall effectiveness of the treatment plan.

Table 3–3   **The Use of Thermal Agents in the Clinical Setting for the Accomplishment of Treatment Goals**

Treatment Goal	Heat	Cold	Comments
Pain reduction	X	X	
Reduction of muscle guarding	X	X	
Increasing tissue extensibility	X	X	If the restriction is caused by spasticity

DISCUSSION QUESTIONS

1. Explain the differences between conductive heat transmission from a hot pack and the continuous immersion technique for a paraffin application.

2. Which of the heating agents discussed in this chapter would feel the hottest after about 5 minutes, plateau, and then cool off? Why?

3. Which of the heating agents discussed in this chapter may continue to feel hotter throughout the treatment time? Why?

4. What factors should be considered before applying superficial heat to a patient?

5. When would ice or cryotherapy be contraindicated and heat be indicated?

6. When would heat be contraindicated and cryotherapy potentially be indicated?

7. How would you explain the sensations that a patient should expect to feel during an application of superficial heat?

8. How would you explain the sensations that a patient should feel during cryotherapy?

REFERENCES

1. Wessman, MS and Kottke, FJ: The effect of indirect heating on peripheral blood flow, pulse rate, blood pressure and temperature. Arch Phys Med Rehabil 48:567, 1967.

2. Lehmann, JF and de Lateur, BJ: Therapeutic heat. In Lehman, JF (ed): Therapeutic Heat and Cold, ed 3. Williams and Wilkins, Baltimore, 1982.

3. Moritz, AR and Henriques, FC, Jr: Studies in thermal injury II. The relative importance of time and surface temperature in causation of cutaneous burns. Am J Pathol 23:695, 1947.

4. Henriques, FC, Jr: Studies in thermal injury V. The predictability and the significance of thermally induced rate processes leading to irreversible epidermal injury. Am J Pathol 23:489, 1947.

5. Abramson, DI, et al: Changes in blood flow, oxygen uptake and tissue temperatures produced by the topical application of wet heat. Arch Phys Med Rehabil 42:305, 1961.

6. Abramson, DI, et al: Indirect vasodilation in thermotherapy. Arch Phys Med Rehabil 46:44112, 1965.

7. Fischer, E and Solomon, S: Physiological responses to heat and cold. In Licht, S (ed): Therapeutic Heat & Cold, ed 2. Waverly Press, Baltimore, 1965.

8. Cummings, J and Kloth, LC: Role of light, heat, and electromagnetic energy in wound healing. In McCullough J, Kloth, LC, and Feedar, JA (eds): Wound Healing: Alternatives in Management, ed 2. FA Davis, Philadelphia, 1995.

9. Melzack, R and Wall, PD: Pain mechanisms: A new theory. Science 150:971, 1965.

10. Gammon, GD and Starr, I: Studies on the relief of pain by counter imitation. J Clin Invest 20:13, 1941.

11. Benson, TB and Copp EP. The effects of therapeutic forms of heat and ice on the pain threshold of the normal shoulder. Pheum Rehabil 1974, 13:101.

12. Coseutino, AB, et al: Ultrasound effects on electroneuronuyographic measures in sensory fibers in the median nerve. Phys Ther 63:1789, 1983.

13. DeVries, H: Quantitive electromyographic investigation of the spasms theory of muscle pain. Am J Phys Med 45:119, 1966.

14. Harris R: Physical methods in the management of rheumatoid arthritis. Med Clin North Am, 52:707, 1968.

15. Weidenbacher, RA and Smith, C: Does heat cause relaxation? Phys Ther Rev 40:261, 1960.

16. Mense, S: Effects of temperature on the discharges of muscle spindles and tendon organs. Pflugers Arch 374:159, 1978.

17. LeBann, MM: Collagen tissue: Implications of its response to stress in vitro. Arch Phys Med Rehabil 47:345, 1966.

18. Enneking, WF and Horowitz, M: The intra-articular effects of immobilization on the human knee. J Bone Joint Surg [Am] 5:973, 1972.

19. Kottke, FJ, Pauley, DL, and Ptok RA: The rationale for prolonged stretching for correction of shortening of connective tissues. Arch Phys Med Rehabil 47:345, 1966.

20. Warren, GC, Lehmann, JF, and Koblanski, JN: Heat and stretch procedures: An evaluation using rat tail tendon. Arch Phys Med Rehabil 57:122, 1976.

21. Light, KE, et al: Low-load prolonged stretch vs high-load brief stretch in treating knee contractures. Phys Ther 664:330, 1984.

22. Backlund, L and Tiselius, P: Objective measurement of joint stiffness in rheumatoid arthritis. Acta Rheum Scand, 13:275, 1967.

23. Greenberg, RS: The effects of hot packs and exercise on local blood flow. Phys Ther 52:273, 1972.

24. Chastain, PB: The effect of deep heat on isometric strength. Phys Ther 58:543, 1978.

25. Edwards, HT, et al: Effect of temperature on muscle energy metabolism and endurance during successive isometric contractions, sustained to fatigue of the quadriceps muscle in man. J Phys 220:335, 1972.

26. Wickstrom, R and Polk, C: Effect of whirlpool on the strength endurance of the quadriceps muscle in trained male adolescents. Am J Phys Med 40:91, 1961.

27. Abramson, DI, et al: Changes in blood flow, oxygen uptake and tissue temperatures produced by the topical application of wet heat. Arch Phys Med Rehabil 42:305, 1961.

28. Greenberg, RS: The effects of hot packs and exercise on local blood flow. Phys Ther 52:273, 1972.

29. Lehmann, JF, et al: Temperature distributions in the human thigh produced by infrared, hot packs and microwave applications. Arch Phys Med Rehabil 47:291, 1966.

30. Whyte, HM and Reader, SB: Effectiveness of different forms of heating. Ann Rheum Dis 10:449, 1951.

31. Borrell, RM, et al: Comparison of in vivo temperatures produced by hydrotherapy, paraffin wax treatment and Fluidotherapy. Phys Ther 60:1273, 1980.

32. Borrell, RM, et al: Fluidotherapy: Evaluation of a new heat modality. Arch Phys Med Rehabil 58: 69, 1977.

33. Kloth, LC and Ziskin, MC: Diathermy and pulsed electromagnetic field. In Michlovitz, SL (ed). Thermal Agents in Rehabilitation, ed 2. FA Davis, Philadelphia, 1990.

34. Lewis, T: Observations upon the reactions of the vessels of the human skin to cold. Heart 15:177, 1930.

35. Fox, RH and Whyatt, HT: Cold-induced vasodilatation in various areas of the body surface in man. J Physiol 162:289, 1962.

36. Downey, JA: Physiologic effects of heat and cold. J Am Phys Ther Assoc 44:713, 1964.

37. Clarke, RSJ, Hellon, RF, and Lind, AR: Vascular reactions of the human forearm to cold. Clin Sci 17:165, 1958.

38. Clarke, RSJ and Hellon, RF: Hyperemia following sustained and rhythmic exercise in the human forearm at various temperatures J Physiol 145:447, 1959.

39. Behnke, R: Cold therapy. Athlet Train 9:178, 1974.

40. Behnke, R: Cryotherapy and vasodilation. Athlet Train 8:106, 1973.

41. Grant, AE: Massage with ice (cryokinetics) in the treatment of painful conditions of the musculoskeletal system. Arch Phys Med Rehabil 45:233, 1964.

42. Hayden, C: Cryokinetics in an early treatment program. J Am Phys Ther Assoc 44:11, 1964.

43. Knight, KL, Aquino, J, Johannes, SM, and Urbano, CD: Reexamination of Lewis cold induced vasodilation in the finger and the ankle. Athlet Train 15:248–250, 1980.

44. Moore, R, Nicolette, R, and Behnke, R: The therapeutic use of cold (cryotherapy) in the care of athletic injuries. Athlet Train, 2:6, 1967.

45. Moore, R: Uses of cold therapy in the rehabilitation of athletes, recent advances, Proceedings of the 19th American Medical Association National Conferences on the Medical Aspects of Sports. San Francisco, June 1977.

46. Murphy, AJ: The physiological effects of cold application. Phys Ther Rev 40:1112, 1960.

47. Olson, JE and Stravino, U: A review of cryotherapy. Phys Ther 52:840, 1972.

48. Michlovitz, SL: Cryotherapy. In Michlovitz, SL (ed): Thermal Agents in Rehabilitation, ed 2. FA Davis, Philadelphia, 1990.

49. Matsen, FA, Questad, K, and Matsen, AL: The effect of local cooling on post fracture swelling. Clin Orthop 109:201, 1975.

50. Jezdinsky, J, Marek, J, and Ochonsky, P: Effects of local cold and heat therapy on traumatic oedema of the rat hind paw. I: Effects of cooling on the course of traumatic oedema. Acta Universitatis Palackianae Olomucensis Facultatis Medicae 66:185, 1973.

51. Marek, J, Jezdinsky, J, and Ochonsky, P: Effects of local cold and heat therapy on traumatic oedema of the rat hind paw. II: Effects of various kinds of compresses on the course of traumatic oedema. Acta Universitatis Palackinanae Olomucensis Facultatis Medicae 66:203, 1973.

52. McMaster, WC and Liddle, S: Cryotherapy influence on post traumatic limb edema. Clin Orthop 150:283, 1980.

53. Smith, TL, et al: New skeletal muscle model for the longitudinal study of alterations in microcirculation following contusion and cryotherapy. Microsurgery 14:487, 1993.

54. Basur, R, Shephard, E, and Mouzos, G: A cooling method in the treatment of ankle sprains. Practitioner 216:708, 1976.

55. Levy, AS and Marmar, E: The role of cold compression dressings in the postoperative treatment of total knee arthroplasty. Clin Orthop and Rel Res 297:174, 1993.

56. Helay, WL, et al: Cold compressive dressing after total knee arthroplasty. Clin Orthop Rel Res 299:143, 1994.

57. Knuttsson, E and Mattsson, E: Effects of local cooling on monosynaptic reflexes in man. Scand J Rehabil Med 1:126, 1969.

58. Newton, M and Lehmkuhl, D: Muscle spindle response to body heating and localized muscle cooling: Implications for relief of spasticity. Phys Ther 45:91, 1965.

59. Miglietta, O: Electromyographic characteristics of clonus and influence of cold. Arch Phys Med Rehabil 45:508, 1964.

60. Miglietta, O: Action of cold on spasticity. Am J Phys Med 52:198, 1973.

61. Eldred, E, Lindsley, DF, and Buchwald, JS: The effect of cooling on mammalian muscle spindles. Exp Neurol 2:144, 1960.

62. Hartvikksen, K: Ice therapy in spasticity. Acta Neurol Scand 38:79, 1962.

63. Waylonis, GW: The physiologic effect of ice massage. Arch Phys Med Rehabil 48:37, 1967.

64. Boyer, JT, Fraser, JRE, and Doyle, AE: The haemodynamic effects of cold immersion. Clin Sci 19:539, 1980.

65. Claus-Walker, J, et al: Physiological responses to cold stress in healthy subjects and in subjects with cervical cord injuries. Arch Phys Med Rehabil 55:485, 1974.

66. Austin, KD: Diseases of immediate type hypersensitivity. In Isselbacher, KJ, et al (eds): Harrison's Principles of Internal Medicine, ed 9. McGraw-Hill, New York, 1980.

67. Day, MJ: Hypersensitive response to ice massage: Report of a case. Phys Ther 54:592, 1974.

68. Horton, BT, Brown, GE, and Roth, GM: Hypersensitiveness to cold with local and systemic manifestations of a histamine-like character: Its amenability to treatment. JAMA 107:1263, 1936.

69. Schumacher, HR (ed): Cryoglobulinemia. In Primer on Rheumatic Diseases, ed 9. Arthritis Foundation, Atlanta, 1988, p 82.

70. DeRosa CP, Porterfield JA: A physical therapy model for the treatment of low back pain. Phys Ther 72:261, 1992.

APPENDIX: Temperature Conversions for Fahrenheit and Centigrade*

To convert Centigrade to Fahrenheit: $\frac{9}{5}C + 32$

°C	°F	°C	°F
46	114.8	22	71.6
45	113.0	21	69.8
44	111.2	20	68.0
43	109.4	19	66.2
42	107.6	18	64.4
41	105.8	17	62.6
40	104.0	16	60.8
39	102.2	15	59.0
38	100.4	14	57.2
37	98.6	13	55.4
36	96.8	12	53.6
35	95.0	11	51.8
34	93.2	10	50.0
33	91.4	9	48.2
32	89.6	8	46.4
31	87.8	7	44.6
30	86.0	6	42.8
29	84.2	5	41.0
28	82.4	4	39.2
27	80.6	3	37.4
26	78.8	2	35.6
25	77.0	1	33.8
24	75.2	0	32.0
23	73.4		

To convert Fahrenheit to Centigrade: $\frac{5}{9}$ (F $-$ 32)

°F	°C	°F	°C
120	48.9	76	24.4
119	48.3	75	23.9
118	47.8	74	23.3
117	47.2	73	22.7
116	46.7	72	22.2
115	46.1	71	21.7
114	45.6	70	21.1
113	45.0	69	20.6
112	44.4	68	20.0
111	43.9	67	19.4
110	43.3	66	18.9
109	42.8	65	18.3
108	42.2	64	17.8
107	41.7	63	17.2
106	41.1	62	16.7
105	40.5	61	16.1
104	40.0	60	15.5
103	39.4	59	15.0
102	38.8	58	14.4
101	38.3	57	13.9
100	37.8	56	13.3
99	37.2	55	12.8
98	36.7	54	12.2
97	36.1	53	11.7
96	35.5	52	11.1
95	35.0	51	10.6
94	34.4	50	10.0
93	33.9	49	9.4
92	33.3	48	8.9
91	32.8	47	8.3
90	32.2	46	7.8
89	31.7	45	7.2
88	31.1	44	6.6

°F	°C	°F	°C
87	30.6	43	6.1
86	30.0	42	5.6
85	29.4	41	5.0
84	28.9	40	4.4
83	28.3	39	3.9
82	27.8	38	3.3
81	27.2	37	2.8
80	26.7	36	2.2
79	26.1	35	1.7
78	25.6	34	1.1
77	25.0	33	0.6
		32	0

*From Michlovitz, SL (ed): Thermal Agents in Rehabilitation, ed 2. FA Davis, Philadelphia, 1990, pp 286–287, with permission.

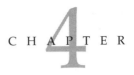

Therapeutic Ultrasound

Ethne L. Nussbaum MEd, BSc, PT

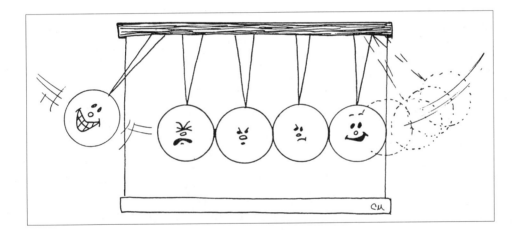

CHAPTER OBJECTIVES

- Discuss the theory and rationale for the application of therapeutic ultrasound.
- Outline and differentiate between the parameters for therapeutic ultrasound.
- Discuss the application of therapeutic ultrasound.
- Outline current research trends in the utilization of ultrasound.
- Discuss clinical decision making in the determination of the appropriate treatment parameters for ultrasound.

CHAPTER OUTLINE

Acoustic principles have been used for detection since early in this century. During development of underwater detection apparatus in the 1920s, it was observed that extremely high pressure waves were damaging to living tissues. This led to the first use of ultrasound in medicine, initially for its tissue-destructive potential in cancer treatment.[1] During the 1930s, low intensities of ultrasound were used for the first time in physical medicine to treat soft tissue conditions with mild heating.

In therapeutic ultrasound a mechanical pressure wave is applied to tissues at a level of intensity that is so low and at a frequency that is so rapid, that the pressure itself cannot be detected by the person receiving it. We encounter larger-scale pressure waves of different types in many everyday events. For example, a water wave, which radiates out in all directions from the point where a pebble is dropped into a pond, is large enough to see. Beating a drum causes the drumhead to vibrate, which produces a sound wave in air. Sound waves are not visible but they can be heard. Audible sound lies in the range of frequencies between 30 hertz (Hz) and 20 kilohertz (kHz). Ultrasound lies in the range beyond audible sound. In ultrasound treatment streams of pressure waves are transmitted to a small volume of tissue, which causes the molecules of the tissue to vibrate.

BIOPHYSICS OF ULTRASOUND

PHYSICAL PRINCIPLES AND TERMINOLOGY OF ULTRASOUND

The goal of this section is to provide the clinician with sufficient background knowledge to promote effective and safe practice with ultrasound. For more detailed information on waves and energy, the text by Sternheim and Kane[2] is recommended.

Sound Propagation

During the positive-pressure phase of a wave, called the compression or condensation phase, molecules in the path of a wave are "squeezed" together. This is followed by a negative-pressure phase, called *rarefaction*, during which molecules are spread out more than before the pressure was applied. A wave cycle includes both a compression and a rarefaction phase (Fig. 4–1). When a pebble is dropped in water it generates only a single wave, which travels away from the source of the wave in an expanding circle until the wave energy is dissipated. The peak and trough of the wave reflect the phases of compression and rarefaction, respectively. When waves are generated in rapid succession, as in ultrasound therapy, molecules in the wave path are jostled to and fro by the rapidly alternating phases of successive waves.

A principle common to all wave formation is that matter in a wave does not itself travel; only the wave energy is transmitted. Each energized particle bumps into the next, transferring momentum in a chain reaction, until the wave runs out of energy. A mobile table ornament, sometimes called Motion Balls, illustrates some principles of this type of energy transfer. The mobile consists of a frame with five metal balls suspended on thin rods from a horizontal bar. The balls touch each other when the mobile is motionless. The mobile is energized initially by manual lift and release of the first ball. When released, the ball swings back into place and bumps the next ball. Energy is transferred in an instant from ball to ball along the

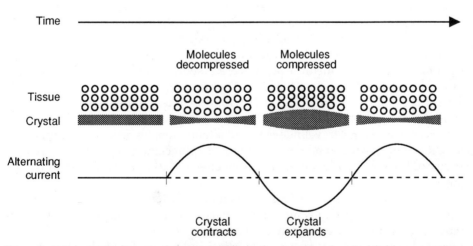

Figure 4–1. Schematic diagram showing the effect of a changing electrical field on crystal size and the effect of changing pressure on tissue molecules in the sound field.

row. The last ball swings out into space because it is unopposed. When it falls back into line, it sets a new cycle in motion. The mobile will continue to oscillate for a long period of time before the system runs out of energy and comes to a standstill.

Waves require a medium for transmission. This is understandable because waves travel by transfer of energy. The medium can consist of the particles of a gas, liquid, or solid. Waves travel in two modes. When the particles of a medium are compressed and decompressed in the direction that the wave travels it is called *longitudinal wave*. When the particle movement is at right angles to the direction of wave propagation, it is called *shear* or *transverse wave*. Shear waves occur more readily in solids, and longitudinal waves occur in liquids and gases (a wave traveling on the surface of water is a shear wave and is therefore an exception to the rule). In human tissues both modes of travel occur but a notable effect of shear waves really occurs when pressure waves reach bone, at which point waves are generated along the periosteum, the outer covering of the bone.

Absorption and Penetration

The velocity of wave travel depends on the closeness of the molecules of a medium; the closer the molecules, the quicker they collide with each other and the sooner they respond to a disturbance. This is unlike electromagnetic radiation, which travels independently of the medium through which it passes. Acoustic impedance is the term that denotes the relative resistance of a medium to wave energy; the more dense or heavy the molecules and the less compliant they are to be being squeezed, the greater the impedance. Energy is consumed as a wave travels. More work has to be done to transmit a wave against high impedance. It follows that over any given distance that a wave travels, the more dense the medium, the greater the energy loss from the wave and the furthest point the wave reaches is accordingly reduced. There is an inverse relationship between absorption and penetration.

Sound has relatively low velocity in air because the molecules of gases are widely dispersed. The speed of light (an electromagnetic wave) is not similarly affected, which explains why during an electric storm you experience an interval between seeing a flash of lightning and hearing the roll of thunder. There is also relatively low absorption of sound energy through air because gas molecules are easily compressed; this explains the long distance that sound travels through air. By contrast, in a dense medium such as brick, sound velocity is relatively high because the molecules are close together. The wave energy, however, is quickly absorbed because dense molecules resist compression—so the wave travels only a short distance. The acoustic absorption coefficient describes the way in which energy is consumed in a traveling wave and attenuation describes the rate of energy loss. Readers may have had the experience of appreciating the high absorptive capacity of brick walls when there has been effective attenuation of sound from an adjacent room.

Tissue is a medium more dense than air but less dense than brick. Tissue, however, is not a homogeneous medium; it consists of interspersed layers and compartments of quite different density. Each tissue layer transmits and absorbs ultrasound according to its specific acoustical properties. Fluid elements, such as blood and water, have the lowest impedance values and lowest acoustic absorption coefficients. This means that these elements are poor absorbers of ultrasound. Bone, the most dense of all tissues, has the highest impedance value and highest acoustic absorption coefficient. This implies that bone is a good absorber of ultrasound. The energy absorbed by tissues from an ultrasound wave leads to physiologic changes and, with higher energy levels, heating of tissues.

Reflection and Refraction

The behavior of waves at boundaries is an important concept of ultrasound. When a wave crosses a boundary, it undergoes a loss of energy because some of the wave power is reflected back into the original medium (Fig. 4–2). In human tissues ultrasound encounters boundaries repeatedly. The acoustic properties of skin, fat, blood vessels, and muscle are similar. When ultrasound crosses boundaries from one to another of these layers, for example, from fat to muscle, the amount of reflection is insignificant to treatment outcome. However, reflection increases in proportion to the difference in acoustic impedance of the materials on either side of a boundary. The amount of reflection at a metal-air interface is about 99%, which means that the amount of ultrasound transmitted from a metal transducer to air is negligible. This is the reason for using a coupling medium in ultrasound treatment between the transducer and the skin. At a tissue-bone interface, some of the incident energy is reflected back into the tissue (see Fig. 4–2). If a wave arrives on a perpendicular path to a boundary, the line of travel for the transmitted and reflected portions remains on the perpendicular. Waves arriving at an angle from the perpendicular travel away from the boundary on a new path (see Fig. 4–2).

If the source of a wave is kept stationary opposite a boundary and the path of the incident and reflected waves coincide, the resultant energy along the path is the algebraic sum of the two waves. If the waves are also exactly in phase so that the high and low peaks of the inbound wave reinforce the high and low peaks of the returning wave, very intense peaks and lows of power result and the position of the wave is stationary. This is called a *standing wave*. To prevent the formation of standing waves in ultrasound treatment the ultrasound applicator must be continuously moved.

When waves arrive at boundaries on a nonperpendicular path, the transmitted portion of the wave changes direction (see Fig. 4–2). This is known as refraction, and it is one of the reasons for the gradual divergence of an ultrasound beam in the tissues. Refraction is proportional to the difference in acoustic impedance of

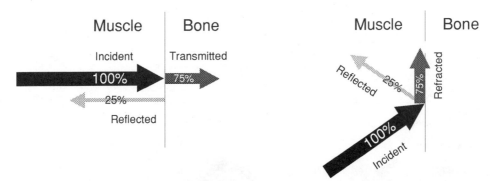

Figure 4–2. Schematic diagram showing reflection and refraction of ultrasound at a muscle-bone interface. (*A*) A wave arriving perpendicular to the boundary; (*B*) a wave arriving at an angle of 34° from the perpendicular.

the boundary materials and to the incident angle of the wave. Refraction at any combination of skin, fat, blood, or muscle interfaces is very small. At a tissue-air boundary, however, the transmitted wave changes direction by 90°. This means the wave travels along the boundary on the original side instead of crossing it. The clinical implication is that ultrasound energy is turned back into the tissues at an air-filled space, such as a sinus, and ultrasound does not leave the body. For example, ultrasound applied to one surface of the hand will penetrate the tissue and at the opposite surface the remaining energy will be reflected back into the hand.

Frequency

Frequency is an aspect of electronic waves that can be selected. Frequency describes the number of complete wave cycles generated each second. The duration of each cycle and wavelength necessarily decreases as the number of cycles per second increases. Therapeutic ultrasound units usually operate in the range of 0.75 million cycles per second (megahertz, MHz) to 3 MHz, but frequencies up to 5 MHz are available in some countries.

The frequency of ultrasound influences the amount of energy absorbed by the tissues. Higher frequency, with a correspondingly faster rate of molecule oscillation, entails more work and a greater amount of energy is absorbed. Absorption and attenuation are inversely related; therefore, higher frequencies also result in more limited penetration. Within the range of therapeutic equipment, it follows, therefore, that treatment using a frequency of 3 MHz will lead to more superficial effect than a treatment using a frequency of 1 MHz.

We have seen previously that tissue impedance also influences depth of penetration. The penetration of ultrasound is commonly described in terms of the distance at which 50% of the original intensity remains in the beam. This distance is called the *half-value depth* of ultrasound. The combined influences of frequency and tissue density on attenuation of ultrasound are shown in Table 4–1.

Intensity

Intensity is the term used to describe the magnitude of the force in a sound wave. As intensity increases so does excursion of molecules in the wave field. Intensity of an ultrasound treatment is the most significant factor in determining tissue re-

Table 4–1 **Attenuation of Energy in an Ultrasound Beam***

	ENERGY REMAINING (PERCENT OF ENERGY AT FRONT OF TISSUE LAYER) AT DIFFERENT THICKNESSES OF TISSUE					
Frequency of Ultrasound	FAT		MUSCLE			BONE
	1.0 cm	2.0 cm	1.0 cm	2.0 cm	4.0 cm	1.0 cm
3 MHz	65	53	41	17	3	0
1 MHz	87	76	74	55	30	1

*Approximate values through homogeneous tissue layers. Based on amplitude attenuation coefficients from Repacholi,[2] p 27.

sponse. Total power emitted by a transducer is measured in watts. A watt is a unit of electrical power. The area of the emitting surface is measured in square centimeters. Intensity is reported in watts per square centimeter (W/cm^2), which is the amount of power (in watts) from the transducer per effective radiating area of the transducer.

THERAPEUTIC EQUIPMENT

Generators and Transducers

Therapeutic ultrasound machines generate a pressure wave by causing a crystal to vibrate. The crystal is made of natural quartz or a synthetic material that responds to an alternating electric current by contracting during one phase of the current and expanding, when polarity is reversed, during the alternate phase (see Fig. 4–1). Thus when a rapidly alternating current is applied, the effect is a vibrating crystal. The crystal is housed inside an applicator called a *transducer*. The treatment surface of the transducer consists of a metal plate that acts as an interface between the vibrating crystal and the patient's tissues. Greater detail on the construction of ultrasound machines can be found in the text by Wells.[3]

Continuity between the crystal, metal plate, and tissues is essential for transmission of the pressure wave to the tissues. Reflection at a metal-air boundary is about 99%; therefore, an air gap between the transducer face and skin will prevent the pressure wave from leaving the transducer. This results in heating of the transducer, which is potentially damaging to the crystal.[4] An acoustically conductive couplant, oil or water based, is used between the transducer face and skin to improve continuity. Ultrasound units may feature a light-emitting diode (LED) on the transducer head, or some other type of signal that warns the operator when skin contact is inadequate. At the same time, power is interrupted and the unit timer waits in a hold mode until skin contact is resumed.

The electronic circuitry of an ultrasound unit is matched to the natural vibration frequency of the crystal. This means that transducers are not interchangeable among units of different manufacturers. Crystals are delicate and can be damaged by a hard blow and it is difficult, without sophisticated measuring equipment, to check when only part of a crystal is vibrating.

It has been noted that ultrasound treatment is applied at different frequencies. In older machines a separate transducer had to be purchased for each frequency. Recent technology has made it possible to switch to different frequencies on a single transducer head. Ultrasound units can be set to generate a pressure wave continuously or in very short pulses (pulsed ultrasound).

Therapeutic transducers are available in a variety of sizes from 1 cm^2 to 10 cm^2, with 5 cm^2 the most frequently used. The appropriate size, however, should be selected according to the anatomic area to be treated. For example, a 5-cm^2 applicator may be more appropriate for treatment in the axilla than a 10-cm^2 applicator. Whereas to access the web space between the thumb and first digit of the hand, a 1-cm^2 applicator may be indicated in order to maintain skin contact.

Ultrasound units are manufactured with different options. Flexibility is desirable because setting ultrasound characteristics specific to the tissue condition will lead to better treatment outcome. Options should be available for the following characteristics:

Frequency (1 or 3 MHz)

Various transducer sizes (effective radiating areas and external dimensions)

Continuous or pulsed modes (with several options for pulsed modes)

Dosage (intensity) from 0.1 to 3.0 W/cm^2

Features should include:

Intensity display (meter or digital type)

Treatment timer

Electronic contact monitor (LED or other indicator or thermistor monitor to protect the head from overheating)

Measurement of Intensity in an Ultrasound Field

Understanding of the spatial and temporal patterns of energy distribution within the ultrasound field underlies an understanding of the measurement terms.

Spatial Distribution of Energy   Characteristically an ultrasound transducer produces a pressure wave in the tissues confined to a near cylindrical beam, with a cross-sectional area similar to the diameter of the crystal (Fig. 4–3). The spread of the ultrasound field is modified by the frequency and size of the crystal. A lower frequency gives a more divergent beam than a higher frequency. If frequency is constant and the crystal is made smaller, for example, by changing from a 5-cm^2 to a 1-cm^2 transducer, again the field diverges more.

Variation of energy *within* an ultrasound field has clinical importance. The energy is unevenly distributed (1) because pressure waves radiating from different

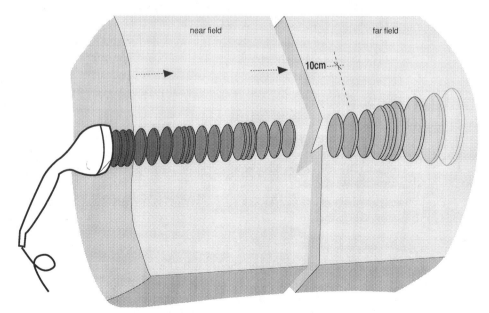

Figure 4–3. Schematic diagram showing transmission of ultrasound through a large homogeneous tissue with progressive loss of energy in the beam and divergence of the beam in the far field.

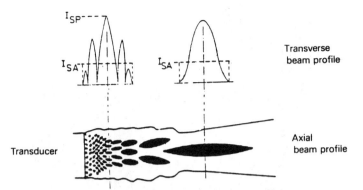

Figure 4–4. Intensity, spatial distribution. (*From Hekkenberg et al,[5] p 390, with permission.*)

points on the surface of the crystal interfere with each other, and (2) because vibrations around the circumference of the crystal are mechanically blocked by adhesive bonding of the crystal in the transducer cap. Energy distribution in a typical therapeutic sound field is shown schematically in Figure 4–4 and in scans of an ultrasound beam at two distances from the transducer face, in Figures 4–5 and 4–6. The noteworthy points are as follows:

1. Pressure is not evenly distributed over the cross-sectional area of the field.
2. A very high percentage of the applied intensity lies in the central one third of the beam. The remaining percentage is distributed in the surrounding two thirds of the beam.
3. The interference effect occurs closest to the transducer, in the portion of the field called the *near field*. The near field is of most interest to clinicians because the greatest amount of energy is absorbed by the tissues from this portion of the beam.

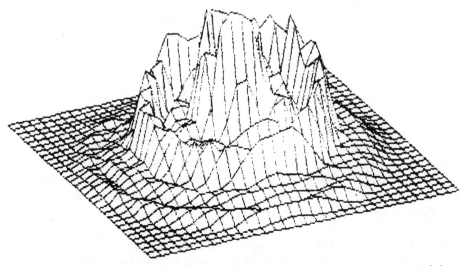

Figure 4–5. Hydrophone scan of an ultrasound beam in water showing uneven spatial distribution of energy. Characteristics: frequency 1 MHz; distance from transducer 0.5 cm; ERA 5.2 cm^2; BRN 4.2. (*Courtesy of Excel Tech Ltd., Mississauga, Canada.*)

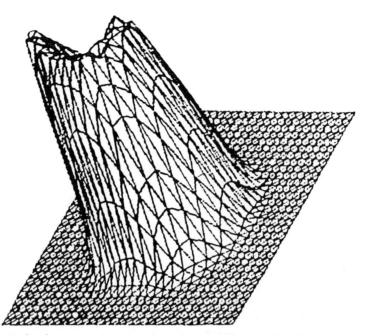

Figure 4–6. Hydrophone scan in water of an ultrasound beam of 1 MHz taken at a distance 10.0 cm from the transducer face. (*Courtesy of Excel Tech Ltd., Mississauga, Canada.*)

4. Energy is more evenly distributed across the beam area in the field furthest from the transducer. But the far field is less important clinically because the field is diverging and energy is rapidly attenuating.
5. Dividing the total power in the beam by the cross-sectional area of the crystal provides the average intensity of the treatment. Clearly average intensity does not reflect the uneven distribution in the near field.

The characteristic uneven spatial distribution of ultrasound has given rise to more specific measurement terms. Spatial peak intensity (SP_I) refers to the maximum intensity appearing at any point in the beam. Spatial average intensity (SA_I) is the intensity measured within 0.5 mm of the transducer and averaged out over the radiating area of the transducer. These new terms have been used increasingly over the last decade to describe ultrasound dosage.

The relationship between the spatial peak intensity and the spatial average intensity is called the *beam nonuniformity ratio* (BNR). BNR is a required labeling term in the specification of ultrasound machine characteristics. BNR informs the clinician what the highest intensity would be, within the beam, for the given transducer. For example, if the BNR of a crystal is 6:1, when the intensity is set by the clinician at 1.0 W/cm² there is a portion within the beam where the intensity of the treatment is at 6.0 W/cm². At a BNR higher than this, discomfort may be elicited during treatment.

Temporal Distribution of Energy   In continuous-mode ultrasound, the set intensity level remains constant throughout the treatment period. This means that the peak intensity equals the average intensity. If ultrasound power is intermittent during the treatment, as occurs in pulsed ultrasound, the average intensity over the treatment time is less than the peak intensity that occurs during the pulse. Figure 4–7 illustrates the difference between temporal average intensity (TA_I) and temporal peak intensity (TP_I).

The pulse ratio denotes the relationship between the pulse on and off periods. For example, a 1:1 ratio implies equal periods on and off. A common on time is 2 ms. A 1:1 ratio and a 1:4 ratio would then mean that in milliseconds the pulse is on 2 ms and off 2 ms, and on 2ms and off 8 ms, respectively. Ratios vary from 1:1 to 1:10, depending on manufacturer specifications of the machine.

The percentage of time that the ultrasound is on in each on-off period can be calculated from the pulse ratio and it is called the *duty factor* (cycle) of the treatment. In a 1:1 ratio, power is on for half of each on-off period, giving a duty factor of 50%. In a 1:4 ratio, power is on for one fifth of each period, giving a duty factor of 20%.

When pulsed doses of ultrasound are very low, the intensity during the pulse can still be quite high. In fact, the lower the duty factor, the higher the TP_I intensity. The relationship between TA_I and TP_I when TA_I is constant and the pulse ratio is varied, is shown in Figure 4–8. It should be recalled that energy is not evenly distributed in the beam and the combined effect of temporal and spatial energy variations can result in instantaneous doses of ultrasound in excess of 30.0 W/cm^2 ($SPTP_I$).

Manufacturing Trends and Technical Advancements

Technical advancements are constantly occurring. In one of the latest developments the clinician can use computer-controlled treatment duration. The clinician selects on the menu their requirements for treatment in regard to temperature (no heat, mild, moderate, or vigorous heat) and penetration depth, and keys in the size of the transducer and coupling medium they will be using. Intensity level is increased by the clinician. Ultrasound frequency and treatment duration are then controlled by the unit for treatment of a prescribed area (two times the effective radiating era [ERA]). The computation is based on a limited amount of research on normal tissue. The unit automatically extends treatment duration to compen-

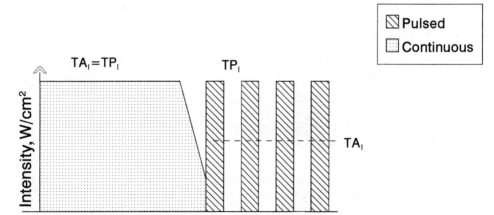

Figure 4–7. Schematic diagram showing the relationship between temporal average and temporal peak intensity in continuous versus pulsed-mode ultrasound.

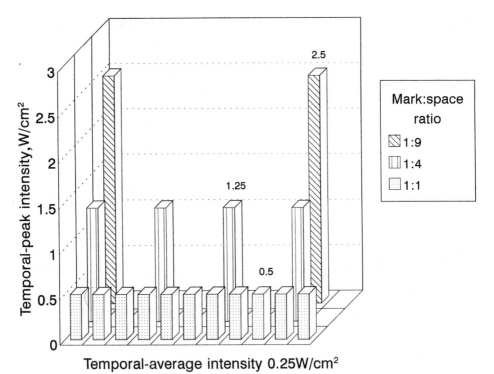

Figure 4–8. Schematic diagram showing the effect on temporal peak intensity of three different pulse ratios when the temporal average intensity is constant at 0.25 W/cm².

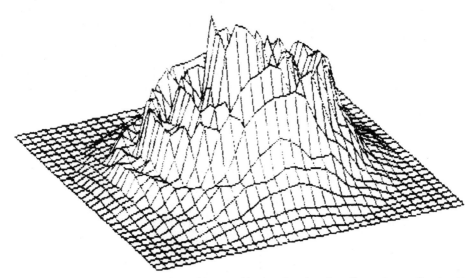

Figure 4–9. Hydrophone scan of an ultrasound beam showing the effect of appodization on spatial distribution of energy. Characteristics: frequency 1 MHz; distance from transducer 0.5 cm; ERA 5.5 cm²; total power 22.1 W; intensity 4.0 W/cm²; peak intensity 12.6 W; BNR 3.1. (*Courtesy of Excel Tech Ltd., Mississauga, Canada.*)

sate for inadequate coupling (a response to heating of the transducer). Such a device is certainly user-friendly, but it has limitations (Fig. 4–9).

Another development called *appodization* is already used by many ultrasound manufacturers. In this process the crystal is made with a tiny central hole, which dampens vibrations in the center of the crystal. The result is that the peak intensity in the beam is reduced and BNR has a lower value (approaching 2). Pressure distribution in the beam of a crystal with appodization is shown in Figure 4–10. It should be compared with Figure 4–5.

What are the implications for the future? Innovations such as the types mentioned above are likely only the beginning of a new generation of transducers and ultrasound controllers. Their value must be considered in terms of treatment outcome and usefulness to clinicians. What is clinically important is to establish if there is improved outcome for patients when dosages can be precisely set and ultrasound energy can be delivered with low spatial peak intensities. To date this has not been determined. These and future innovations need to be evaluated.

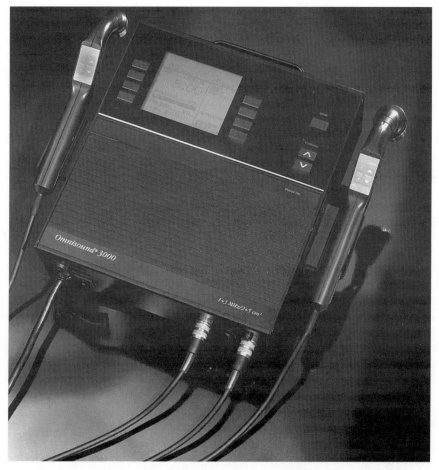

Figure 4–10. Photograph of an ultrasound unit with two transducers, dual frequency capability for each transducer, preprogrammed temperature increase settings, and both intensity and frequency controls located on each of the transducers. (*Courtesy of PTI, Topeka, KS.*)

Safety Regulations

There has been frequent criticism of therapeutic ultrasound machines for failing to meet testing standards on various characteristics.

Effective Radiating Area Ultrasound machines are calibrated by measuring the power of the transducer in watts in degassed water and dividing the power by the known ERA of the crystal in square centimeters. The ERA is calculated at or close to the transducer face. ERA includes all points of the cross-sectional beam area through which the radiated power has an intensity at least 5% of the maximum intensity in that plane. The ERA is less than the geometric area of the crystal. If the crystal is in some way defective and the actual ERA is not equal to the ERA measured at time of manufacture, the displayed dose is then an inaccurate reflection of the actual dose being received by the patient.

The finding of discrepancies between actual and nominal ERA in supposedly functioning units is reported in the literature.[5,6]

Beam Nonuniformity Ratio The BNR is the ratio of the maximum spatial intensity in the beam to the average spatial intensity (see Fig. 4–4). An acceptable value lies in the range of 6:1 or lower. There are reports of BNR values of 8 and even as high as 15.[7] That means that as the transducer is applied over the tissue there is a spot in the tissues receiving ultrasound at an intensity 8 to 15 times higher than the prescribed intensity. This "spot" occurs whether the applicator is moved or held stationary. There is substantial evidence that high doses of ultrasound and hot spots can be hazardous to regenerating tissue.[7,8]

Intensity Intensity of 3.0 W/cm^2 is often stated as the safe limit for treatment, based on the World Health Organization guidelines.[9] Lower intensities, however, are usually effective. A prudent approach to using any form of applied energy is to use the lowest dosage that achieves the desired effect.

Accurate determination of dosage is necessary for effective treatment and also to ensure patient safety. The intensity dial operated by a clinician controls the amount of electrical signal delivered to the transducer. If the efficiency of the crystal or its housing is impaired, the electrical signal is not converted to ultrasound energy and the patient does not receive the dose registered on the meter.

Machines are calibrated by using the measured power of the beam in degassed water at room temperature and the transducer ERA. A common approach is to measure the total power (W) using a radiation force balance and calculate intensity (W/cm^2) using the nominal ERA (at time of manufacture). A radiation force balance does not measure ERA. An acoustic hydrophone (underwater microphone) is utilized to scan transducers to determine the precise values for ERA and BNR (see Figs. 4–5 and 4–6). A plot is obtained from thousands of points in a plane parallel to the transducer face, which shows pressure variations in the field and will allow identification of total power, peak power, ERA, and BNR values. Ideally, dosage of an ultrasound unit should be calibrated annually using scanning techniques, with interim checks using a radiation force balance method.

Intensity is a critical factor in applying effective treatment with ultrasound. It is a measure dependent on the area of the crystal that generates pressure waves. Faulty equipment forces the clinician into errors that they cannot detect and can make the difference between effective and noneffective dosage. A discrepancy of 20% between the displayed dosage and actual value is the limit of acceptability.[5]

BIOPHYSICAL EFFECTS

The effects of ultrasound that predominate depend on whether the intensity delivered is high enough to cause heating of the tissues or whether heating is minimized or eliminated by use of low-intensity and pulsed-mode delivery.

Thermal Ultrasound

The heat that develops in the tissues from continuous-mode ultrasound is generated within the tissues. The ultrasound beam does not itself transmit heat. Heat accumulates by conversion of kinetic energy absorbed from the ultrasound beam. You can crudely mimic this effect by rubbing back and forth with a fingertip over a small area of your skin. The skin becomes heated. If you try to make the oscillations faster, keeping the distance the same, there is a greater amount of energy in the movement, with the result that heating is greater. These principles are true for delivery of ultrasound; the amount of energy absorbed from a wave is greater for higher frequency at the same displacement intensity. When energy is absorbed, penetration is reduced. The reason for the more rapid absorption and more superficial effect of ultrasound at 3 MHz, compared with ultrasound at 1 MHz, now becomes clear. Ultrasound at 3 MHz is not appropriate for heating deep-seated lesions, such as plantar fasciitis or adhesive capsulitis of the shoulder, as the heating takes place superficially.

In a high-intensity ultrasound field, tissue temperature is also raised as a result of unstable cavitation. Cavitation is the term for the stimulated behavior of micron-sized gas bubbles in the fluids in a sound field. Bubbles contract and expand, as they lose air and gain air, during the compression and rarefaction phases, respectively, of a sound wave. Cavitation activity increases as wave intensity increases. A number of conditions most coexist for unstable cavitation to occur. If intensity is high enough and the duration for expansion is long enough, bubbles become progressively larger because they tend to take in more air during the rarefaction phase than they lose in the compression phase. If there is sufficient repetition of cycles for bubbles to reach a critical size, they can collapse violently under pressure; this is called *unstable cavitation*. The "implosion" sends shock waves through the tissues and the released energy raises the overall tissue temperature. Frequency and cycle duration are inversely related; therefore, the duration for bubble growth is longer for lower-frequency waves. This explains why unstable cavitation occurs more readily at 1-MHz ultrasound rather than at 3 MHz.[10]

Energy is absorbed from an ultrasound beam in proportion to the density of the tissue. Different tissues will therefore become heated in proportion to their density. This is the basis of the statement often seen in the literature that protein structures "selectively" absorb ultrasound. It is probably more correct to state that ultrasound provides clinicians with an opportunity to deliver heat selectively to dense tissues, such as scar tissue, joint capsule, ligament, and tendon.

General principles of heat transfer apply to heating with ultrasound. This means that the ultimate temperature in the tissues will be the net effect of absorbed mechanical energy that is converted to heat, and heat transfer, to or from the tissue, by conduction and convection. It was noted previously that ultrasound is rapidly absorbed by periosteum, which becomes significantly heated. As a result, structures adjacent to bone gain additional heat in an ultrasound treatment by conduction of heat from the periosteum. Convection currents exist both within tissues, via circulating blood and lymph, and external to tissues, via air and water currents acting on the skin. Clinically this means that relatively dense tissues, such as scar tissue, capsule, ligament, tendon, and bone, which accumulate more heat from ultrasound, also retain heat better than more vascular tissue. Muscles, on the other hand, especially large "red" postural muscles, have an abundant capillary network so that they give up heat to adjacent cooler tissue from convection and conduction. When treatment is applied in water, heating of superficial tissue is limited by the loss of heat to the water, through convection and conduction.

Effects of tissue heating are the same for equivalent temperatures, regardless of the modality used. Thus a heating dose of ultrasound may diminish pain perception, by slowing nerve conduction velocity; raise the metabolic rate; increase blood flow, which assists in resolution of swelling; stimulate the immune system; increase extensibility of soft tissue and decrease viscosity of fluid elements in the tissues, in the temperature range of 40° to 45°C.[11] Temperatures above 45°C are noxious to tissues and can cause nonreversible tissue changes. Pain is normally felt before dangerous temperatures are reached.

Nonthermal Ultrasound

When heating effects of ultrasound are reduced, either by application of very low intensity or by pulsing the ultrasound, changes in cell function are noted. Mechanical vibration and acoustic streaming are mechanisms that initiate the nonthermal changes.

Mechanical Vibration and Acoustic Streaming The initial effect appears to occur at the cell membrane.[12] The membrane may be sensitive to the distortions that cells are subjected to in an ultrasound field. The mechanism of the distortion is twofold. The compression phase of an ultrasound wave deforms tissue molecules. The deformation is called radiation force but is sometimes referred to by the slang term "micromassage." Radiation force also affects gas bubbles in the tissue fluids and the bubble effects add further stress to cell boundaries. When bubbles expand and contract, without growing to critical size, the activity is called *stable cavitation*.[10] Cavitation sets up eddy currents in the fluid surrounding the vibrating bubble and eddy currents in turn exert a twisting motion on nearby cells. In the vicinity of vibrating gas bubbles intracellular organelles are also subjected to rotational forces and stresses.[13] The fluid movement in a sound field is generally known as *acoustic streaming*, but in an ultrasound field in living tissue the scale of the events is microscopic, and so it is sometimes called *microstreaming*.

To summarize the role of bubble activity (cavitation) in ultrasound mechanisms, it appears that gas bubbles are readily generated in an ultrasound field in living tissue even at low intensities.[14] Bubble activity augments the mechanical effect of a pressure wave. The scale of cavitation depends on the ultrasound characteristics; bubble growth is limited by low-intensity, high-frequency, and pulsed ultrasound. Higher frequency means shorter cycle duration, so that the time for bubble growth is restricted. Pulsed ultrasound restricts the number of successive cycles for growth and allows the bubble to regain its initial size during the off period. The risk of unstable cavitation is reduced when using 3 MHz, pulsed, low-intensity ultrasound for treatment. Cavitation is a phenomenon that must be considered both in thermal and nonthermal mechanisms of ultrasound.

Second-Order Effects of Athermal Ultrasound The primary site of ultrasound interaction is the cell membrane.[12] Destabilization of membranes leads to increased permeability, which allows various ions and molecules to diffuse into cells, where they precipitate a series of secondary events. Research on ultrasound has particularly focused on influx of calcium ions because calcium is a known second messenger for other cell functions, including protein synthesis. Histamine has also drawn attention because of its influence on circulation and stimulating effect on protein synthesis. Clinically it has been demonstrated that ultrasound facilitates tissue repair, and researchers are exploring various events that could explain the clinical benefits.[15]

Histamine and other vasoactive substances are released from granules in mast cells and from circulating platelets.[16] The extent of mast cell degranulation is in proportion to the ultrasound intensity. It is important to keep treatment intensity low as there is some indication from animal research that high-intensity ultrasound could produce too much histamine, which can potentially prolong inflammation rather than giving the desired effect of a stimulus to healing. Prolonged inflammation can potentially occur with any heat treatment given during the inflammatory stage post injury.

Increased plasma and cells for repair appear in the extravascular tissues after ultrasound. Histamine increases vascular permeability but it is hypothesized that ultrasound may enhance this. The result is an enhanced inflammatory response. Inflammation is an essential step in tissue repair because it brings cells that are normally in the circulation into the injury site. For example, monocytes arrive at the wound site and are turned into macrophages; they cleanse the wound. The macrophages release factors that attract fibroblasts.

Phagocytic activity of macrophages is increased. Accompanying this is an increase in the concentration and activity of lysosomes; lysosomes are the enzymes that break down foreign material. Clearing of tissue debris and bacteria is essential for tissue regeneration to begin.

Fibroblasts increase in number and show increased motility, a response which has been linked to macrophage release factors.[18] The stimulated fibroblast activity may provide a better basis for the subsequent step of fibroblast attachment and proliferation.

Protein synthesis by fibroblasts increases. Protein synthesis is the basis of collagen production. There are ultrastructural changes in the cell that may also be signs of increased activity in protein synthesis pathways.

Angiogenesis is enhanced.[18] This is the process of endothelial cell "budding" and growth into newly formed collagen to form blood vessels. The mechanism by which ultrasound stimulates this process is not clearly identified. It may be secondary to enhanced macrophage activity.

Capillary density is increased in ischemic tissue after repeated treatment with ultrasound. The effect, though, is only evident after repeated doses. The same effect is not seen in nonischemic tissue.[19]

Wound contraction is enhanced.[18] Contraction is an advantage in tissue repair since less scar tissue is required to fill the wound gap. There is a centralizing pull on healthy collagen fibers at the edge of the lesion that pulls the wound together. This process is attributed to myofibroblast activity. Ultrasound has been shown to increase smooth muscle cell activity and this may be the mechanism through which ultrasound enhances wound contraction.

In summary, the effects of ultrasound have been examined on different stages of tissue repair. Benefits have been demonstrated for various components of inflammation, proliferation, and maturation processes. Research is ongoing to identify the mechanisms and interactions that occur.

PRINCIPLES OF THERAPEUTIC APPLICATION

A HISTORICAL PERSPECTIVE

Ultrasound was used therapeutically as early as 1930.[9] The machines of the time only provided continuous-mode output and it was thought that treatment benefit was due entirely to heating effects. In the sixties, when pulsed ultrasound was available, the common dosage for treatment was still in the range 0.5 to 1.5 W/cm^2 SA$_I$. Clinical research in physical therapy was scarce up until this point but then the development of focused ultrasound for medical diagnostics, and continuing interest in ultrasound hyperthermia for treatment of cancer, promoted intensive medical research. The main interest of biophysicists doing the research was in intensities much lower at one end and much higher at the other end of the scale than were used in physical therapy. The by-product of this early research was the finding that beneficial results could be effected with lower doses than had been previously considered for treatment. The information generated by medical research filtered through to physical therapy literature in the early eighties and had a spin-off effect on treatment dosages. The medical research also gave impetus to research activities directed specifically toward therapeutic use of ultrasound.

A Current Perspective: Research on Therapeutic Ultrasound

Research through the eighties was most commonly conducted by scientists who were not themselves users of therapeutic ultrasound.[10,14,19] This trend has been recently reversed. The research in the early eighties concentrated mainly on low-intensity pulsed ultrasound to promote tissue healing. Current work also includes studies that evaluate heating doses of ultrasound. What is clear from a review of the literature is the wide gulf between dosages that promote healing and dosages that heat tissues.

Heating Tissues with Continuous-Wave Ultrasound

The literature on heating human tissues is scarce because invasive procedures are required to measure temperature at depth.[20–22] Some researchers have used a pig model to simulate heating in humans.[23,24] Studies on heating effects of ultrasound have used dosages from 0.5 to 3.0 W/cm^2 SA$_I$. Numerous studies have reported the heating effects of ultrasound, often reporting temperature changes as measured by inserted or implanted thermistors at various tissue depths.[20–25] It is not the purpose of this text to review all of the literature; the reader is encouraged to consult the reference list provided at the end of the chapter for additional information. Table 4–2 outlines some important points for treatment that can be deducted from the research to date.

Further research on tissue heating with ultrasound is essential. It appears from the present literature that ultrasound is not an efficient modality for heating large muscles such as gastrocnemius and quadriceps, probably because muscles have low absorptive capacity in the first instance and good blood supply to dissipate heat. Ultrasound in contact is effective for subcutaneous tissue and adjacent-to-bone tissue. Other modalities should be considered when muscle heating is required: shortwave preferentially heats vascular tissue and may be a more effective approach to muscle heating than ultrasound.

Clinical Studies Using Ultrasound as a Heating Agent

There are a few controlled clinical studies that evaluate ultrasound for treatment of chronic inflammatory connective tissue conditions, including lateral epicondylitis[26–28] and osteoarthritis.[29] The signs and symptoms of these conditions include soft tissue swelling, decreased range of movement, loss of strength, pain, and impaired function. The conditions have different etiology but there are some common underlying problems, including chronic inflammatory changes, with fibrosis, tissue contracture, and possibly adhesion development.[26–30]

Clinically, ultrasound is not used on its own for treatment of chronic conditions. When tissues are heated to increase extensibility, stretch must be applied and exercise through the range of motion must follow. What then can be learned from studies that treat chronic conditions with heating levels of ultrasound but without appropriate adjunctive treatment? Can ultrasound in combination with other treatment be properly evaluated? A dilemma is apparent for the researcher and clinician. For the reader it is clear: the literature must be approached critically. We need to be able to justify what we do with modalities. At the same time we do not want to discard treatments based on the negative findings of research when the research is problematic, the number of subjects in the study is small, and the treatment might yet be beneficial.

Clinical Studies Using Ultrasound to Facilitate Tissue Repair

The difficulty in studying effects of ultrasound on human tissue wounds is obvious, with the result that most of the research has been carried out on experimen-

Table 4–2   Important Points for Treatment Deduced from the Research to Date

1. The area of tissue that can be realistically heated using ultrasound is an area equivalent to twice the size of the radiating area of the transducer, i.e., $2 \times$ ERA

2. Water-immersion techniques considerably diminish *skin* and *subcutaneous* heating to a depth of at least 3 cm, due to the fact that water quickly absorbs heat. Despite the superficial cooling, effective deep heating occurs.

3. One should expect that patients would report little sensation of warmth during underwater treatments.

4. At 1 MHz and 1.0 W/cm² SA_I, using a stroking technique at a rate of 3.2 cm/s, a change in temperature of 4° to 6°C can be anticipated close to bone.

5. Therapeutic temperatures (40°C) are achieved with 8 to 15 minutes of ultrasound treatment using dosages between 1 to 1.5 W/cm².[20,21]

tal animal wounds. Animal studies often draw criticism because loose-skinned animals, typically rats and guinea pigs, and to a lesser extent pig skin, heal differently than human skin. While there are drawbacks to using animal models for ultrasound research, valuable information has emerged, which can and should be extrapolated to clinical practice, albeit with discretion.

Various animal studies looked at rate of wound contraction,[31] rate of wound healing,[32–36] rate and quality of tendon healing,[37–40] formation of new blood vessels,[41] activity of the phagocyte system,[42] and the role of calcium ions.[43] Ultrasound delivered at intensities between 0.1 and 0.5 W/cm^2 (SATA$_I$—spatial average temporal average intensity), usually pulsed in 20% duty cycle, consistently appeared to benefit healing, whether the experimental model was an open wound, a tendon repair, or closed trauma. Pulsed treatments at intensities of 0.8 W/cm^2 and higher, either proved no better than controls or retarded healing.[37] Recently a new area of interest has emerged, with the research finding that bone healing is enhanced with low-intensity ultrasound (0.1 W/cm^2 SATA, pulsed 1:4).[44]

There are a number of clinical studies that looked at the healing effects of ultrasound on venous ulcers[45–48] and pressure ulcers.[49] Treatments using intensities higher than 0.5 W/cm^2 SATA in continuous mode did not always provide benefit.[46] Treatments using lower dosages in continuous mode and the dosage 0.5 W/cm^2 SATA$_I$ in a pulsed mode 1:4 were beneficial.[45,48] It should be noted that when 0.5 W/cm^2 SATA$_I$ was used in a pulsed-mode 10% duty cycle, no benefit was seen.[47] What is the optimum pulse ratio for stimulation of tissue healing? It has been shown that when the intensity is extremely high, even though the pulse is short (2 ms), the occurrence of unstable cavitation is enhanced,[50] which may explain the lack of benefit using a 10% duty cycle.

In contrast to the facilitation of human tissue repair demonstrated by use of low-dose pulsed ultrasound, a study using high-intensity ultrasound to treat damaged tissues demonstrated a worsening of subjects' symptoms. Muscle inflammation and pain (delayed-onset muscle soreness) were induced in human volunteers and then ultrasound was applied to the muscle at 1 MHz, 1.5 W/cm^2 SA$_I$ for 5 minutes using a 10-cm^2 transducer size.[51] Compared with controls, the treatment increased subjects' symptoms of pain. The results of this work suggest that such high-intensity ultrasound can aggravate tissue injury during the acute phase. Important points for treatment that can be deduced from the research are outlined in Table 4–3.

Reliability and Efficiency of Ultrasound Equipment

There are a number of studies that have assessed the function of ultrasound equipment.[4–7] Authors appear to be in agreement that equipment is not reliable and clin-

---

Table 4–3 **Treatment Techniques for the Facilitation of Tissue Healing**

1. Lower dosages of 0.1 and 0.2 W/cm^2 SATA$_I$, pulsed in 20% duty cycle, are beneficial for tissue healing.

2. Brief treatment durations are sufficient to stimulate healing processes. Each area of tissue equivalent to the radiating area of the transducer should be treated for 30 to 60 seconds, i.e., 30 to 60 seconds per ERA.

3. Treatment should be repeated daily or every 48 hours to enhance healing.

ical units should be checked regularly. Researchers have found units with BNR values[7] and ERA characteristics[5] that do not agree with values reported by the manufacturer. The availability of suitable technology (since about 1980) and increasing awareness of the importance of BNR and accurate measurement of ERA have promoted this area of research.

Transmission Properties of Ultrasound Couplants

Some studies have compared transmission properties of ultrasound coupling media to determine their relative acoustic transmission efficiency.[52–54] The comparator is usually degassed water. The results show that acoustic conductivity differs among products. Docker[52] notes that the properties required of a couplant are that it lubricates the skin, absorbs very little ultrasound, has sufficient viscosity not to "run off," has no odor, does not stain clothing, and is not susceptible to bubble formation. A sterile semisolid gel dressing (Geliperm, Geltech Sons Ltd, Newton Bark, Chester, England) 3.3 mm thick, has been tested for efficiency and it transmitted 95% of ultrasound power.[55] The testing was done underwater with the adhesive dressing applied directly to the transducer face. It would be difficult to apply a dressing to skin without trapping air, significantly decreasing the acoustic conductivity. The purpose of the dressing is to allow treatment directly over abrasions and wounds, using water or gel lubricant between the dressing and transducer. The authors who tested the product recommended using a syringe to fill shallow wounds with sterile saline before applying the dressing in order to eliminate air gaps between the tissue and dressing. An adhesive transparent wound dressing available in North America (Opsite, Smith & Newphew, Inc., Lachne, Quebec, Canada) transmitted less than 10% of radiated ultrasound power when tested using similar procedures.[56]

Phonophoresis and Phonophoretic Products

Phonophoresis is the practice of applying ultrasound through a medicated couplant. The mechanism by which phonophoresis may enhance uptake of drugs is not known.[57] One theory is that ultrasound pressure drives the drug into the skin. An alternative theory is that heating of superficial tissue causes vasodilation of dermal capillaries, which speeds up the rate at which drugs are absorbed into the circulation. Another theory suggests that increased permeability of cell membranes enhances diffusion of the drug into the cell, which is the site of the chemical interactions. The studies on phonophoresis reflect all three theories.

The goal of some earlier studies[58,59] and more recent work[60] was to determine the depth that drugs were driven by ultrasound. Investigative procedures such as muscle sectioning in rabbits and joint aspirations in dogs were carried out as soon as 10 minutes after phonophoresis. Whereas drugs appeared in greater amounts at the depth of muscles, no benefit was found at the depth of the canine knee. It remains uncertain whether the drug needed more time to diffuse to greater depth or if in fact benefit is limited to the depth of muscle.

It is unclear from a review of the literature whether drugs that normally diffuse through the skin diffuse in greater amounts after ultrasound.[51,57,61] Early noncontrolled clinical trials[62–64] showed that patients with a variety of inflammatory conditions benefited from phonophoresis using hydrocortisone preparations; implying, as with the above depth studies, that the drug was successfully transmitted through skin by the ultrasound. However, in two recent controlled studies on epicondylitis,[65,66] hydrocortisone preparations of 10% and 1% were used without significant benefit compared with ultrasound alone. A topical nonsteroidal anti-inflammatory drug was rubbed on the skin in another study and the same amount of drug was absorbed whether ultrasound was added or not.[67] In preliminary testing it was shown that less than 1% of ultrasound power was transmitted when 10% hydrocortisone acetate was mixed in gel and used as a couplant. Poor transmission qualities of some preparations may account for lack of benefit.[57]

The question of how much ultrasound is transmitted through phonophoretic preparations[54,68–70] was only studied after the early clinical trials. A variety of topical creams, ointments, and gels were generally found to be less efficient than regular gels and water for transmission. For most products tested, transmission was better at a frequency of 1.5 MHz and 3 MHz than at 0.75 MHz, and there was no difference in transmission between intensities of 0.3 W/cm^2 SA$_I$ and 1.0 W/cm^2 SA$_I$.[68] Preparations tested at 1.5 W/cm^2 SA$_I$ suggested that drug-containing media that transmitted 80% ultrasound power could be considered good media. There was a choice of corticosteroids, local anesthetics, and nonsteroidal anti-inflammatory and salicylate drugs that met this criteria. The products tested included a variety of creams, ointments, gels, other media, and mixed media (Table 4–4). Conflicting findings have been reported on some preparations.[70] Transmission through hydrocortisone cream has been reported as 47%[69] and 1%.[57] Neither level is satisfactory and it makes it difficult to explain the earlier clinical successes of hydrocortisone phonophoresis.

The confusion in this field may be because of lack of uniformity in research methods. There are differences in preparation of phonophoretic products, especially in concentration of active ingredients, in the type of base (gel, ointment, or cream), and in the dosage and number of ultrasound treatments. It seems that in preparation for phonophoretic treatment a clinician should at the least do a crude underwater test on the medicated product to see if it transmits any ultrasound.

Indications for Treatment

Apart from ultrasound there are other modalities to stimulate tissue healing, such as pulsed shortwave diathermy, laser and low-frequency transcutaneous electrical currents (TENS). There are also alternatives for heating tissues, such as continuous shortwave diathermy, hot packs, and other superficial agents. A series of questions may assist the inexperienced clinician in deciding whether ultrasound is indicated.

1. Has a tissue problem been clearly identified? Ultrasound is not a global treatment for undiagnosed pain and impairment of function. The clinician should have determined specific treatment goals when ultrasound is being considered.
2. Is stimulation of tissue repair indicated? Acute and subacute inflammation from strains and sprains, bruising, muscle tears, burns, superficial and deep skin wounds, crush injuries, and other similar types of conditions, respond positively to low-intensity pulsed ultrasound.
3. Is heat and stretch indicated? Restriction of movement, with or without pain, because of muscle spasm, chronic edema, fibrosis, connective tissue contracture, adhesions, unresolved hematoma, and similar conditions of a chronic inflammatory nature are indications for high-intensity continuous-mode ultrasound.
4. Is ultrasound a time-effective approach to the problem? The clinician has to be with the patient for the duration of treatment. Ultrasound in excess of

Table 4–4   **Ultrasound Transmission by Phonophoresis**

Good Transmitting Media	Percentage Transmission Relative to Water (%)
Lidex gel, fluocinonide 0.05%	97
Thera-Gesic cream, methyl salicylate 15%	97
Mineral oil	97
Ultrasound gel (U*)	96
Ultrasound lotion (Polysonic)	90
Betamethasone (Pharmfair) 0.05% in gel (U*)	88
Poor Transmitting Media	
Diprolene ointment, betamethasone 0.05%	36
Hydrocortisone powder 1% in gel (U*)	29
Hydrocortisone powder 10% in gel (U*)	7
Cortril ointment, hydrocortisone 1%	0
Eucerin cream	0
Hydrocortisone cream 1% (EF†)	0
Hydrocortisone cream 10% (EF†)	0
Hydrocortisone cream 10% (EF†) in equal weight gel (U*)	0
Myoflex cream, trolamine salicylate 10%	0
Triamcinolone acetonide cream 0.1% (EF†)	0
Velva hydrocortisone cream 10% (Purepac Pharm.)	0
Velva hydrocortisone cream 10% in equal weight gel (U*)	0
White petrolatum ointment	0
Other Preparations	
Chempad-L, lidocaine 2%, menthol 1%	68
Polyethylene wrap (Saran wrap)	98

*Ultraphonic
†E. Fougera & Co.
Source: From Cameron et al,[70] p 145, with permission.

12 to 15 minutes is not time efficient and a shortwave diathermy approach should be considered. Ultrasound is indicated for treatment of well-defined localized tissue areas.

5. Is the target tissue accessible? Ultrasound is preferentially absorbed by dense tissue; therefore, bone and joint structures should not lie between the problem and the path of the ultrasound beam. For example, this would mean selecting an alternative modality if swelling is inside a joint, whereas swelling outside a joint may be an indication for ultrasound. If the patient

is unable to maintain a posture that makes the tissue accessible, another modality should be considered. For example, a contracture of the inferior portion of the shoulder joint capsule may be better heated with shortwave diathermy if a patient is unable to abduct the arm sufficiently for an ultrasound approach.

6. Is delivery of ultrasound practical? Either direct contact or a water-immersion technique has to be used. Skin breakdown, risk of infection, tenderness, and presence of dressings, casts, and splints may preclude the use of ultrasound.

7. Is the treatment goal to enhance delivery of topical medication? If difficult tissue contours preclude ultrasound delivery, iontophoresis may be an alternative, for example, over the lateral epicondyle of the humerus or the calcaneal bursa in "bony" individuals.

8. Is ultrasound medically safe for the patient? There are some contraindications that would immediately preclude ultrasound as a choice of treatment. Screening of patients is essential.

SAFETY CONSIDERATIONS WITH THE APPLICATION OF ULTRASOUND

Precautions

Precautions are necessary to protect patients, clinicians, and equipment. Discomfort should not be experienced during treatment. Pain is usually a sign of too much periosteal heating, and treatment settings must be adjusted by decreasing intensity or moving the transducer more quickly. It is possible to cause a burn with ultrasound,[32] and this is the reason why some national radiation councils have regulated output limits for ultrasound.[9]

A stationary transducer technique is not safe; there is a great risk of overheating at "hot spots" in the field and there is an added risk of standing wave formation. This caution especially applies when there are implanted materials in the tissues.[71,72] Metal reflects about 90% of incident ultrasound,[8,15] and therefore the chance of standing wave formation is increased. Plastic responds like periosteum and it absorbs a large percentage of ultrasound.[71,73] Generally, treatment over implanted materials is safe provided proper technique is used.

Skin integrity is not essential for ultrasound treatment; however, direct contact with gel may be inappropriate over traumatized skin and in dermatologic conditions. A water-immersion technique can be used provided infection control procedures are followed. Clinicians should protect themselves during all water-immersion techniques; gloves serve the purpose well, because they trap air that reflects ultrasound, thus at the same time they prevent self-treatment and contamination.

Transducer crystals are fragile and transducers should be handled with care. Intensity should only be increased when the transducer is in contact with a suitable medium, because a metal-air interface prevents transmission of the pressure wave. When energy cannot flow from the transducer, the metal cap itself becomes heated. Heat may affect the bonding of the crystal within the transducer. Repeated careless use of the transducer will eventually damage the crystal.

Contraindications

Ultrasound promotes cell proliferation and cell activity. Abnormal cell division occurs in many serious medical conditions, including cancer and tuberculosis, and in non–life-threatening diseases such as psoriasis. Ultrasound is contraindicated over or close to the site of any abnormal growth. The clinician should be extraordinarily cautious in treating undiagnosed pain in patients with a past history of malignancy.[74] Tissue being treated with radiation therapy should not be treated with ultrasound.

Rapid cell division and growth is also a feature of fetal development and, as yet, the effect of therapeutic ultrasound on the human fetus is unknown. For safety, ultrasound treatment is never given over the lower back or abdomen of a pregnant woman. Diagnostic ultrasound, at 2.5 MHz, is used at significantly lower doses than therapeutic ultrasound (less than 0.1 W/cm^2).

The contraindication to treatment over epiphyseal plates in children has been passed on as part of the tradition of ultrasound. These plates give rise to new bone cells. The original work that gave rise to concern was done on legs of dogs at very low frequency (0.8 MHz) and high intensity (0.5–3.0 W/cm^2 SA) using a stationary transducer. These characteristics would have caused high absorption and intense heating of bone. Subsequent work on animal bone by Dyson[75] and others[76] suggests that healing fractures in fact benefit from ultrasound at low doses. In view of the adverse treatment characteristics of the early work and advantages found in recent work, treatment over epiphyseal plates in children is not considered a contraindication at the present time. It is suggested that low treatment intensity be used and that the course of treatment should not be prolonged.[8,15]

Treatment of the orbits of the eyes and directly over the gonads is contraindicated. Ultrasound should not be applied over the area of a thrombus.[77] Treatment of the calf after a deep vein thrombosis also is contraindicated; it is thought that ultrasound might dislodge a thrombus, which could have catastrophic consequences.

Pain and temperature awareness must be checked before treatment with continuous-mode ultrasound. Sensation must be intact to proceed with heating dosages.

Infection that is enclosed under tension, i.e., abscesses, should not be treated with ultrasound. Infection with open drainage can be treated using very low pulsed dosages, but should be discontinued if there are any signs of increased redness, heat, or pain.

Ultrasound vibration may interfere with operation of any implanted medical device, such as a pacemaker, and should be avoided directly over the device. Ultrasound should not be applied below the ribs directed at the heart.[78]

Ultrasound should not be used when there is uncontrolled bleeding. It is ideal for enhancing reabsorption of hemorrhage in soft tissue, but treatment should begin after bleeding has ceased or after replacement factor has been administered in conditions such as hemophilia.

THERAPEUTIC APPLICATION

PROBLEM ANALYSIS AND GOAL SELECTION

A successful outcome with ultrasound is best assured when treatment settings are carefully matched to treatment goals. History taking and a hands-on assessment of the patient is required to identify the tissues involved in the problem, and to define the tissues in terms of location, extent of involvement, textural changes, and interference with function. Stimulation of tissue repair would be an appropriate goal if the problem were an acute or resolving tissue injury. Heating tissue prior to stretch could be the treatment goal if examination revealed a tissue contracture. Ultrasound has a sedative effect on pain and pain control could be the treatment goal in certain conditions, for example, herpes zoster (shingles).

Some or all of the following information may be used in analysis of the problem.

1. History of the injury
2. Relevant medical history
3. History of oral and injected drugs
4. History of previous modality use
5. Swelling and discoloration
6. Findings upon palpation
7. Range of movement
8. Pain (as measured on a pain scale)
9. Skin and wound appearance
10. Comparison with the contralateral side

Figure 4–11 depicts an ultrasound treatment for a chronic lateral epicondylitis.

Acute, Resolving, or Chronic Condition

The problem may be considered acute or resolving for a period up to 3 to 4 months after injury. Repetitive injuries, for example, "tennis elbow," are characterized by acute bouts superimposed on a chronic problem and the underlying chronic condition must also be addressed.

Inflammatory swelling feels spongy, fluid, and mobile on palpation. Chronic edema is dense, organized, usually restrictive, and immobile. Swelling may be dif-

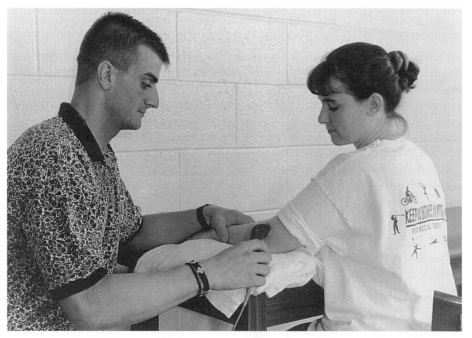

Figure 4–11. Photograph of an ultrasound treatment to the lateral epicondyle.

fuse or consist of well-defined thickened bands around ligaments and tendons. Restraining bands are best identified by palpation during movement. Skin bruising and chronic brown discoloration are evidence of acute and chronic swelling, respectively. Brownish pigmentation, as seen in chronic venous disease, is caused by pigment release from red blood cells.

Swelling seldom remains localized. Depending on the extent of swelling and available space at the injury site, extravascular fluid tracks with gravity and settles in loose-connective-tissue areas where if it is not reabsorbed it becomes progressively more organized by invading fibroblasts. For example, a patient who had a fractured patella may have limited knee extension with obvious indurated swelling around the patella. Assessment is not complete until the popliteal fossa has been examined; it may reveal thickened tissue restricting the capsule and flexor tendons. All involved tissue must be treated for optimum outcome. Bony prominences, for example, the lateral malleolus, and surfaces that preclude good contact, such as the dorsum of the hand, should be noted.

For most conditions time is an indicator of the state of tissue repair. Exceptions occur. Nonhealing wounds, often called chronic wounds, may have a history of months or years, but as noted previously, wounds respond to healing doses of ultrasound. Hematomas of 1 to 2 weeks duration may be very dense and organized. A low-dose approach can be tried on hematomas for one to two treatments, and if no benefit is found, a mild heating approach should be used. A history of previous unsuccessful ultrasound treatment may be a reason for choosing an alternative modality.

Steroids are anti-inflammatory drugs. Low-dose ultrasound is proinflammatory. The effects of ultrasound may be inhibited in patients who take oral steroids, for instance, patients with rheumatoid disease. This is not a contraindication to ultrasound treatment but expectations should be realistically adjusted.

Ultrasound Parameter Selection

The purpose of an assessment is to reach a decision regarding the treatment goals for that patient. At the outset, the clinician has to decide whether to stimulate healing or to heat the tissues. The judicious approach is to select a specific dose, one that is low enough to benefit healing tissues or high enough to heat tissues. A model for clinical decision making is shown in Table 4–5.

Sequence of Ultrasound in a Treatment Plan

Stimulation of tissue healing by ultrasound is effected through a cascade of events triggered by the treatment and the benefit is not immediately evident. Ultrasound may be sequenced prior to any other activities in a treatment plan to take advantage of the pain-relieving effects of the modality.

The purpose of thermal treatment with ultrasound is to increase tissue length; therefore, stretch must be imposed on the tissue immediately after ultrasound. Without proper sequencing, thermal doses of ultrasound are pointless.

There are numerous methods of stretching tissues and clinicians generally have individual approaches they prefer. The important point is not how the stretch is achieved, but that heated tissues should be stretched gently through the full available range of motion, without increasing pain levels. Independent or assisted exercise using mechanical devices (see Chapter 8), proprioceptive neuromuscular

Table 4–5 **Ultrasound Treatment Parameters: A Model for Clinical Decision Making**

Treatment Parameter	Healing Tissue	Heating Tissue	Rationale
Frequency	3 MHz norm; 1 MHz > 4.5 cm depth, e.g., wound sinus, hip, lower spine	1 MHz norm; change to 3 MHz if patient reports pain	Frequency effects penetration; cavitation risk ↑ as frequency ↓,
			Deep penetration enhances heating by: (1) reflection off bone; (2) heating of periosteum; (3) conduction
Mode and duty factor	Pulsed 1:4, i.e., 20%		Pulsed mode → ↓ heat and ↓ cavitation risk; duty factor 20% enhances tissue repair; ? effect duty factor < 20%
		Continuous mode	Conserve heat by no off periods
Intensity	0.1–0.2 W/cm² (SATA)		Sufficient to stimulate tissue repair
		≥ 0.8 W/cm² if bone is superficial; ≥ 1.5 W/cm² if bone is deep; ↑dose until skin warmth is reported	Heating occurs at lower dose if bone is superficial
			Skin and deep heating occur simultaneously

Continued

facilitation techniques, or end-of-range mobilization techniques are all appropriate methods of applying stretch.

Research shows that optimum results are achieved if the stretch is maintained during the cooling period.[79–81] There is little information on the time it takes for human tissues to cool after ultrasound heating. Judging from Lehmann et al.'s[39] studies on human thighs, full-range stretching activities should continue for a duration of 8 to 10 minutes. Strengthening through *full* range is appropriate during the cool-down period, but strengthening and other activities in *smaller* ranges should be postponed until after the cool-down period.

It is the practice of some clinicians to apply ice in combination with ultrasound. The reason for applying ice is not clear. Cooling changes the depth at which ultrasound is absorbed because attenuation increases as temperature decreases.[82] Prior cooling results in more superficial absorption of ultrasound. In fact, ice and

Table 4–5   **Ultrasound Treatment Parameters: A Model for Clinical Decision Making** *(Continued)*

Treatment Parameter	Healing Tissue	Heating Tissue	Rationale
Treatment time	30–60 s per ERA		Stimulates repair via second messengers, e.g., calcium
		Minimum 5 minutes from reported skin warmth; 8–10 minutes total; 10–12 minutes under water	5 minutes at 40°–45°C → ↑ extensibility; inefficient if area > 10 cm^2; water cools tissue
Transducer size	5 cm^2 norm; 10 cm^2 for large flat areas	5 cm^2 norm; 10 cm^2 for large flat areas	ERA ↓ → penetration ↓; 1 cm^2 only if area is inaccessible
Contact media	Gel or water		Depends on pain and tissue integrity
		Gel preferred;	Water ↓ heat to ≤ 3 cm depth
		Products tested for phonophoresis	Transmission qualities vary
Treatment repetition	Until resolution; or response falls off		No cumulative effect; treat maturation stage for improved scar tissue
		Until resolution; or response falls off	Assess before and after treatment—for carry-over and transient effect; 3–4 treatments without benefit → change ultrasound settings or discontinue

ultrasound appear to have contradictory effects. Ice causes vasoconstriction, decreases cell activity, and overall has an anti-inflammatory effect. Low-dose ultrasound is a proinflammatory agent. Ice effectively restricts bleeding and swelling in acute tissue trauma; low-dose ultrasound initiated 24 hours after injury promotes resolution of the swelling and repair of tissue. Application of ice after ultrasound would likely inhibit the effects of the ultrasound.

The use of ice and thermal doses of ultrasound also appears to be contradictory. Decreasing tissue temperature, and thereby increasing stiffness, prior to or after using ultrasound to heat the tissues in order to resolve the stiffness appears to be indefensible! Moreover, there is no advantage to rapid cooling of tissues during or after stretch.[83] Applying any heating modality when sensory nerves have been numbed is a dangerous practice and for this reason ice should not be applied before ultrasound.

The use of ice for pain control at the end of a treatment session that included thermal ultrasound may be seen clinically. There seems to be no conflict in this practice, as long as the ice is used briefly. Research shows that for an application of under 8 minutes, the effect of ice is very superficial (less than ½ inch or 1 to 2 cm).[84] Therefore, a 5-minute ice pack will relieve posttreatment pain[85] without counteracting the benefit achieved from deep heating ultrasound, stretch, and exercise.

Ultrasound Treatment Procedures

A minimum amount of preparation is required for ultrasound treatment, which probably accounts for its high favor among clinicians. No discomfort is experienced during treatment with ultrasound, which no doubt explains why it is well accepted by patients.

1. Preparation for Treatment   Before uncovering the body part to be treated and positioning the patient, all accessory items should be collected. If choosing in-water coupling, the treatment container should be plastic or rubber, as metal reflects stray ultrasound. Treatment in a whirlpool or in water that has been vigorously stirred is not recommended. Air bubbles on the patient's skin should be gently smoothed away before underwater treatments.

Air bubbles are also trapped on the skin under gel; they are just less obvious and get overlooked. When skin is generously covered in hair, trapped air cannot be so easily overlooked. Modern machines, with electronic contact monitors, confirm this by switching off power. Transmission improves if air is removed by smoothing down hair with a wet cloth before gel is applied.

2. Patient Education and Consent to Treat   Patient consent implies that the patient has been advised of the benefits and risks of the procedure, as well as the sensations they should expect during the procedure.

In the case of pulsed ultrasound there should be no sensation other than the gliding of the transducer on the skin. When ultrasound is given in a continuous mode, mild skin heating occurs, usually at doses above $0.8 \text{ W/cm}^2 \text{ SA}_I$. Pain is a sign of excess periosteal heating. Patients should be instructed that the appropriate sensation is mild warmth and that excess heat, or pain, should be reported immediately.

For patient safety, and to ensure delivery of effective treatment, inability to report skin warmth should be an exclusion criterion for continuous-mode ultrasound. Potential to cooperate should be considered when patients are very young, very old, or have limited understanding.

3. Preparation of Equipment   The treatment space must be organized for safety, comfort, and access. Clinicians should be seated with back support, and positioned so that the tissues being treated and dials of the equipment are simultaneously visible and within easy reach.

Time and intensity dials should be at zero before the main power is switched on and returned to zero after treatment. A reminder is appropriate at this point that the clinician checks on the ultrasound unit that the intensity meter is set at W/cm^2 (not total watts).

4. Patient Position Patient comfort is basic to treatment with any modality. Support is required for trunk and limbs, whether the patient is lying or sitting. Injured limbs need the additional support of pillows or rolled towels, and elevation should be provided for acute swelling even though treatment periods are short.

Specific positioning must be considered in addition to general principles. For example, the supraspinatus tendon lies partly under the acromion. If the arm is passively extended, the humeral head rotates forward from underneath the acromion, and the tendon can be reached where it inserts into the greater tuberosity of the humerus; otherwise this tendon is not accessible. The patient can be seated in a high-backed chair with his or her arm resting on padding over the chair back to achieve the required position.

5. Technique Gel is applied to the skin or to the surface of the transducer. There should be a 1- to 2-mm layer that would be sufficient to allow gliding of the soundhead without creating a mess. The soundhead is moved in overlapping circles or linear paths from the moment power is increased. Overlap ensures even distribution of energy to the treated tissue (recall that maximum intensity is distributed in the central one third of the ultrasound beam). The rate of transducer movement is slow, maximum 3 to 4 cm/s. If the transducer is "raced" over the skin, ultrasound effects may be reduced.

To ensure maximum penetration, the soundhead should be parallel to the tissue surface, which means adjusting the angle of the soundhead to the contours of the part being treated. In other words "point" the transducer toward the target tissue. This applies to treatment given in contact, when air gaps must not be allowed between the transducer and skin, and to water-immersion techniques, when treatment is applied at a distance of 1 to 2 cm from the skin.

6. Adjustment of Parameters During Treatment If a patient reports pain during a thermal mode treatment with ultrasound, the clinician must immediately lower intensity. There are two options for proceeding: the treatment can be delivered at a lower intensity, provided the patient still feels skin warmth, or the intensity can be delivered at a higher frequency, which will result in less periosteal heating and should eliminate pain. If pain persists in spite of taking one of the above steps or the patient complains of increased pain associated with the condition, treatment should be terminated.

7. Repetition of Treatment There is no limit to the number of ultrasound treatments that can safely be applied, but treatment should only continue if measurable and sustained benefits are noted.

Observation and Documentation After Ultrasound Treatment

Assessment after treatment and prior to the next treatment is essential to demonstrate to the patient, as well as to satisfy the clinician and any third-party payer, that ultrasound is effective for the patient's problem. Some immediate benefits can be expected.

Ultrasound has a soothing effect on pain, possibly from stimulation of mechanoreceptors in the skin acting via a gate control mechanism, and also from the sedative effect of heat. The "feel" of tissues is a subjective measure, and as such is difficult to document. Palpation will provide one of the surest signs of posttreatment improvement. An example is the softening of an unresolved hematoma after ultrasound.

Documentation of Ultrasound Treatment

Incomplete documentation makes it difficult to repeat successful treatment or to determine how to modify treatment. Good documentation includes details of the patient's position; the treatment area; the technique; the transducer size; the machine settings for frequency, pulse ratio, intensity, and duration of treatment; and the nature and sequence of other activities.

CARE OF THERAPEUTIC ULTRASOUND EQUIPMENT

BIOMEDICAL DEPARTMENT INSPECTION

Electrical safety checks should be left to technical experts who may be available through institutional biomedical departments or through manufacturers or distributors of equipment. Specialized equipment is required to measure the total power, spatial distribution of power, and ERA of the ultrasound beam to recalibrate machines. In view of the fact that displayed dosage tends to be unreliable[5–8,15] recalibration every 6 months is advisable.

CLINICAL MONITORING

Clinicians should watch for signs of damaged or worn equipment. When the metal face of a transducer is old it becomes dull or ridged and may not transmit ultrasound adequately. Undue heating of the transducer is a sign that energy is being lost within the transducer instead of being transmitted to the patient. The most common damage is inflicted by dropping the head. A dent in the transducer casing is a sign that the crystal might be damaged.

A water displacement test can be performed to see if the unit is emitting any sort of pressure wave. The head is held under water with the face at an angle of 45° to the surface, which will protect the crystal from the beam being reflected back from the water air boundary; intensity is turned up to 1.0 W/cm^2. The beam should cause a cone-shaped displacement of the water surface opposite the transducer face. The displacement should change appearance as the intensity is changed. These simple tests do not replace checks by qualified technicians.

The conductivity of gels and medicated topical agents for phonophoresis can be tested in a similar manner. The height and shape of the water displacement is compared with and without a 1- to 2-mm layer of the couplant spread over the transducer face.

SUMMARY

An understanding of the physical properties and physiologic effects of ultrasound are fundamental to effective use of the modality. Distribution of energy in an ultrasound beam is dependent on frequency and radiating area of the beam. When the BNR is higher than 8, damaging "hot spots" can occur in tissues. A moving head technique is required to distribute the points of maximum intensity evenly through the treated tissue. Distribution of ultrasound also varies in time, dependent on pulsing ratio. The lower the percentage duty cycle, the higher the temporal-peak intensity. Penetration depends on frequency and density of the medium.

Good clinical outcomes using ultrasound are achieved by careful treatment planning. Low-intensity pulsed ultrasound stimulates cellular activities that then trigger a chain of events leading to enhanced tissue repair. Benefit is obtained at dosages of 0.1 to 0.2 W/cm^2 $SATA_I$ (pulse ratio 1:4) for 30 seconds per 5 cm^2 of treatment area. Heating of tissue by ultrasound is for the treatment of chronic inflammatory conditions that restrict movement. Heating occurs with continuous-mode ultrasound using intensities between 0.8 to 1.5 W/cm^2 SA and higher. Tissue stretching should be performed during or immediately following heating. Appropriate timing is an important aspect of treatment.

DISCUSSION QUESTIONS

1. The patient is a 50-year-old woman with chronic venous swelling of the lower legs. She has an ulcer 20 cm^2 in area and 2 cm deep on the anteromedial aspect of one leg. The ulcer has not healed in 10 months despite excellent wound cleansing by a visiting nurse and use of moist dressings.

   a. Select ultrasound parameters that would be suitable to stimulate healing of the ulcer.

   b. Draw on paper a representative 20-cm^2 ulcer. Calculate the time it would take you to apply ultrasound around the perimeter of the ulcer at the rate of 30 seconds per 5 cm^2 of treatment area. If you have a 5-cm^2 transducer face you can count exactly the number of 5-cm^2 areas that fit around the ulcer perimeter.

   c. The patient's skin circulation is also compromised in areas close to the ulcer because of severe tissue swelling. How can you use ultrasound to improve the condition of these other areas?

2. A 30-year-old patient suffered a whiplash injury 10 days ago. The present problems are painful muscle-guarding spasm of the upper trapezius, limited range of neck movement, and headache that the patient reports starts at the back of the head. As part of the current treatment session you plan to use ultrasound.

   a. Select ultrasound parameters that would be suitable for treating the muscle spasm.

   b. Would you also consider using ultrasound over the spinal joints at the level of the injury? If so, what parameters would you use?

REFERENCES

1. Hill, CR: Ultrasound biophysics: A perspective. Br J Cancer 45(suppl V):46, 1982.

2. Sternheim, MM and Kane, JW: General Physics, ed 2. Wiley and Sons, New York, 1991.

3. Wells, P: Biomedical Ultrasonics. Academic Press, London, 1977.

4. Allen, KGR and Battye, CK: Performance of ultrasonic therapy instruments. Physiotherapy 64:174, 1978

5. Hekkenberg, RT, Oosterbaan, WA, and van Beekum, WT: Evaluation of ultrasound therapy devices. Physiotherapy 72:390, 1986.

6. Fyfe, MC and Bullock, MI: Acoustic output from therapeutic ultrasound units. Austr J Physiother 32:13, 1986.

7. Hekkenberg, RT, Reibold, R, and Zeqiri, B: Development of standard measurement methods for essential properties of ultrasound therapy equipment. Ultrasound Med Biol 20:83, 1994.

8. Williams, R: Production and transmission of ultrasound. Physiotherapy 73:113, 1987.

9. Repacholi, M: Standards and recommendations on ultrasound exposure. In Repacholi, MH, Grandolfo, M, and Rindi, A (eds): Ultrasound: Medical Applications, Biological Effects and Hazard Potential. Plenum Press, New York, 1987, p 233.

10. Apfel, RE: Acoustic cavitation: A possible consequence of biomedical uses of ultrasound. Br J Cancer 45(suppl V): 140, 1989.

11. Lehmann, JF, Warren, CG, and Guy, AW: Therapy with continuous wave ultrasound. In Fry, FJ (ed): Ultrasound: Its Applications in Medicine and Biology. Elsevier, New York, 1978, p 561.

12. Dinno, MA, et al: The significance of membrane changes in the safe and effective use of therapeutic and diagnostic ultrasound. Phys Med Biol 34, 1989.

13. Nyborg, WL: Ultrasonic microstreaming and related phenomena. Br J Cancer 45(suppl V):156, 1982.

14. ter Haar, G, et al: Ultrasonically induced cavitation in vivo. Br J Cancer 45(suppl V):151, 1982.

15. Williams, AR: Ultrasound: Biological Effects and Potential Hazards, Academic Press, London, 1983, p 177.

16. Williams, AR: Release of serotonin from human platelets by acoustic streaming. J Acoust Soc Am 56:1640, 1974.

17. Fyfe, MC and Chahl, LA: Mast cell degranulation. A possible mechanism of action of therapeutic ultrasound. Ultrasound Med Biol 8 (suppl 1):62, 1982.

18. Dyson, M: Role of ultrasound in wound healing. In McCullough, JM, Kloth LC, and Feedar, JA (eds): Wound Healing: Alternatives in Management, 2d ed. FA Davis, Philadelphia, 1995.

19. Hogan, RD, Burke, KM, and Franklin, TD: The effect of ultrasound on microvascular hemodynamics in skeletal muscle: Effects during ischemia. Microvas Res 23:370, 1982.

20. Lehmann, JF, DeLateur, BJ, and Silverman, DR: Selective heating effects of ultrasound in human beings. Arch Phys Med Rehabil 47:331, 1966.

21. Lehmann, JF, et al: Temperatures in human thighs after hot pack treatment followed by ultrasound. Arch Phys Med Rehabil 59:472, 1978.

22. Draper, DO, et al: A comparison of temperature rise in human calf muscle following applications of underwater and topical gel ultrasound. J Orthop Sports Phys Ther 17:247, 1993.

23. ter Haar, GR and Hopewell, JW: Ultrasonic heating of mammalian tissues in vivo. Br J Cancer 45(suppl):65, 1982.

24. Forrest, G and Rosen, K: Ultrasound: Effectiveness of treatments given under water. Arch Phys Med Rehabil 70:28, 1989.

25.   Lehmann, JF: Therapeutic temperature distribution produced by ultrasound as modified by dosage and volume of tissue exposed. Arch Phys Med Rehabil Dec:662, 1967.

26.   Haker, E and Lundeberg, T: Pulsed ultrasound treatment in lateral epicondylalgia. Scand J Rehabil 23:115, 1991.

27.   Binder, A, et al: Is therapeutic ultrasound effective in treating soft tissue lesions? Br Med J 290:512, 1991.

28.   Lundeberg, T, Abrahamsson, P and Haker E: A comparative study of continuous ultrasound, placebo ultrasound and rest in epicondylalgia. Scand J Rehabil 20:99, 1988.

29.   Falconer, J, Hayes, K, and Chang, R: Effect of ultrasound on mobility in osteoarthritis of the knee. Arthritis Care Res 5:29, 1992.

30.   Hashish, I, et al: Reduction of post-operative pain and swelling by ultrasound treatment: A placebo effect. Pain 33:303, 1988.

31.   Dyson, M and Smalley, DS: Effects of ultrasound on wound contraction. In Millner, R, Rosenfeld, E, and Cobet, U (eds): Ultrasound Interactions in Biology and Medicine. Plenum Press, New York, 1983, p 151.

32.   Shamberger, RC, et al: The effect of ultrasonic and thermal treatment on wounds. Plast Reconstr Surg 68:860, 1981.

33.   Byl, N, et al: Incisional wound healing: a controlled study of low and high dose ultrasound. J Orthop Sports Phys Ther 18:619, 1993.

34.   Young, SR and Dyson, M: Effect of therapeutic ultrasound on the healing of full-thickness excised skin lesions. Ultrasonics 28:175, 1990.

35.   Dyson, M, et al: The stimulation of tissue regeneration by means of ultrasound. Clin Sci 35:273, 1968.

36.   El-Batouty, MF, et al: Comparative evaluation of the effects of ultrasonic and ultraviolet irradiation on tissue regeneration. Scand J Rheumatol 15:381, 1986.

37.   Roberts, M, Rutherford, JH, and Harris, D: The effect of ultrasound on flexor tendon repairs in the rabbit. Hand 14:17, 1982.

38.   Enwemeka, CS, Rodriquez, O, and Mendosa, S: The biomechanical effects of low-intensity ultrasound on healing tendons. Ultrasound Med Biol 16:801, 1990.

39.   Turner, SM, Powell, ES, and Ng, CSS: The effect of ultrasound on the healing of repaired cockerel tendon: Is collagen cross-linkage a factor? J Hand Surg 14B:428, 1989.

40.   Stevenson, JH, et al: Functional, mechanical, and biochemical assessment of ultrasound therapy on tendon healing in the chicken toe. Plast Reconstr Surg 77:965, 1989.

41.   Young, SR and Dyson, M: The effect of therapeutic ultrasound on angiogenesis. Ultrasound Med Biol 16:261, 1990.

42.   Saad, AH, and Williams, AR: Effects of therapeutic ultrasound on the activity of the mononuclear phagocyte system in vivo. Ultrasound Med Biol 12:145, 1986.

43.   Al-Karmi, A, et al: Calcium and the effects of ultrasound on frog skin. Ultrasound Med Biol 20:73, 1994.

44.   ter Haar, G: Recent advances and techniques in therapeutic ultrasound. In Rapacholi, MH, Grandolfo, M, and Rindi, A (eds): Ultrasound: Medical Applications, Biological Effects and Hazard Potential. Plenum Press, New York, 1987, p 333.

45.   Dyson, M, Franks, C, and Suckling, J: Stimulation of healing of varicose ulcers by ultrasound. Ultrasonics Sep:232, 1976.

46.   Eriksson, SV, Lundeberg, T, and Malm, M: A placebo controlled trial of ultrasound therapy in chronic leg ulceration. Scand J Rehabil Med 23:211, 1991.

47.   Lundeberg, T, et al: Pulsed ultrasound does not improve healing of venous ulcers. Scand J Rehabil Med 22:195, 1990.

48.   Callam, MJ, et al: A controlled trial of weekly ultrasound therapy in chronic leg ulceration. Lancet 2(8582):204, 1987.

49.   Nussbaum, EL, Biemann, I, and Mustard, B: Comparison of ultrasound/ultraviolet-C and laser for treatment of pressure ulcers in patients with spinal cord injury. Phys Ther 74:812, 1994.

50.   Pickworth, MJW, et al: Studies of the cavitational effects of clinical ultrasound by sonoluminescence: 2. Thresholds for sonoluminescence from a therapeutic ultrasound beam and the effect of temperature and duty cycle. Phys Med Biol 33:1249, 1988.

51.   Ciccone, CD, Leggin, BG, and Callamaro, JJ: Effects of ultrasound and trolamine salicylate phonophoresis on delayed-onset muscle soreness. Phys Ther 71:666, 1991.

52.   Docker, MF, Foulkes, DJ, and Patrick, MK: Ultrasound couplants for physiotherapy. Physiotherapy 68:124, 1982.

53.   Balmaseda, MT, et al: Ultrasound therapy: A comparative study of different coupling media. Arch Phys Med Rehabil 67:147, 1986.

54.   Benson, HAE and McElnay, JC: Transmission of ultrasound through topical pharmaceutical products. Physiotherapy 74:587, 1988.

55.   Brueton, RN and Campbell, B: The use of geliperm as a sterile coupling agent for therapeutic ultrasound. Physiotherapy 73:653, 1987.

56.   Nussbaum, EL: Personal communication. August, 1994.

57.   Byl, NN et al: The effect of phonophoresis with corticosteroids: A controlled pilot study. J Orthop Sports Phys Ther 18:590, 1993.

58.   Griffin, JE and Touchstone, JC: Ultrasonic movement of cortisol into pig tissue—movement into skeletal muscle. Am J Phys Med 42:77, 1963.

59.   Novack, EJ: Experimental transmission of lidocaine through intact skin by ultrasound. Arch Phys Med Rehabil 45:231, 1964.

60.   Muir, WS, et al: Comparison of ultrasonically applied vs. intra-articular injected hydrocortisone levels in canine knees. Orthop Rev 19:351, 1990.

61.   Davick, JP, Martin, RK, and Albright, JP: Distribution and deposition of tritiated cortisol using phonophoresis. Phys Ther 68:1673, 1988.

62.   Griffin, JE, et al: Patients treated with ultrasonic driven hydrocortisone and with ultrasound alone. Phys Ther 47:595, 1967.

63.   Kleinkort, JA and Wood, F: Phonophoresis with 1% vs 10% hydrocortisone. Phys Ther 55:1321, 1975.

64.   Wing, M: Phonophoresis with hydrocortisone in the treatment of temporomandibular joint dysfunction. Phys Ther 62:33, 1982.

65.   Stratford, P, et al: The evaluation of phonophoresis and friction massage as treatments for extensor carpi radialis tendinitis: A randomized controlled trial. Physiother Can 41:93, 1989.

66.   Holdsworth, LK, and Anderson, DM: Effectiveness of ultrasound used with a hydrocortisone coupling medium or epicondylitis clasp to treat lateral epicondylitis: Pilot study. Physiotherapy 79:19, 1993.

67.   Benson, HA, McElnay, JC, and Harland, R: Use of ultrasound to enhance percutaneous absorption of benzydamine. Phys Ther 69:114, 1989.

68. Benson, HA and McElnay, JC: Topical NSAID products as ultrasound couplants: Their potential in phonophoresis. Physiotherapy 80:74, 1994.

69. Warren, G, et al: Ultrasound coupling media: Their relative transmission. Arch Phys Med Rehabil 57:218, 1976.

70. Cameron, MH and Monroe, LG: Relative transmission of ultrasound by media customarily used for phonophoresis. Phys Ther 72:142, 1992.

71. Lehmann, JF, et al: Ultrasound: Considerations for use in the presence of prosthetic joints. Arch Phys Med Rehabil 61:502, 1980.

72. Skouba-Kristensen, E: Ultrasound influence on internal fixation with a rigid plate in dogs. Arch Phys Med Rehabil 63:371, 1982.

73. Krotenberg, R, Ambrose, L, and Mosher, R: Therapeutic ultrasound effect on high density polyethylene and polymethyl methacrylate. Arch Phys Med Rehabil (abstr) 67:618, 1986.

74. Sicard-Rosenbaum, L, et al: Effects of continuous therapeutic ultrasound on growth and metastasis of subcutaneous murine tumors. Phys Ther 73:3, 1995.

75. Dyson, M: Therapeutic applications of ultrasound. In Nyborg, WL and Ziskin, MC (eds): Biological Effects of Ultrasound (Clinics in Diagnostic Ultrasound). Churchill Livingstone, New York, 1985, p 121.

76. Duarte, LR: The stimulation of bone growth by ultrasound. Arch Orthop Trauma Surg 101:153, 1983.

77. Frizzel, LA, Miller, DL, and Nyborg, WL: Ultrasonically induced intravascular streaming and thrombus formation adjacent to a micropipette. Ultrasound Med Biol 12:217, 1986.

78. Williams, AR: Effects of ultrasound on blood and the circulation. In Nyborg, W and Ziskin, MC (eds): Biological Effects of Ultrasound. Churchill Livingstone, New York, 1985, p 49.

79. Lehmann, JF, et al: Effects of therapeutic temperatures on tissue extensibility. Arch Phys Med Rehabil 41:481, 1970.

80. Warren, CG, Lehmann, JF, and Koblanski, JN: Elongation of rat tail tendon: Effect of load temperature. Arch Phys Med Rehabil 52:465, 1971.

81. Sapega, AA, et al: Biophysical factors in range of motion exercise. Physician Sports Med 9:57, 1981.

82. Gammell, PM, LeCroissette, DH, and Heyser, RC: Temperature and frequency dependence of ultrasonic attenuation in selected tissues. Ultrasound Med Biol 5:269, 1979.

83. Lentell, G, et al: The use of thermal agents to influence the effectiveness of a low-load prolonged stretch. J Orthop Sports Phys Ther 16:200, 1992.

84. Low, J and Reed, A: Cold therapy. In Electrotherapy Explained Principles and Practice. Heinemann Medical, Oxford, 1990, p 202.

85. Waylonis, GW: Physiologic effects of ice massage. Arch Phys Med Rehabil 48:38, 1967.

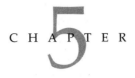

Therapeutic Use of Light: Ultraviolet and Cold Laser

Barbara J. Behrens, BS, PTA

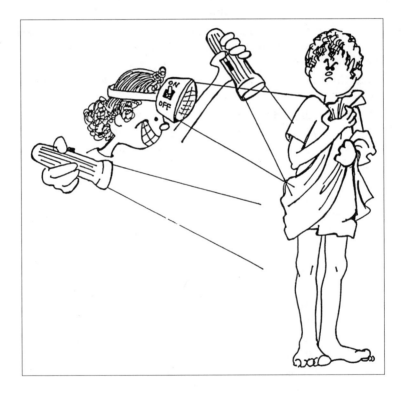

CHAPTER OBJECTIVES

- Define the uses of light in clinical practice.
- Outline the physical properties of light.
- Outline the electromagnetic spectrum in terms of therapeutic light sources.
- Describe the application of ultraviolet light.
- Discuss the production of laser light.
- Discuss the potential uses for laser light.
- Discuss the regulatory guidelines involving investigational devices.

CHAPTER OUTLINE

Sunlight is perhaps one of the most primitive examples of a physical agent. It provides illumination in the dark and warmth from the cold. Continuous study of its differentiating characteristics has led to the development and refinement of several forms of treatment modalities that utilize different forms of light, namely ultraviolet (UV) and laser.

This chapter will discuss and outline the uses of both cold laser and UV light in terms of their indications, application techniques, and safety considerations. It is not intended to be an in-depth study of the theoretical basis for either modality. It is merely an overview for clinicians should they have the opportunity to utilize the techniques in the future.

UV and laser represent two modalities that are not commonly in use in clinical facilities in the United States today, for very different reasons. Lasers are considered "investigational devices" by the Food and Drug Administration (FDA), and are therefore restricted in their use with humans. Investigational status of a modality is a classification assigned to any "new" modality application for human use. There is a process that any new modality introduced within the United States must go through to ensure both the safety and the efficacy for human use. Laser will be discussed in terms of the process involved with an investigational modality, as well as its applications as reported in the literature. UV light or radiation represents a modality utilized primarily for the treatment of skin conditions, many of which are now treated pharmacologically and under the auspices of a dermatologist. It will be discussed in terms of its application considerations.

LIGHT AS A THERAPEUTIC MODALITY

Both laser and UV can be administered to a patient to accomplish a specific set of treatment goals. Light has very specific characteristics that differentiate it from other forms of energy. These characteristics will be discussed in this section.

CHARACTERISTICS OF LIGHT

Light is defined in part by its wavelength and frequency. Techniques utilizing light take into consideration the physical properties of reflection, refraction, and absorption.

Wavelength

The spectrum of visible light is made up of light of many different wavelengths, each represented by its own specific color. Wavelength is the distance between the beginning and the end of a single wave cycle. The wave cycle referred to is the oscillation of electromagnetic energy, which occurs in an orderly and predictable pattern of a sine wave (Fig. 5–1).

Wavelengths are measured in nanometers (nm), or billionths of a meter. The visible spectrum of wavelengths occurs between 400 and 800 nm. All visible colors from violet to red have wavelengths within this range. Wavelengths from 180 to 400 nm represent UV nonvisible light and wavelengths from about 800 to 1500 nm are considered infrared. Ultraviolet occurs on the electromagnetic spectrum just adjacent to visible violet light. Infrared occurs just beyond the visible red wavelengths (Fig. 5–2).

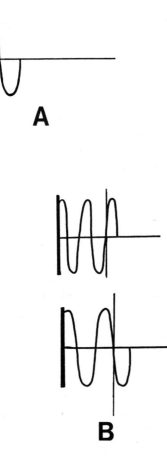

A

B

Figure 5–1. *(A)* A sine wave. *(B)* As the wavelength is longer, there are fewer wavelengths occurring within a given time.

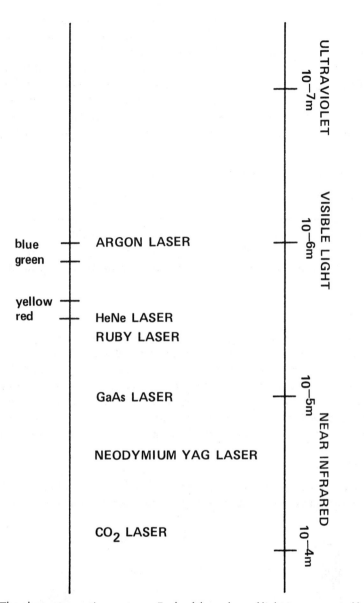

Figure 5–2. The electromagnetic spectrum. Each of the colors of light is represented by a specific wavelength, which is measured in nanometers (nm). The visible range is indicated.

Frequency

The frequency of a color of light is inversely proportional to its wavelength. The higher the frequency, the shorter the wavelength. The frequency and resultant wavelength influence the absorption of the light source. Higher-frequency, shorter-wavelength light has a tendency to be absorbed at a more superficial level than light of longer wavelengths.[1,2]

Two bands of UV are commonly used. They are referred to as UV-A and UV-B. The difference between the two forms of UV is in their frequency and wavelength.

UV-B has a higher frequency and therefore a shorter wavelength (250 to 320 nm) than UV-A (320 to 400 nm). Both UV-A and UV-B are used clinically with different responses.[4] UV-B from unfiltered sunlight or simulated sunlight can potentially be harmful to human skin. UV-B may cause degenerative and neoplastic changes in the skin and modification of the immunologic system of the skin. Therefore prolonged unmonitored exposure is not recommended.[6] UV-C is a third band of UV that has been discussed in the literature. UV-C, which has a wavelength of 250 nm, has been utilized to promote wound debridement bactericidal effects and tissue regeneration.[7]

PHYSICAL PROPERTIES OF LIGHT

Reflection

Light, like sound, travels in a sine wave pattern and has specific properties such as reflection, refraction, and absorption. Reflection refers to the phenomenon of throwing back a ray of radiant energy from a surface. Light has the ability to "bounce off" different surfaces. The degree of reflection is reduced as the treatment angle approaches 90°.[2]

Refraction

Refraction refers to a "bending" of energy that is related to the source of the energy, referred to as the incident angle of the energy delivered. The light source may be redirected off a surface at an angle. Example: if a flashlight is pointed at a mirror, it will *reflect* the light back to the flashlight if the flashlight is perpendicular to the surface of the mirror. If the angle is not perpendicular, the light will be *refracted* or "bent" in another direction. The incident angle determines the direction of the redirected light; it also influences the delivery of energy to the treatment tissue (Fig. 5–3).

Absorption

Absorption is a substance's ability to take in light or radiant energy. The intensity of the light source will reduce as it passes through a substance. Window blinds

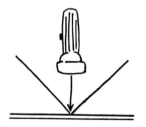

A

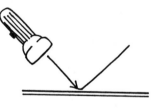

B

Figure 5–3. Light from a flashlight directed at a reflective surface. When the incident angle is 90°, most of the light is bounced off the reflective surface back to the incident source. When the incident angle is less than 90°, the beam bounces back at an angle in another direction. The body is not a reflective surface. In order for penetration to occur in a predictable area, the incident source of light needs to be at a 90° angle. When the angle is less than 90°, part of the energy may be refracted, or "bent," so that it enters the tissue in an unpredictable manner.

typically absorb a great deal of light and only allow a small amount of light through, which is at a much lower intensity once it passes through into a room. Absorption is inversely related to penetration. If an energy source is absorbed by whatever it is passing through, then it will not penetrate deeply. If the energy source is not absorbed, reflected, or refracted, it may penetrate to a much greater depth. In order for a light source to have a physiologic effect, it must be absorbed by the tissue.

Incident Angle and Dosage

Light may be either reflected, refracted, or absorbed, depending on its wavelength, the incident angle of the source, and the type of material receiving the light source. If the given wavelength can be absorbed by a substance or tissue, the absorption intensity will also depend upon the distance from the source. Doubling the distance with radiant light sources typically increases the spread of the light source so that it covers a larger area. By increasing the size of the area but not changing the intensity of the source, it is the same as decreasing the intensity per unit area. If, for example, the treatment area was 1 cm^2, and the source was 10 cm away from the surface, moving the source a distance of 20 cm from the surface will increase the coverage to 4 cm^2 and provide 25% of the intensity per given area. This is known as the *inverse square law*: doubling the distance will decrease the intensity to 25% of the original amount. If the intensity of a radiant heat source is too great, increasing the distance from the patient will significantly decrease the intensity (Fig. 5–4).

This becomes an important consideration in the use of light as a therapeutic modality. If the dosage is to be constant, then the distance from the source must be constant. If a patient is being treated with a radiant source of energy such as a heat lamp and feels uncomfortable, then increasing the distance from the source of the energy will make him or her more comfortable. It is important to note that the increase in distance will significantly alter the delivered dosage.

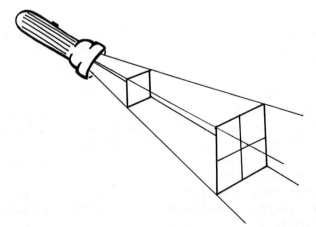

Figure 5–4. The inverse square law: Increasing the distance will decrease the intensity by the square of the distance. If the distance from the flashlight is doubled, then the light will cover four times the area but be one-fourth of the brightness or intensity of the original source.

ULTRAVIOLET (UV)

UV light has been utilized as a treatment modality for dermatologic conditions such as psoriasis. UV falls just beyond the visible portion of the electromagnetic spectrum and is therefore not visible to the naked eye. UV follows the principles that have been described for light. The absorption of UV is also dependent upon the wavelength, with absorption being greater for shorter wavelengths. Shorter wavelengths tend to penetrate less than longer wavelengths, but this is also dependent upon the thickness of the epidermis and the amount of melanin in the skin.[1] Melanin is a significant factor in the protection of human skin from the effects of UV.[5]

PHYSIOLOGIC EFFECTS OF UV

UV is used predominantly to promote an erythemal response, which occurs within 12 hours of exposure to the UV. Photon energy is absorbed by pigmenting molecules of the skin such as melanin. The absorbed energy may induce photochemical reactions and release chemical energy into the surrounding molecules of the skin, promoting chemical reactions, potentially impacting the immune system.[1,6–8]

AN OVERVIEW OF THE APPLICATION TECHNIQUE FOR UV

The following information is intended to serve as a guide to the application of the modality, potential reasons for its application, and safety considerations for its application. It is not intended to be an in-depth study of UV.

Treatment Goals with UV

- Erythemal response within 12 hours of initial exposure
- Pigmentation-thickening of the stratum corneum of the skin
- Destruction of bacteria in wounds and ulcers

Safety Considerations

- Patients who are photosensitive should not be treated with UV. (UV is a photon energy source that may not be tolerated well by individuals who are specifically photosensitive. These individuals typically burn easily when exposed to sunlight.)
- Patients with pellagra, a niacin-deficiency dermatitis, should not receive UV (UV exposure may reduce the effectiveness of Langerhans cells of the epidermis. The Langerhans cells are capable of activating T lymphocytes and may be involved in the promotion of contact dermatitis.)[6]
- Patients who have dermatitis secondary to systemic lupus erythmatosus (SLE) should not receive UV. (Sunlight is said to induce skin lesions in patients with SLE and to exacerbate the systemic manifestations of the disease.[8,9])
- Patients with active tuberculosis should not receive UV, as it may exacerbate the disease process.[2]
- Patients with a fever or acute diabetes should not receive UV, as it may exacerbate the disease process.[2]

- Skin rarely exposed to light may respond more dramatically to UV. (Areas such as the genitals may respond adversely to UV and therefore should receive one third to one half the dosage of the rest of the body.)[4]
- Some medications are photosensitizing and cause reactions to UV. Topical antihistamines, phenothiazine, sulfonamides, hexachlorophene, and topical bleaches are considered photocontact allergens that will respond adversely to UV.[10] Some antibiotics and some diuretics photosensitize the patient. Patients who are taking these medications should not receive UV if the medication has been identified as a photosensitizing drug.[4]
- Both the patient and the clinician should wear protective eye gear with UV (unprotected exposure to UV may promote the formation of cataracts and conjunctivitis).

Dosage

In order to establish a minimal erythemal dosage (MED)—the exposure time necessary to produce a mild erythema that lasts up to 48 hours—the UV lamp should be placed approximately 60 to 90 cm from the patient at a 90° angle to the surface being treated. The steps involved in determining the dosage level are illustrated in Figure 5–5 and outlined in Table 5–1.

Because of the application techniques of UV and the importance of accurate dosimetry, patient education is important. A patient must understand that the purpose of the MED test is to determine just how much exposure time is necessary based on their skin sensitivity. The UV used in the clinic is not for "tanning" pur-

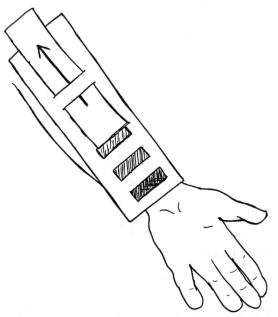

Figure 5–5. A method that can be used to determine a minimal erythemal dosage (MED). The patient would be draped so that no skin was exposed except for the forearm. This piece of cardboard is made so that there are several openings, as well as a slide cover that can be pulled up to reveal one opening at a time. The most distal opening would receive the longest exposure time, and the most proximal opening would receive the least amount of exposure time.

Table 5–1   **Minimal Erythemal Dosage (MED) Procedure**

1. Drape patients so that only a small area of the forearm is exposed.

2. Give patients protective polarized goggles to wear and instruct them not to look at the UV lamp when it is ON.

3. Cover the exposed forearm with a prepared piece of UV opaque cardboard that has a total of four to six openings in it. Each of the openings should be about 1 cm^2 and 1 cm apart, preferably of different shapes. Cover the openings with an additional piece of UV-opaque cardboard of equal size.

4. Allow the lamp to warm up according to the manufacturer's instructions.

5. Place the lamp perpendicular to the area being tested and a distance of 60 to 80 cm from the site.

6. Open the shutters of the lamp and expose the first opening for 30 seconds, then expose the second opening for another 30 seconds, etc.

7. Close the shutters of the lamp.

8. Turn the lamp OFF.

9. Instruct the patient to monitor the forearm every 2 hours and note which opening or shape appeared pink/red first and when it faded.

Dosimetry:

MED   = time necessary to produce erythema

1° dose = 2.5 MED to produce erythema for up to 48 hours

2° dose = 5 MED to produce erythema, edema for up to 72 hours

3° dose = 10 MED to produce erythema and blistering (limit to small surface area of exposure)[3–5]

poses, and exposure should be carefully monitored. Proper patient education is outlined in Table 5–2.

Improper dosage may cause either no therapeutic effect or potential skin damage. Appropriate documentation is also an important part of the treatment. Details that should be included in the documentation are outlined in Table 5–3.

LASER

PRODUCTION OF LASER LIGHT

The use of light for therapeutic purposes is not new to clinical practice, but the technology that enables the light source to have such specific characteristics as laser is relatively new. *Laser* is an acronym for *l*ight *a*mplification by the *s*timulated *e*mission of *r*adiation. It consists of photons moving in the same direction at the same frequency and same wavelength.[12]

Stimulated emission of radiation involves a contained chamber that houses an active medium of excitable atoms of either a gas, liquid, or solid. When electrical

Table 5–2   **Patient Education**

1. Wear goggles during entire exposure time (cataracts may develop with ocular exposure to UV).

2. Observe and monitor skin condition.

3. Keep skin moisturized following exposure to UV.

4. Pigmentation changes are to be expected and are a normal response. The time of the appearance of the pigmentation change should be recorded and reported to the therapist at the next visit.

5. Prolonged and repeated exposure to UV may promote premature aging of the skin.

Table 5–3   **Documentation for Treatment with UV**

1. Record patient's response to previous exposures to UV (time of appearance of erythema, any adverse sensitivities to the UV or applied agents).

2. Indicate the UV lamp that was utilized by recording its brand name, model and serial number if there is more than one UV lamp in the department. Age of the lamp and manufacturer specification differences may produce variations in the predictability of results.

3. Record the distance from the patient (consistently indicating centimeters or inches).

4. Record the incident angle of the lamp to the patient (which should be 90° to promote uniformity and predictability of the response).

5. Draping procedures should be noted, listing the exact area of exposure and any irregularities of the surface of the skin, e.g., bony prominences or other contouring of the treatment area.

6. Record the exposure time in seconds.

7. Record the appearance of the skin following exposure to the UV.

8. Record the use of any topically applied moisturizers or medications following exposure to UV.

energy is introduced into the active medium, a molecular excitation occurs. Electrons in the outermost energy level of the active medium are elevated to the next level, resulting in an unstable molecule. This unstable molecule needs to shed energy to accommodate the degradation of the electrons to their original and stable position. The energy released in the process is in the form of photons of energy, which pass through the active medium, further exciting it and creating a situation known as "population inversion" or an active photon emission process.[13,14]

The chamber that houses the active medium is sometimes referred to as the resonant cavity. This resonant cavity is mounted with mirrors at each end that are virtually parallel to each other. One of the mirrors is completely reflective, and the other is partially reflective, allowing a small percentage of the photon energy (light) to be emitted from the cavity or chamber.

CHARACTERISTICS OF LASER LIGHT

Laser light has unique characteristics that further differentiate it from "white light." Laser light is monochromatic, coherent, and exhibits low beam divergence.

Monochromaticity

Laser light is of one specific wavelength and therefore one color, that is, mono-chromatic. Because the photon emission is the result of the excitation of an isolated active medium, the emitted light has one specific wavelength. White light is made up of many different wavelengths, or many different colors, as evidenced by re-fracting white light through a prism; it exits the prism as a rainbow of colors of the visual spectrum. Laser light entering a prism would be identical on exit because it is monochromatic.

Coherence

Coherence refers to the precise nature of the laser wavelength in the way it trav-els. Each individual photon emitted from a laser is emitted precisely in phase with every other photon. Laser light is a phase-related form of energy. All emitted pho-tons travel in the same direction, creating a parallel beam profile (Fig. 5–6). The significance is that all the peaks and valleys of the sine wave pattern are occurring at precisely the same time.

Beam Divergence

Beam divergence refers to the relative parallelism of the beam. The more parallel, or collimated, the beam, the greater the concentration of energy in a localized area. There is a minimal divergence or spreading apart of the photons from a laser. They are easily focused into well-contained areas.[4,14] This property of laser light enabled the first accurate measuring system for recording the distance to the moon. Astro-nauts placed a mirror on the moon's surface, and a pulsed laser from the earth was focused on it, reflecting the light back to the incident source. Because the speed of light is known, the distance could be calculated based on the time required for the laser beam to return. After having traveled almost a quarter of a million miles of

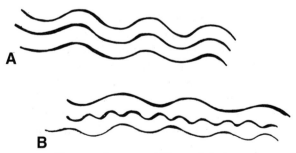

Figure 5–6. The property of beam coherence. *(A)* Laser light is a coherent light source of one specific wavelength. Therefore, the sine waves occur completely parallel to each other. *(B)* White light is made up of many different colors of light, so it is physically impossible for the sine waves to be perfectly parallel.

space, the laser beam had spread out to a diameter of only 2 miles because of its low beam divergence[4,12,13] (Fig. 5–7).

These characteristics enable lasers to be focused into microscopic points, yielding enormous energy densities in the area of the focus for many medical and non-medical applications. The combination of fiber optic and laser technologies has enabled clinicians to easily handle and direct the incident beam regardless of the dimensions of the resonant cavity of the active medium. Gaseous lasers such as carbon dioxide (CO_2) and carbon dioxide YAG lasers utilize fiber optics to transmit the laser beams for arthroscopic surgical procedures.[15]

LOW-POWER LASERS IN CLINICAL PRACTICE

Clinicians in the United States have reported beneficial effects from two specific lasers, helium neon (HeNe) and gallium arsenide (GaAs). Both of these lasers are considered low-power (cold) lasers, because their maximum power levels are not capable of producing a thermal response. HeNe lasers produce a wavelength of 632.8 nm, and fall within the visible spectrum of light, emitting a brilliant red light. GaAs semiconductor diode chip lasers produce a wavelength of 910 nm, which does not fall within the visible spectrum of light. For this reason GaAs lasers are referred to as infrared lasers (IR) (910 nm is considered IR in the electromagnetic spectrum).[4,11,16–18]

HeNe and GaAs lasers are considered low-power lasers since typically the total peak power is less than 1 milliwatt (mW), and they produce no significant heat in the treated tissues. Surgical lasers are considered high-power lasers and their effects are associated with damaging changes to cells and tissues through thermal effects.[4] The power of a laser device is preset within the device along with the wavelength, based on the active medium or type of laser and power source.

Lasers have been utilized in a wide variety of applications since their development in the early 1960s.[4] Their uses range from industrial applications, such as very accurate drills, scanning devices in supermarkets, and compact disc (CD) players, to medical applications in many fields including but not limited to: dermatology, ophthalmology, gynecology, urology, dentistry, and physical medicine.[24] Lasers are considered investigational devices in the United States and therefore certain protocols for permission to use the devices must be followed. The investigational status also restricts claims that can be made regarding the applica-

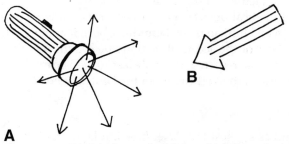

Figure 5–7. Beam divergence. *(A)* Light from a flashlight, which is made up of many different wavelengths, will spread out in all directions. *(B)* Laser light has very low divergence properties; it does not tend to spread out.

tion of the devices until such time as low-power lasers receive full premarket approval from the FDA. This approval process will be referred to throughout this section.

Proposed Indications

Low-power lasers have been reported in the literature to have specific therapeutic effects for tissue healing and pain management for both acute and chronic pain.[25–27]

Safety Considerations

Lasers utilized for physical rehabilitation have few contraindications since they are low-power lasers with low emitted energy. The FDA has classified these devices as insignificant risk devices that are generally safe. Despite this, there are some precautions to the use of the devices because of the potential for the enhancement of the growth of tissues on a cellular level, sometimes referred to as biostimulation. The following list outlines the additional precautions.

- Pregnant women should not be treated with biostimulative lasers.
- Unclosed fontanels of children should not be treated with biostimulative lasers.
- Areas with cancerous lesions should not be treated with biostimulative lasers.
- Direct laser application over the cornea is to be avoided.

Regulatory Processes and Safety of Low-Power Lasers The FDA classifies low-power lasers as Class III medical devices, which are devices represented to be life sustaining or life supporting, those implanted in the body, those presenting potential or unreasonable risk of illness or injury, or those new or modified devices not substantially equivalent to any devices marketed before May 28, 1976 (date of enactment of the Medical Device Amendments).[19]

Lasers were introduced to American clinicians in the early 1980s for the treatment of pain and the enhancement of tissue healing.[11] Lasers are among the first medical devices proposed for use by therapists to go through the premarket approval (PMA) process for safety and efficacy, as outlined by the Center for Devices and Radiological Health (FDA). Lasers were introduced after May 28, 1976. Many clinical trials to date have been poorly designed.

This chapter addresses the laser modality and the regulatory issues surrounding its use, to inform clinicians of the process required for the use of the devices. It is ultimately the responsibility of the clinician to make sure that any newly introduced modality has met the regulatory guidelines set forth by the FDA, despite what a manufacturer of the device may claim.

As Class III medical devices, low-power or cold lasers require PMA prior to mass distribution and human use. Claims have been made regarding the benefits of laser biostimulation for the acceleration of tissue healing and the reduction of pain by numerous European researchers for the last 10 to 15 years. These claims are in the process of being tested today throughout the United States, Canada, and China.[19]

Proposed Effects

Preliminary studies suggest that laser biostimulation has an effect on type I and type III procollagen mRNA levels, which seem to enhance wound healing by optimizing scar formation.[20–22] Researchers have also reported favorable results for pain relief, improvement in grip strength and tip pinch strength in the treatment of patients with rheumatoid arthritis, enhancement of experimental pain thresholds[25,26] and tissue repair.[16–18] Despite the reports of favorable findings by numerous investigators, analysis of the research designs has indicated that some of the studies were poorly controlled or monitored.[31]

Biostimulative lasers have not yet satisfied the requirements of the FDA for PMA. At the time of this writing, they are considered investigational devices, which have specific requirements for use with human subjects.

Institutional Review Board (IRB)

Clinicians who wish to conduct research with low-power lasers are required to submit a protocol to an Institutional Review Board (IRB), or Human Subject Committee, who will review the use of the technique with humans. The IRB is a committee or group assembled to approve the initiation of new research protocols and conduct periodic review of biomedical research involving human subjects. Their primary purpose is to assure the protection of the rights and welfare of human subjects. Studies may be sponsored or funded by a facility or a manufacturer. The sponsor of the investigation bears the responsibility for the conduct of the investigation, but does not actually perform the investigation. Manufacturers of the devices have served in this capacity over the last 10 to 12 years. If the devices are being utilized under the supervision of an IRB, with a well-defined protocol, then the device is considered investigational and can be used with human subject participant within the scope of the study as an Investigational Device Exemption (IDE).[23]

Low-power lasers have been considered non-significant-risk devices since their output is not capable of causing a burn. They are, however, investigational devices that require the approval of an IRB for use within a well-defined protocol with informed consent of the patient before they can be utilized.[19]

Documentation for IRBs

Each institution has its own procedure designed to protect the human subjects in the study. General guidelines for information submitted to an IRB include:

- A well-defined protocol outlining the diagnoses and patient population
- Members of the research team and any financial relationship to the manufacturer
- Plan for periodic review of the results of the investigation
- Informed consent forms for patients describing the purpose of the study and potential risks

The future of low-power laser as a therapeutic modality is uncertain because of the conflicting reports in the literature regarding potential benefits.[28–30] Until uniformity of dosage documentation exists and more well-controlled clinical trials have been performed, clinicians are encouraged to keep an open but critical eye and mind on the use of the modality.

TREATMENT TECHNIQUE WITH LASER

Protocols are based on the amount of energy delivered to the patient measured in joules per square centimeter, which is calculated by a formula encompassing the time of exposure, the power of the laser, and the size of the treatment area. Low-

Table 5–4   Parameters Recorded in the Documentation of a Laser Treatment

- Type of laser utilized (HeNe, YAG, GaAs, etc.)
- Wavelength of laser (632.8 nm, 1032 nm, etc.)
- Power of the laser (milliwatts or watts)
- Size of the treatment area (number of square centimeters)
- Exposure time (seconds, minutes etc.)

power (biostimulative) lasers provide no sensation to the patient and have no intensity setting, so treatment dosage is determined by the aforementioned factors. Since the devices are still investigational, specific treatment parameters are still being determined at the time of this writing. Clinical trials to date have not demonstrated sufficient evidence to prove the efficacy of low-power lasers.[31]

Documentable Parameters

In order for clinical results to be duplicated with any modality or treatment plan, the parameters of the treatment need to be documented. Each of the individual modalities or techniques will have their own specific sets of variables that must be recorded. Laser is no different from other modalities in terms of the need for accurate documentation for reproducibility of results. The specific parameters that must be recorded for a laser treatment are listed in Table 5–4.

THERAPEUTIC USES OF LIGHT: ACTINOTHERAPY

This chapter has outlined two very different sources of therapeutic light. Their use in clinics will vary greatly depending on many factors, including the patient population, the types of conditions treated most often within the facility, and whether or not the facility is participating in an investigational study.

For lasers to become clinically acceptable, well-designed, controlled studies must demonstrate effectiveness. These studies, whether negative or positive, need to be published and reviewed. Proven efficacy of the techniques will facilitate availability of the devices for clinical use.

UV has been utilized for many years, but has seen limited use in the recent past perhaps because of the "cumbersome" nature of determining the appropriate dosage for a patient and the emergence of new medications. Pharmacologic interventions are rarely without side effects, and not all patients can ingest medications without difficulty. UV represents a potential safe treatment option for many patients with skin disorders. It should not be overlooked or discredited as a treatment option.

DISCUSSION QUESTIONS

1. Describe the differences between laser light and UV.

2. Outline the process necessary for the approval of any "new" modality for human use.

3. What are the differences between radiant energy sources and nonradiant energy sources?

4. Describe the production of laser light, and explain why some are visible and some are not visible light sources.

5. Discuss the potential benefits of UV in clinical practice.

6. What are the precautions for the application of a luminous light source?

7. You are treating a patient with UV. The distance from the lamp to the patient is 36 inches, and their exposure time for an MED is 90 seconds. What would potentially be the exposure time necessary to provide an MED if the distance from the lamp was doubled? If the lamp was moved to 18 inches from the patient?

8. Explain the relationship between the incident angle of a light source and the target tissue.

REFERENCES

1. Kitchen, SS and Partridge, CJ: Review of ultraviolet radiation therapy. Physiotherapy, 77:423, 1991.

2. Scott, BO: Clinical uses of ultraviolet radiation. In Stillwell, GK (ed): Therapeutic Electricity and Ultraviolet Radiation, ed 3. Williams & Wilkins, Baltimore, 1983, pp 228–262.

3. Kahn, J: Physical agents—electrical, sonic and radiant modalities. In Skully, RM and Barnes, MR (eds): Physical Therapy. JB Lippincott, Philadelphia, 1989, pp 894–897.

4. Snyder-Mackler, L and Collander, S: Therapeutic uses of light in rehabilitation. In Michlovitz, SL (ed): Thermal Agents in Rehabilitation, ed 3. FA Davis, Philadelphia, 1995.

5. Kollias, N, et al: New trends in photobiology (invited review). Photoprotection by melanin. Photochem Photobiol 9:135, 1991.

6. Baadsgaard, O: In vivo ultraviolet irradiation of human skin results in profound perturbation of the immune system. Arch Derm, 127:99, 1991.

7. Nussbaum, EL, Biemann, I, and Mustard, B: Comparison of ultrasound/ultraviolet-C and laser for treatment of pressure ulcers in patients with spinal cord injuries. Phys Ther 74(9):812–823, 1994.

8. Nived, O, Johansson, I, and Sturfelt G: Effects of ultraviolet irradiation on natural killer cell function in systemic lupus erythematosis. Ann Rheum Dis 51:726, 1992.

9. Golan, TD, et al: Enhanced membrane binding of autoantibodies to cultured keratinocytes of systemic lupus erythmatosus. Clin Invest 90:1067, 1992.

10. Taber's Cyclopedic Medical Dictionary, ed 17. FA Davis, Philadelphia, 1993, p 1501.

11. Kleinkort, JA and Foley, RA: Laser: A preliminary report on its use in physical therapy. Am J Acupunct 12:51, 1984.

12. Asimov, I: Understanding Physics. Dorset Press, 1988, pp 99–101.

13. Nave, CR and Nave, BC: Physics for the Health Sciences, ed 3. WB Saunders, Philadelphia, 1985, pp 348–352.

14. Miller, F: College Physics, ed 4. Harcourt Brace Jovanovich, New York, 1977, pp 680–684.

15. Corson, SL: Uses of the YAG laser in laporoscopic gynecologic procedures. Obstet Gynecol Clin North Am 18:619, 1991.

16. Goldman, JA, et al: Laser therapy of rheumatoid arthritis. Lasers Surg Med 1:93, 1980.

17. Gogia, PP, Hurt, BS, and Zirn, TT: Wound management with whirlpool and infrared cold laser treatment—A clinical report. Phys Ther 68:1239, 1988.

18. King, CE, et al: Effect of helium-neon laser auriculotherapy on experimental pain threshold. Phys Ther 70:24, 1990.

19. FDA: Fact sheet—laser biostimulation. Clin Manag 7:40, 1987.

20. Lam, TS, et al: Laser stimulation of collagen synthesis in human skin fibroblast cultures. In Lasers in the Life Sciences, Harwood Academic Publishers, 1:61, 1986.

21. Lyons, RF, et al: Biostimulation of wound healing in vivo by helium-neon laser. Ann Plast Surg 18:1987.

22. Sapiera, D, et al: Demonstration of elevated type I and type II procollagen mRNA levels in cutaneous wounds treated with helium-neon laser—proposed mechanisms for enhanced wound healing. Biochem Biophys Res Commun 138:1123, 1986.

23. US Department of Health and Human Services Public Health Service, Food and Drug Administration: Investigational Device Exemptions, Division of Small Manufacturers Assistance, Office of Training and Assistance, Rockville, MD, February 1986.

24. Enwemeka, CS: Laser photostimulation. Clin Manag 10:24, 1990.

25. Snyder-Mackler, L, et al: Effects of helium-neon laser irradiation on skin resistance and pain in patients with trigger points in the neck or back. Phys Ther 69:336, 1989.

26. King, CE, et al: Effect of helium-neon laster auriculotherapy on experimental pain threshold: Phys Ther 70:24, 1990.

27. Snyder-Mackler, L and Bork, CE: Effects of helium-neon laser irradiation on peripheral sensory nerve latency. Phys Ther 68:223, 1988.

28. Kramer, JF and Sandrin, M: Effect of low-power laser and white light on sensory conduction rate of the superficial radial nerve. Physiother Can 45:165, 1993.

29. Basford, JR, et al: Low-energy helium neon laser treatment of thumb osteoarthritis. Arch Phys Med Rehab 68:794, 1987.

30. Waylonis, GW, et al: Chronic myofascial pain: Management by low-output helium-neon laser therapy. Arch Phys Med Rehab, 69:017–1020, 1988.

31. Beckerman, H, et al: The efficacy of laser therapy for musculoskeletal and skin disorders: A criteria-based meta-analysis of randomized clinical trials. Phys Ther 72:483, 1992.

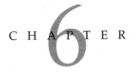

HYDROTHERAPY: WHIRLPOOLS TO AQUATIC POOLS

Robert Babb, PT
Elaine Muntzer, PT, CHT

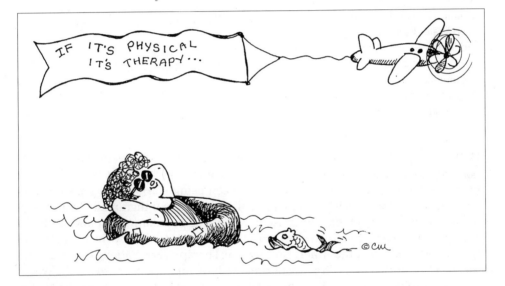

CHAPTER OBJECTIVES

- Describe the physical principles of water.
- Describe the therapeutic benefits of hydrotherapy.
- Describe the components and care for a whirlpool.
- Describe the benefits of aquatic exercise as a modality.
- Differentiate between the benefits of land and water activities.
- Describe the benefits of hydrotherapy for wound management.
- Describe the techniques for wound care with hydrotherapy.
- Differentiate between the benefits and potential problems of utilizing hydrotherapy for wound care.

Hydrotherapy has ancient roots and is one of the oldest forms of therapy. Hippocrates, the Greek father of medicine, used contrast baths of hot and cold water to treat various diseases. Europeans have been using warm-water spas for hundreds of years and developed a great deal of the original therapeutic water regimens that are utilized today. Exercise in water was popular in the polio era and a resurgence of interest has occurred in the 1990s as evidenced by the formation of the Aquatic Section of the American Physical Therapy Association, which defines *aquatic physical therapy* as "treatment time with therapeutic exercises in the water, utilizing supine, prone, vertical, or reclined positions."[1] Today thousands of clinicians utilize water for therapeutic purposes every day in their practices. This utilization has evolved into two different areas, hydrotherapy and aquatic therapy. This chapter will define, discuss, and differentiate between the wide variety of therapeutic applications of water.

HYDROTHERAPY VERSUS AQUATIC THERAPY

Hydrotherapy utilizes tanks of water such as a whirlpool or Hubbard tank. These tanks come in a variety of depths and sizes dependent on the amount of immersion required for the treatment.[2] Hydrotherapy involves the treatment of one patient at a time in an individual tank. Aquatic therapy refers to the utilization of larger pools with more body immersion and potential treatment of more than one patient at a time. Individuals with a true phobia of the water would potentially be able to tolerate hydrotherapy, but not aquatic therapy, treatment techniques.

PHYSICAL PRINCIPLES AND PROPERTIES OF WATER

BUOYANCY

Buoyancy is a force that works in the opposite direction to gravity. Gravity pulls downward, buoyancy pushes upward from the bottom. When an object is placed in water, water displacement will occur because of the upward pressure of buoyancy. The amount of displacement has been described by Archimedes, who stated that an immersed body will experience an upward thrust equal to the weight of the liquid displaced.[3] Water is more supportive than air because of buoyancy. There will be greater buoyant forces acting on larger objects, creating more water displacement, than on smaller objects, which will experience less water displacement and less buoyancy. A relative "weightlessness" occurs when a body is immersed in water. The amount of weightlessness depends on the percentage of the body that is below the surface of the water (Fig. 6–1). Buoyant forces support the body, giving the sensation of weightlessness. This will also be affected by body density, postural alignment, and vital capacity of the lungs. When a patient fully inflates his or her lungs, he or she will be much more likely to float than if the lungs were not inflated. Buoyancy can offer enough support to the extremities, reducing the compressive forces that would be experienced out of the water. Buoyancy can provide opportunities for patients to perform squatting exercises without back pain, or run with reduced joint compression.

CENTER OF BUOYANCY

The center of buoyancy (COB) and center of gravity (COG) are functionally similar. COB refers to a point when a body is underwater and the COG refers to a point out of the water. They represent points or locations on the human body that need to be maintained within a base of support (BOS) to establish and maintain an up-

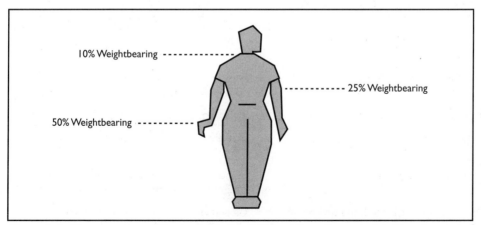

Figure 6–1. The percentage of body weight that will be relieved by varied depths of water immersion.

right and stable posture. The COG is located just anterior to the sacral vertebrae, the COB is located in the chest region. While submersed in the water, the forces of buoyancy and gravity act in opposite directions to each other. Buoyancy devices or flotation devices can be utilized to help a patient maintain his or her COB within the BOS to maintain an upright position in the water. Anteriorly placed buoyancy devices will tend to cause extension of the spine to assist in maintaining proper body alignment.

HYDROSTATIC PRESSURE

Hydrostatic pressure is pressure exerted by water on an object immersed in the water. It will assist in venous return, heart rate reduction, and a centralization of peripheral blood flow.[4] Pascal's law states that the pressure of a liquid is exerted equally on an object at a given depth, and the object will experience pressure that is proportional to the depth of immersion.[5] Pressure increases 0.433 lb/in^2 for each foot of depth. This pressure is thought to help control inflammation with water exercise. There is less inflammation when patients who have had anterior cruciate ligament repairs perform their exercises in the water as compared to performing their exercises out of the water.[6] Perhaps this is because of reduction of joint compression and shear forces.

Because hydrostatic pressure is proportional to the depth of immersion, exercises will be easier to perform closer to the surface of the water where the pressure is less. For example, a patient who has had a total hip replacement needs to be able to perform buoyancy-supported hip abduction before he or she would be able to perform standing hip abduction (Table 6–1).

Table 6–1   **Documentation and Progression of Hip Abduction in Aquatic Exercise**

EXERCISE TYPE	ACTIVITY
Buoyancy-supported passive (supine in water)	Provider provides passive stretch.
Buoyancy-supported active assist (supine in water)	Provider assists movement of the motion while in buoyancy-supported position.
Buoyancy-supported active (supine in water)	Active range of motion.
Buoyancy supra assist	Standing, abduction with buoyancy-assist device on ankle.
Buoyancy-assisted	Standing, abduction.
Buoyancy resist	Standing, abduct with increasing speed against resistance.
Buoyancy supra resist	Standing, resistive boot secured, abduct against resistance.
Buoyancy-supported, manual resist (supine in water)	Closed chain, body moves over fixed extremity (fixed by provider)

SPECIFIC GRAVITY

Specific gravity is the weight of a particular substance compared with the weight of an equal volume of water. It is related to the density of an object and is therefore also referred to as relative density. The specific gravity of a person increases when there is increased bone mass and muscle mass and decreases when there are greater amounts of adipose tissue. An object with a low specific gravity or specific gravity of less than 1.0 will float; an object with a high specific gravity or greater than 1.0 will sink. Water has a specific gravity of 1.0. The human body has a specific gravity of 0.87 to 0.97; therefore, the human body will tend to float just beneath the surface of water. For example, children with chronic debilitating diseases do well in water therapy since they spend little energy to stay afloat, and the buoyant forces assist in reducing weight bearing. Men tend to have lower percentages of body fat than women[7] and may require more buoyancy-assistive devices than women to keep them afloat. The lower extremities will have larger bones than the upper extremities and therefore will tend to sink more than the upper extremities.

VISCOSITY AND RESISTANCE

Viscosity is a measure of the frictional resistance caused by cohesive or attractive forces between the molecules of a liquid.[5] Resistance is created by the viscosity of the liquid and is proportional to the velocity of movement through the liquid. Water has a higher viscosity than air but less than oil, so it would be easiest to move through air, then water, then oil. Exercise training in an aquatic environment can result in increased strength, improved cardiovascular responses, and improved VO^2 maximums.[8,9] The amount of resistance in water can be adjusted in several ways to vary the training regimen. Decreasing the length of the lever arm will decrease the resistance in a buoyancy-resisted movement, a movement down toward the bottom of the pool. Adding a "boot" or "paddle" will increase the resistance of an activity, since increasing the surface area of the part to be moved will also increase the resistance.

SPECIFIC HEAT

Specific heat is defined as the amount of heat, in calories, required to raise the temperature of 1 gram of a substance 1°. The specific heat of water is 1.0 and it is used as the standard for setting specific heat units of other substances. When heat is added to an object, the change in temperature depends on its mass and specific heat. The specific heat or thermal capacity of water is greater than that of air. This will cause more heat loss in the water as compared to out of water at the same temperature. Cool or tepid water temperature is best for a long exercise session, whereas warm water is indicated for short-duration exercise and manual techniques. Patients diagnosed with multiple sclerosis will perform better in cooler water, which will assist in keeping their inner core body temperature low, preventing an exacerbation of their symptoms that might be seen if the exercise were performed out of the water. Patients with arthritis will benefit from warmer water temperatures. Warm-water exercise may increase the core body temperature of obese patients, since adipose tissue acts as an insulator, limiting proper heat exchange. Therefore, warmer water temperatures may be inappropriate for obese patients if they will also be exercising in the water, which would also increase the core body temperature.

HYDROMECHANICS OF WATER

Hydromechanics is a term used to refer to movement through water. It is a function of velocity of movement, surface area of the moving object, and direction of the movement of the immersed object. Turbulence is a product of several forces acting on an object immersed in water. Laminar flow, drag, and resistance to forward movement all act on the body moving in the water (Fig. 6–2). Frontal resistance is encountered initially as a body moves through the water, creating a positive pressure. The resistance is proportional to the velocity. The faster the movement, the greater the resistance.[3] Progressive resistance in aquatic exercise can be increased by increasing the velocity of movement, increasing the surface area, or by moving closer to the surface of the water where the turbulence is greater.[10]

Frontal resistance, proportional to the surface area, will offer resistance to initiation of movement as inertial forces are overcome. The greater the surface area, the greater the amount of water is moved; therefore, more drag will be created. Drag inhibits movement by resisting forward motion. Quick changes in the direction of movement in water will also encounter greater resistance.

Laminar flow is the horizontal flow of water passing over a body part in motion that creates drag. The more irregular the laminar flow, the greater the drag of a part. Irregular shapes will alter the laminar flow of the water. Increasing the velocity, surface area, and change in direction will raise the level of effort needed to accomplish a task in the water. Depending on the effort exerted, energy requirements in an aquatic environment have been reported to be 33% to 42% greater at any given workload when compared with land exercises (Table 6–2).

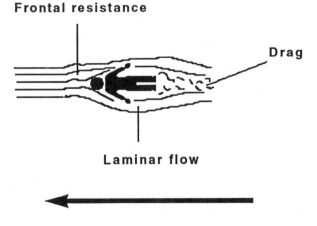

Figure 6–2. The various forces that will act on an object as it moves through the water.

Table 6–2 Comparison of Treatment Goals for "Land" Versus Aquatic Exercise

	Land	Aquatic
Improving range of motion	Manual stretching	Manual stretching
Improving arthrokinematics	Joint mobilizations	Joint mobilizations
Improving strength	Open-chain manual resistive Resistive equipment	Closed-chain manual resistance Paddles, boots, boards
Improving balance	Unilateral stance, mini-tramp	Unilateral stance, turbulence challenge
Improving endurance	Bike, treadmill	Deep water walk, run, bicycle
Improving ambulation status	Parallel bars to crutches to cane	Deep water to shallow water to land

WATER TEMPERATURE

Temperature regulation is more difficult in water in part because of diminished body surface area to lose heat. Conversely, cold water could produce a significant amount of heat loss because water conducts heat 25 times faster than air.[12] Therapeutic warmth is considered to be 94°F, which is appropriate for performing therapeutic exercises. Warm water may act as a superficial heating agent and has been reported to elevate pain threshold and decrease muscle spasm.[2] Inappropriate temperature selection could decrease the effectiveness of the therapeutic intervention and possibly cause adverse responses (Fig. 6–3).

EQUIPMENT

Equipment for hydrotherapy involves the use of whirlpools with stainless steel or fiberglass tanks that may be movable or stationary (depending on their size and configuration) and have a turbine, drain, and thermostatically controlled

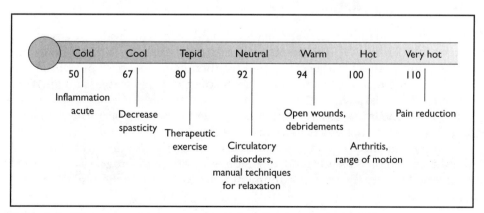

Figure 6–3. Water temperatures and potential applications for hydrotherapy.

water supply. Whirlpools vary in size, and one is selected for treatment depending on the treatment goal and extremity or area to be treated. The smallest tanks are extremity tanks, which hold approximately 25 gallons of water depending on the manufacturer. They vary in depth from 20 to 25 inches and have one turbine. Full-body tanks are called "low boys," and they resemble a bathtub resting on the floor with enough room for patients to "long sit" in the tank with their legs outstretched in front of them. Low-boy tanks may hold as much as 200 gallons of water and they too have a turbine for aeration of the water. Both extremity and low-boy tanks have been utilized in the treatment of open wounds, peripheral joint stiffness, and postoperative joint replacements (Fig. 6–4).

Hubbard tanks are whirlpool tanks that were created to accommodate a patient in a supine position, and allow range of movement in both the upper and lower extremities with support from the water. These tanks may have a deep trough in the center of the tank with parallel bars for in-water ambulation. Patients who cannot be transferred into a low boy or who have too large a surface area for treatment in an extremity tank or low boy are candidates for the Hubbard tank. There are several turbines on Hubbard tanks that can be moved to different positions around the tank so that the turbulence can be directed to more than one area at a time. These tanks have a lifting device to transfer the patient from a gurney into the pool and out. Often these lifts are hydraulically controlled and may be intimidating to certain patients. It is important to remember this when transferring a patient into any pool.

TURBINES

Turbines mix air and water to provide agitation and turbulence to the water in a tank. The mechanical stimulation from the agitation to the skin receptors may promote an analgesic effect. Turbines have several adjustable features including: height, direction of flow, and strength of the aerated flow. The more air that is mixed with the water, the more turbulence will be created in the water. Turbulence may assist in nonspecific debridement of an open wound if indicated. Wound management with hydrotherapy is discussed later in this chapter.

THERAPEUTIC AQUATIC POOLS

Therapeutic aquatic pools vary in depth and size with water temperature ranges from 86 to 94°F. The therapeutic treatment goals for aquatic pools can be the same goals as those established for therapeutic exercise out of the water. Water immersion eliminates the effects of gravity, so water is an ideal environment for early interventions for many musculosketal and neurologic conditions. The initial assessment of the patient should be performed on land and then again in the water to assure that the medium is capable of assisting the patient in meeting negotiated treatment goals. Aquatic rehabilitation should be combined with land techniques in order to progress the patient functionally, since the land environment will ultimately be the goal (Table 6–3 and Fig. 6–5).

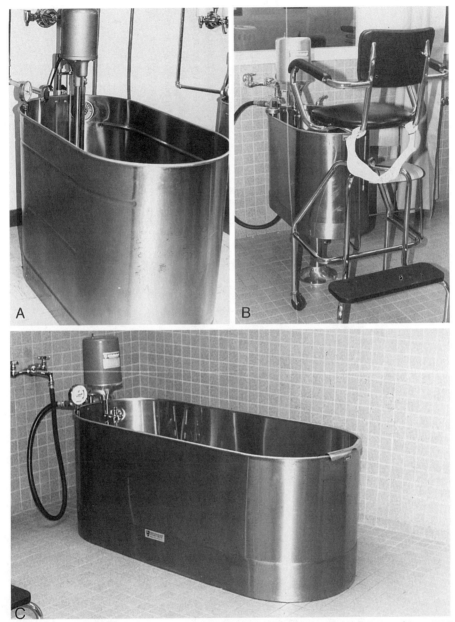

Figure 6–4. Various types and styles of whirlpools. *(A)* "High boy" for knees or hips. *(B)* Extremity tank for distal upper or lower extremities. *(C)* "Low boy." *(From Walsh, MT: Hydrotherapy: The use of water as a therapeutic agent. In Michlovitz, SL (ed): Thermal Agents in Rehabilitation, ed 2. FA Davis, Philadelphia, 1990, p 114, with permission.)*

Table 6–3 **The Relationship Between the Depth of Water in an Aquatic Pool and the Types of Activities That Would Be Possible in That Depth**

Deep Water, 5 ft or > (Unloaded, open chain)	Midlevel Water, Shoulder to Nipple (Minimal load, closed chain)	Shallow Water, Iliac Crest to Nipple (Moderate load, closed chain)	Therapeutic Pool
Cardiovascular with joint protection Unloaded sport specific Ambulation without assistive devices Unloaded exercises for spine/lower extremity injuries	Wall slides Trunk PNF patterns Progressive ambulation to ween from assistive devices Plyometrics General flexibility Sport progressive lateral challenge Balance/proprioceptive challenge using turbulence	Land specific functional movements Progressive ambulation, balance/proprioceptive challenge Sport-specific challenge	Bad Ragaz stretching, isometrics, isotonics, dynamic patterns Closed-chain manual resistive exercises for extremities Massage, mobilizations General buoyancy assistive–resistive exercises

PNF = proprioceptive neuromuscular facilitation.

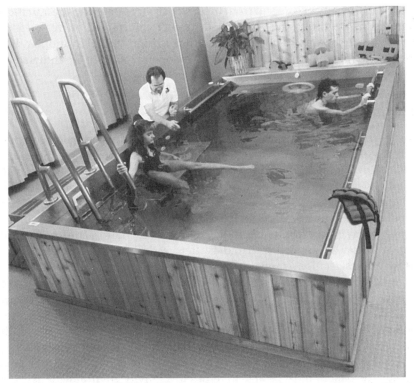

Figure 6–5. Patients performing aquatic exercises in a Therafit therapeutic pool. *(Courtesy of Aqua Therapy Systems, Lafayette Hill, PA.)*

HYDROTHERAPY TREATMENT TECHNIQUES

ADDITIVES TO PREVENT INFECTION

Whirlpools have been utilized for many years in the treatment of open wounds, fractures, and other orthopedic injuries.[13] In order to accomplish treatment goals without spreading infection, the tanks and their turbines must be thoroughly cleaned in between patients. The most common agents used to prevent or reduce the chance of infection are povidone-iodine, chloramine-T, and sodium hypochlorite (household bleach). The size of the tank and the manufacturer's recommendations will guide the clinician toward the appropriate concentration of an additive. It is important to remember that the tank is not the only potential host for infections; the turbine is also a potential source. It is important to run the turbine with a disinfectant agent in the water so that the air intake valves of the turbine are also cleaned.

AQUATIC POOLS AND INFECTION CONTROL

Unlike hydrotherapy treatment tanks, the water is not emptied for a therapeutic pool following every patient treatment. There are also situations where there will be more than one patient in the water at the same time. This presents some different considerations for infection control. First of all, it is recommended that patients shower to remove any excess soil from their skin prior to entering the aquatic pool. These pools have a filtration system that is either chlorinated or treated in some way to minimize the spread of organisms from one individual to another. It is not safe for a patient who is incontinent or with an open wound to be immersed in an aquatic pool.

AQUATIC THERAPY TECHNIQUES

Aquatic therapy is a growing area of interest. The growth in commercial popularity is unfortunately not matched with effectiveness studies to determine the efficacy of the aquatic environment as compared with a land program. Preliminary evidence and intuition lead many clinicians to believe that aquatic therapy is an effective tool for early intervention of acute injuries, for restoring function, for reducing the need for ambulatory assistive devices, for exercise, and for numerous other applications where gravity-resisted exercise and movement are difficult to perform. Therapeutic pools are sometimes equipped with underwater treadmills, stationary bikes, and various other exercise stations similar to what one would see in a therapeutic gym on land. Any of the strengthening or conditioning treatment goals that are worked on in a land environment can also be done in an aquatic environment. The difference between the two is that the aquatic environment will provide the patient with more support and will decrease compressive forces on weight-bearing joints because of the effects of buoyance. Despite this advantage, aquatic therapy cannot completely meet all of the goals, since the ultimate goal of restoring function would be for a land environment. The patient must be able to return to a gravity environment in everyday life. Successive progressions from deep water to shallow water within the aquatic environment will enable patients to prepare for gravity as they recover.

DEEP WATER EXERCISE

Deep water exercises are those that take place in an aquatic pool that is deep enough so that the patient's feet do not touch the bottom. The feet are not "fixed" to the bottom; therefore, the exercises that are capable of being performed are termed *open chain*. Depending on the height of the patient, the depth of the water should be at least 5 to 6 feet so that the patient is suspended in the water without touching the bottom. Buoyancy-assistive devices or tethering devices can be worn by the patient to maintain an upright posture in the water so that the lower extremities are free to move without having to try to maintain flotation. Deep ends of Olympic-size pools or public YMCA pools are effective for deep water unloaded exercise. The water temperature should be tepid, since active and sometimes aggressive exercise is performed for treatment times that may approach 45 minutes. Deep water exercises can be successful and sometimes compare favorably to land exercise, particularly for patients recovering from stress fractures, since the weight-bearing load is decreased.[14]

"Unloaded" deep water exercises may also be an effective exercise medium during late pregnancy, since the pressure will be relieved from the lower back. Caution needs to be taken, though, regarding the length of immersion and water temperature. Generally, the resting heart rate is lowered when patients are immersed in water. This has an important implication when treating pregnant women with back pain, since exercise on land has been reported to increase fetal heart rates.[15] Results from some studies have indicated that there is an increase in oxygen consumption that occurs in the water when compared to the same exercises on land.[10,16,17] This is a critical factor for maintaining levels of function and fitness when recovering from a spinal or extremity injury. Athletes can perform the same amount of cardiovascular work with less strain to their joints because of the increased metabolic demands of exercise in the water, thus maintaining their fitness levels of endurance and VO_2 maximums with "in-water running."[18] Conversely, the cardiac or pulmonary compromised patient may be unduly stressed by in-water exercise.

Full excursion of joints can occur under water without incurring the forces sometimes contraindicated with land or shallow water exercise. In a limited-space immersion deep water tank, tether cords are used to minimize forward movement in the tank. Full movement and forward progression are encouraged with deep water pool walking or running in order to facilitate normal movement patterns of the soft tissues. Many sizes and shapes of buoyancy belts or vests exist today to facilitate floating in an upright position. The devices can be adjusted to promote either lumbar extension or flexion, whichever is indicated for the patient.[19]

MIDDLE-LEVEL TO SHALLOW-LEVEL EXERCISE

Middle-level (T-12 to chin) to shallow-level (knee to T-12) water depths permit the body to move over a fixed distal extremity, promoting some weight bearing. Activities in these depths of water would be considered "closed-chain" activities, since there is weight bearing on the distal extremities. Progression in weight bearing is accomplished through shallower water depths (see Table 6–3). When open-chain exercises are contraindicated, as with an unstable lower extremity or recent joint reconstruction where weight bearing is desired, shallower depths can provide the closed-chain support that is necessary.[20] It has been reported that patients with intra-articular reconstructions had less joint effusion and faster return to perceived functional levels when performing water-based exercise as compared to a similar group of patients performing the land exercises alone.[6]

Significant training effects have been reported with closed-chain water exercises. The findings included improved resting heart rates, improved VO_2 max measurements and improved treadmill endurance tests.[16] Additional studies have reported improved VO_2 responses with water calisthenics and closed-chain exercise. Functionally, low-level patients can practice proper movement patterns of step climbing or upper-extremity reaching with the buoyant support of the water. To treat patients who have trunk weakness, dynamic stabilization of the trunk can be first addressed in middle-level water utilizing buoyancy and hydrostatic pressure forces for support.[23] Pain with exercise can be minimized in an aquatic environment. For example, if shoulder flexion with a weight was painful until the weight is returned to the starting position for a patient on land, in the water, the resistance to movement will stop once movement stops.

BAD RAGAZ TECHNIQUES

Bad Ragaz techniques have been utilized and refined over the last 60 years. They were introduced at the Bad Ragaz Spa in Switzerland during the late 1950s. Bad Ragaz techniques use a buoyant ring to assist the patient in floating in the water. The ring may be placed around the trunk, under the extremities, or it may support the head and neck.[21] As knowledge of exercise and movement patterns increased, diagonal patterns of movement were developed using Voss's patterns of movement and applying them to a water environment.[22] These simple techniques are indicated for many musculoskeletal, neurologic, and arthritic conditions. Manual stretching is performed when there is a restriction in soft tissue movement. The patient's weight can be utilized to offer the overpressure needed to provide for an effective stretch. The patient is in effect lying supported by the buoyant force of the water and his other body weight can act as resistance because of the drag that it creates to movement (Fig. 6–6). Positioning can be in supine buoyancy assisted, prone buoyancy assisted, or sidelying. Manual skills from massage such as soft tissue mobilization have sometimes been incorporated into buoyancy-supported movements. Aggressive stretching using techniques of Shiatsu massage have been incorporated into water techniques. Whatever the stretching technique performed, it should be based on a quantifiable dysfunction and have a desired specific outcome. For example, if the glenohumeral joint is hypomobile and the goal is to increase shoulder ROM, stretching of the joint, long axis distraction, and joint mobilization can all be applied by the clinician to the patient lying supine supported by the water. Bad Ragaz techniques also use isometric and isotonic exercises for the trunk or extremities. Multiple-angle isometrics are performed for the extremities while the clinician moves the patient through the water (Figs. 6–7 and 6–8). Trunk "pelvic neutral" exercises have been described and studied developing proximal trunk stability (Fig. 6–9). Progression involves the addition of distal extremity mobility patterns.[23,24] The Bad Ragaz isometric techniques are often less painful to perform with an unloaded supine position as compared with performance on land. For this reason, these exercises are an appropriate starting point for deconditioned patients, such as those with low back pain. The patient will

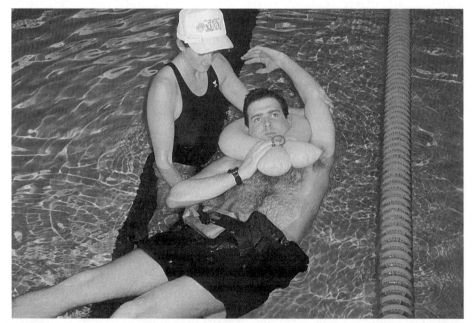

Figure 6–6. Patient supported by flotation devices while performing elongation of the left side of the trunk. Buoyancy is supporting the patient.

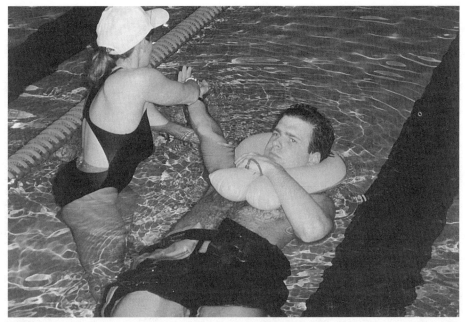

Figure 6–7. The patient is supported by the buoyancy of the water. This picture captures the beginning position for a manual-resisted exercise pattern for extension of the right shoulder.

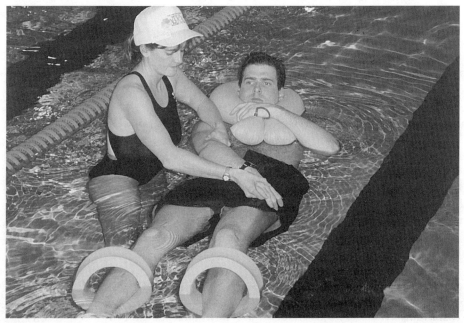

Figure 6–8. The ending position for the exercise pattern from Figure 6-7. The patient's body has moved down into the water during the activity.

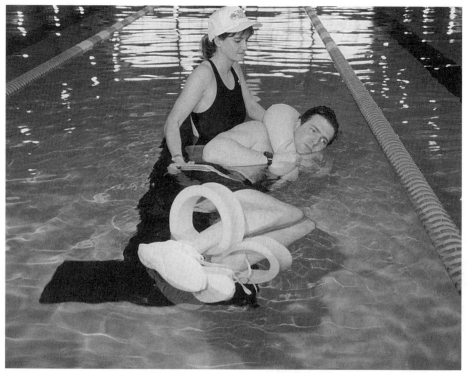

Figure 6–9. Patient performing buoyancy-assisted trunk flexion. He is supported by rings similar to Bad Ragaz rings as flotation devices.

progress appropriately to land activities for functional levels of activity or mobility to return.

DOCUMENTATION

Functional rehabilitation should be carefully documented to record the parameters of care so that its efficacy can be established and the therapeutic program can be adjusted appropriately. A program with progression of exercises from buoyancy-assisted positions to buoyancy-resisted motion are illustrated in Table 6–1. Buoyancy-assisted motions use buoyancy devices to assist agonist muscle groups through the movement; buoyancy-resisted motions are the same motions without the device. These exercises are utilized to improve active motion and function. Buoyancy-resisted motions are performed with the agonistic muscle groups in a direction against the buoyancy of the water, with supraresistive device added to increase the surface area and increase the resistance. It is imperative that the progression from buoyancy-assisted to buoyancy-resisted activities be documented clearly, as well as the depth and temperature of the water.

CLINICAL DECISIONS FOR HYDROTHERAPY AND AQUATIC THERAPY

Consideration should be given for what type of tank should be utilized to conserve water and optimally perform the treatment. If active wrist exercises are needed, a small extremity tank is well suited for this patient. If the patient is being treated for a decubitus ulcer on the ischial tuberosity, a low boy or Hubbard tank would be the most appropriate, since an aquatic pool would be contraindicated for this patient.

The water depth, temperature, and techniques are all important considerations for aquatic therapy. Deep water walking might be appropriate for a total hip replacement after the sutures have been removed, but it would be impossible as a land activity. Midlevel to shallow-level water exercises gradually increase the amount of weight bearing for a patient; activities might include jumping, running, or walking, using the water to assist or resist the activity. Unilateral balance activities can be accomplished in midlevel water depths, and resistance can be increased by adding turbulence to perturb the balance.

HYDROTHERAPY FOR WOUND CARE

The objective of therapeutic intervention for wound care is to provide an optimal wound healing environment. Based on knowledge of the expected progression of wound healing and on thorough assessment of intrinsic and extrinsic factors, treatment should facilitate normal cellular activity. Clinicians need to recognize how treatment will affect cellular function and provide care that will avoid wound trauma.

The objectives of this section are for the reader to (1) understand the effects of hydrotherapy and its clinical indications, (2) be able to describe and document the condition of the wound and surrounding tissues, and (3) clinically utilize hydrotherapy safely and effectively.

CONSIDERATIONS FOR HYDROTHERAPY TREATMENT

In considering hydrotherapy treatment for wound management, the clinician needs to ask:

- What are the effects of the treatment?
- When do the effects facilitate healing and when are they detrimental?
- How should the effects be utilized?
- Are there other treatment options?

Hydrotherapy can be utilized for debridement, cleansing, hydration, circulatory stimulation, and analgesia.

Debridement

Debridement is the rapid removal of necrotic and devitalized tissue to allow re-epithelialization and granulation. Necrotic and devitalized tissue impedes granulation and prevents or slows migration of epithelial cells across the wound.[25,26] Debridement is indicated for wounds with extensive necrotic tissue. This tissue delays healing and provides potential for bacterial growth and infection.[27,28] Hydrotherapy can be utilized to debride, soften, and loosen adherent devitalized tissue in preparation for manual or enzymatic debridement.

Hydrotherapy provides nonselective debridement, with removal of viable tissues along with necrotic devitalized tissue and debris. Nonselective debridement may cause injury to new endothelial and epithelial cells, disrupting the formation of new blood vessels (neovascularization) and the formation of new skin (re-epithelialization).

Cleansing

Cleansing removes dirt, foreign bodies, exudate, or residue from topical agents and bacteria. Excess exudate, bacterial residue, or foreign substances can prolong the normal inflammatory response and delay the proliferative phase of healing.[29] Dirt and foreign bodies provide a medium for promoting bacterial growth and infection. The critical number for bacteria is considered to be 10^5 organisms per gram of tissue;[30] an excess may result in infection. If there is concern of infection, a culture should be obtained.

Removal of residue from topical agents is done to allow topical antibodies or enzymatic preparations, if used, to reach the wound bed. When using cleansing techniques, avoid concentrations of topical agents that might damage new cells.

Hydration

Hydration provides a moist wound bed that will proceed more rapidly through the phases of healing.[25,31,32] Dehydration (desiccation) of the wound may result in an alteration of electrical potentials of skin (e.g., a decreased lateral voltage gradient and adversely affect epidermal migration).[33]

Circulatory Stimulation

Increased circulation obtained with hydrotherapy appears to be the result of thermal rather than mechanical effects.[34] Increasing local circulation can facilitate healing by increasing oxygen levels and metabolite removal.

Increasing circulation in an area of venous insufficiency can facilitate circulatory compromise, increase edema, and impede healing. The blood is entering the area and hydrostatic pressure is increased more than the venous system can compensate.

Mechanical effects of hydrotherapy can be potentially damaging to new endothelial and epithelial cells, slowing healing and decreasing resistance to infection.

Analgesia and Sedation

Mechanical stimulation of skin receptors such as with gentle whirlpool agitation can assist in decreasing pain. Thermal effects can assist with pain relief by increasing circulation in areas of compromised arterial flow.

Intrinsic and Extrinsic Factors

Effective utilization of hydrotherapy for wound healing must consider *intrinsic* and *extrinsic* factors. Information obtained and documented should include status of the patient, condition of tissues other than the wound, and description of the wound.

Patient Status

Important factors in providing treatment include:
- Subjective report, especially of pain and sensory changes
- Duration and intensity of symptoms
- Age
- Occupation
- Alcohol and tobacco use

- Systemic conditions
- Medications
  Previous
  Current
  Allergy
- History of the wound
  Mechanism
  Healing progress or lack of
  Previous treatment
  Location of wound

Condition of Surrounding Tissues

The area around the wound or even an entire extremity environment is important in optimal wound healing. The area around the wound or extremity tissues should be assessed for:

- Color
- Edema
- Temperature
- Areas of pain or sensory changes
- Trophic changes
- Pulses

Attention should be given to areas of swelling, redness, increased temperature, and pain. During the early inflammatory phase, these are not unexpected, but prolongation may indicate potential for delayed healing or infection.

Description of the Wound

Wounds may be classified according to type of closure:

- Primary
- Delayed primary
- Secondary intention
- Grafts or flaps
- Delayed
- Chronic stage I–IV

Open wounds can be classified according to the three-color concept of Marion Laboratory.[35] This uses color description of the wound bed tissue in order of severity: red, yellow, or black. Documentation of color or colors present and percentage of each directs treatment toward the most severe or predominant color.

In addition to the type of closure and description of wound bed, the clinician needs to document and describe the location of the wound; its size, shape, and margins; and the amount, color, consistency, and odor of any exudate.

FACILITATION OF HEALING

Indications

Indications for hydrotherapy include debridement or preparation for debridement in wounds healing by second intention, stable flaps or grafts, and Stage III or IV chronic ulcers with less than 50% necrotic tissue.

Hydrotherapy may also be indicated for cleansing wounds containing excess or malodorous exudate, loose debris or foreign bodies, or localized infection. A venous insufficiency ulcer may benefit from cleansing techniques that avoid dependent positioning and increased tissue temperature. A desiccated wound bed may be moisturized with hydrotherapy techniques. The patient with arterial insufficiency may obtain some pain relief[36] and increased circulation with gentle agitation, warm temperature treatment.

Precautions and Contraindications

Hydrotherapy, especially whirlpool technique, can be overutilized, providing no benefits or even detrimental effects to healing wounds.

The clean, primarily closed, clean re-epithelializing or granulating (red), or the chronic wound with greater than 50% adherent black eschar will usually not benefit from hydrotherapy. A wound with nonlocalized infection or tissues with cellulitis may be further compromised. Whirlpool treatment should not be used with split-thickness skin grafts prior to 3 to 5 days and full-thickness skin grafts prior to 7 to 10 days.

Edematous tissues may incur increased venous compromise with hydrotherapy if the extremity is dependently positioned and provided with increased tissue temperature via warm water. Patient tolerance for treatment, including systemic factors and allergy or sensitivity to additives is an important consideration.

CLINICAL USE OF HYDROTHERAPY TECHNIQUES

Whirlpool may be indicated for debridement or preparation for debridement, cleansing, circulatory stimulation, hydration, or analgesia. Clinical hydrotherapy techniques include whirlpool, irrigation or flushing, rinsing, and soaking. The technique utilized will depend on the desired effect, condition of the patient, and status of the wound and surrounding tissues.

Irrigation or flushing with sterile water or saline in a syringe or Water Pik[37] may be indicated for removing superficial nonadherent cell debris or topical agents. Cleansing of malodorous wounds, removal of exudate, and hydration may also be obtained with alternatives to whirlpool, such as use of a faucet or hose, or soaking in a basin. The amount of pressure delivered to tissues with irrigation, rinsing, or flushing is manually controlled and therefore is not consistent, and care must be taken to avoid tissue and wound trauma.

Cleansing or debridement with irrigation, flushing, rinsing, or soaking techniques can be considered as an alternative to whirlpool, more tolerable to a debilitated patient, with avoidance of prolonged dependent positioning, and more efficient in utilization of time and staff. For example, a cleansing technique other than whirlpool is often appropriate for venous insufficiency ulcers to avoid dependent positioning and increased tissue temperature.

Additives

Bactericidal additives most frequently used are povidone-iodine, sodium hypochlorite and chloramine-T (Chlorazine). These agents, unless properly diluted, can be injurious to fibroblasts.[38] Patients may also have sensitivity or allergy to additives, and the open wound provides entrance for systemic absorption.[39]

The clinician needs to consider the effects of an additive, and if necessary for bacterial control of wound infection, use a concentration that is bactericidal without injuring fibroblasts. Often, use of sterile water or saline for irrigation, flushing, or soaking and avoidance of any whirlpool additive will provide the best wound environment.

Recommended dilutions of povidine-iodine are 1:1000 and of sodium hypochlorite 1:100.[38] Steve and colleagues[40] recommend use of chloramine-T in concentrations of 50 g per 60-gallon tank and 320 g per Hubbard tank.

Temperature

Recommended temperature for hydrotherapy application in wound treatment is in the neutral range of 92 to 96°F (33.5 to 35.5°C),[36] or no greater than 1°C above skin temperature. Temperature will be based on the indications for hydrotherapy, the condition of the patient, and area to be treated.

Duration and Agitation

Duration of treatment and amount of whirlpool agitation or force of irrigation or rinsing is determined by the indications for treatment. Considerations are the desired effects, state of the wound and surrounding tissues, and patient tolerance.

There is no absolute standard duration, with soaking, irrigation, or rinsing varying from 1 to 5 minutes, debridement 10 to 20 minutes, and increasing circulation 20 minutes.[41,42] A venous ulcer may benefit from 5 minutes or less of rinsing or soaking in tepid water.[43]

When utilizing whirlpool agitation, it is important to remember that increased airflow through the turbine results in increased pressure, and that there is increased turbulence toward the water surface.[44] Fragile tissues, such as a split-thickness skin graft at 3 to 5 days or a full-thickness skin graft at 7 to 10 days, should be exposed to only minimal agitation and should not be positioned toward the water surface. Treatment duration initially should be limited to 5 minutes.

Positioning

Patient tolerance and comfort and avoidance of circulatory compromise or nerve compression with posturing or restrictive garments must always be considered when positioning a patient for treatment.

Ambient Temperature

A warm environment is important in ensuring patient comfort and avoiding reflex vasoconstriction and compromised wound healing, which can occur with exposure to cool room air.

Explanation to Patient

Clinicians need to remember the importance of the patient as a member of the health care team. Explanation of the problems, goals, precautions, and treatment plan is a vital component of optimal care.

SUMMARY

Hydrotherapy usage can vary from burn management, active sprains, wound care, and buoyancy-assisted or -resisted exercise. Although specific treatment protocols may vary by facility, the decision to include hydrotherapy for treatment should be based on knowledge of the potential benefits of water as a therapeutic medium and the treatment goals. Wound treatment should be based on knowledge of the biologic events in wound healing, effects of techniques utilized, status of the patient and the wound, and other available options.

DISCUSSION QUESTIONS

1. Use of whirlpool agitation provides which method of debridement?

2. Why is nonselective debridement possibly detrimental to wound healing?

3. What alternative method to whirlpool might be more appropriate for treatment of a venous insufficiency ulcer?

4. Is whirlpool treatment indicated for a wound described as having 100% red granulation bed? Why?

5. What precautions should be considered with use of additives in hydrotherapy treatment?

REFERENCES

1. Framroze, A: Aquatic rehabilitation Q & A: Judy A Cirullo PT. Rehab Manag 8:43, 1995.

2. Walsh, M: Hydrotherapy: The use of water as a therapeutic agent. In Michlovitz, SL (ed): Thermal Agents in Rehabilitation. FA Davis, Philadelphia, 1986.

3. Skinner, AT and Thomson, AM: Duffield's Exercise in Water, ed 3. Bailliere Tindall, London, 1983.

4. Johnson, LB, Stromme, SB, Adamczyk, JW, et al: Comparison of oxygen uptake and heart rate during exercises on land and in water. Phys Ther 57:273, 1977.

5. Bueche, F: Principles of Physics, ed 4. McGraw-Hill, New York, 1982.

6. Tovin, BJ, Wolf, SL, Greenfield, BH, et al: Comparison of the effects of exercise in water and on land on the rehabilitation of patients with intra-articular anterior cruciate ligament reconstructions. Phys Ther 74:712, 1994.

7. Wilmore, J, II: Athletic training and physical fitness. Allyn & Bacon, Boston, 1978.

8. Behlsen, GM, Grigsby, SA, and Winant, DM: Effects of an aquatic fitness program on the muscular strength and endurance of patient with multiple sclerosis. Physiotherapy 64:653, 1984.

9. Hanna, RD, Sheldahl, LM, and Tristani, FE: The effect of enhanced preload with head-out water immersion on exercise response in men with healed myocardial infarction. Am J Cardiol 71:1041, 1993.

10. Hellerbrand, T, Holutz, S, and Eubank, I: Measurement of whirlpool temperature, pressure and turbulence. Arch Phys Med Rehabil 32:17, 1950.

11. Costil, D: Energy requirements during exercise in the water. J Sports Med 11:87, 1971.

12. Bullard, RW and Rapp, GM: Problems of body heat loss in water immersion. Aerospace Med 41:1269, 1970.

13. Abraham, E: Whirlpool therapy for treatment of soft tissue wounds complicated by extremity fractures. J Trauma 4:22, 1974.

14. Clemant, DB, Ammann, W, Taunton, JE, et al: Exercise-induced stress injuries to femur. J Sports Med 14:347, 1993.

15. Katz, VL, McMurray, R, Goodwin, WE, and Cefalo, RC: Nonweightbearing exercise during pregnancy on land and during immersion: A comparative study. Am J Perinatol 7:281, 1990.

16. Routi, RG, Toup, JT, and Berger, RA: The effects of nonswimming water exercises on older adults. J Orthop Sports Phys Ther 19:140, 1994.

17. Cassady, SL and Nielsen, DH: Cardiorespiratory responses of healthy subjects to calisthenics performed in land versus in water. Phys Ther 72:532, 1992.

18. Fyestone, ED, Fellingham, G, George, J, and Fisher G: Effect of water running and cycling on maximum oxygen consumption and two mile run performance. Am J Sports Med 21:41, 1993.

19. Whann, CM, Chung, JK, Gregory, PC, et al: A new improved flotation device for deep-water exercise. J Burn Care Rehabil 12:62, 1991.

20. Shelbourne, KD and Wilckens, JH: Current concepts in anterior cruciate ligament rehabilitation. Orthop Rev 11:957, 1990.

21. Boyle, AM: The Bad Ragaz ring method. Physiotherapy 67:265, 1981.

22. Voss, DE, Ionta, MK, and Myers, BJ: Proprioceptive Neuromuscular Facilitation. Harper & Row, Philadelphia, 1985.

23. Cole, A, Eagleston, RE, Moschetti, M, and Sinnett, E: Spine pain: Aquatic rehabilitation strategies. J Back Musculoskel Rehabil 4:273, 1994.

24. Saal, JA: Dynamic muscular stabilization in the non-operative treatment of lumbar pain syndromes. Orthop Rev 19:691, 1990.

25. Hunt, TK and Van Winkle, W: Wound healing: Normal repair. In Dunphy, JE (ed): Fundamentals of Wound Management in Surgery. Chirugecom, South Plainfield, NJ, 1977, p 40.

26. Feedar, JA: Clinical management of chronic wounds. In McCulloch, JM, Kloth, LC, and Feedar, JA (eds): Wound Healing: Alternatives in Management, ed 2. FA Davis, Philadelphia, 1995, p. 151.

27. Edlich, RF, et al: Technical factors in wound management. In Dunphy, JE and Hunt, TK (eds). Fundamentals of Wound Management in Surgery. Chircurgecom, South Plainfield, NJ, 1977, p 47.

28. Haury, B, et al: Debridement: An essential component of traumatic wound care. Am J Surg 135:238, 1978.

29. Kloth, LC and Miller, KH: The inflammatory response to wounding. In McCulloch, JM, Kloth, LC, and Feedar, JA (eds): Wound Healing: Alternatives in Management. FA Davis, Philadelphia, 1990, p 3.

30. Robson, M: Management of the contaminated wound: Aids in diagnosis and treatment. In Krizek,T and Hoops, J (eds): Symposium: Basic Sciences in Plastic Surgery. CV Mosby, St. Louis, 1976, p 50.

31. Alvarez, OM, Mertz, PM, and Eaglstein, WH: The effect of occlusive dressings on collagen synthesis and re-epithelialization in superficial wounds. J Surg Res 35:142, 1983.

32. Pollack, SV: The wound healing process. Clin Dermatol 2:8, 1984.

33. Kloth, LC: Electrical stimulation in tissue repair. In McCullough, JM, Kloth, LC, and Feedar, JA (eds): Wound Healing: Alternatives in Management, ed 2. FA Davis, Philadelphia, 1995, p 298.

34. Magness, JL, Garrett, TR, and Erickson, DJ: Swelling of the upper extremity during whirlpool baths. Arch Phys Med Rehabil 51:297, 1970.

35. Cazell, JZ: Wound care forum—the new RYB color code. Am J Nursing 1342, 1988.

36. Walsh, MT: Hydrotherapy: The use of water as a therapeutic agent. In Michlovitz, SL (ed): Thermal Agents in Rehabilitation, ed 2. FA Davis, Philadelphia, 1990, p 132.

37. Trelstad, A, et al: Water Piks: Wound cleansing alternative. Plast Surg Nursing 9:117, 198.

38. Linneaweaver, W, et al: Cellular and bacterial toxicities of topical antimicrobials. Plast Reconstruct Surg 75:394, 1985.

39. Aronoff, GR, et al: Increased serum iodide concentration from iodine absorption through wounds treated topically with povidone-iodine. Am J Med Sci 279:173, 1980.

40. Steve, L, Goodhard, P, and Alexander, J. Hydrotherapy burn treatment: Use of choramine-T against resistant micro-organisms. Arch Phys Med Rehabil 60:301, 1970.

41. Abramson, DE, et al: Changes in blood flow, oxygen uptake and tissue temperatures produced by a topical application of wet heat. Arch Phys Med Rehabil 42:305, 1961.

42. Borrell, R, et al: Comparison of in vivo temperature produced by hydrotherapy, paraffin wax treatment, and Fluidotherapy. Phys Ther 60:1273, 1986.

43. McCulloch, JM and Houde, J: Treatment of wounds due to vascular problem. In Kloth, LC, McCulloch, JM, and Feedar, JK (eds): Wound Healing: Alternatives in Management, ed 2. FA Davis, Philadelphia, 1990, p 191.

44. Hellerbrand, T, Holutz, S, and Eubank, I: Measurement of whirlpool temperature, pressure and turbulence. Arch Phys Med Rehabil 32:17, 1950.

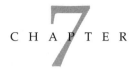
Passive Motion Devices for Soft Tissue Management: Traction

Burke Gurney, MA, PT

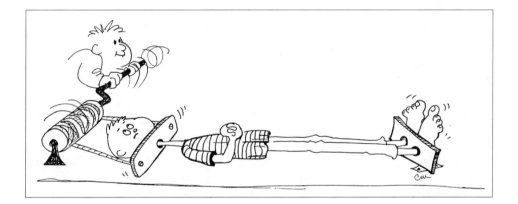

CHAPTER OBJECTIVES

- Define the principles of the therapeutic application of traction.
- Describe the theories of cervical and lumbar traction.
- Describe the theories and application of mechanical forms of traction.
- Discuss the clinical uses and safety considerations regarding the use of traction.
- Outline the clinical decision making in the use of traction as a treatment modality.

CHAPTER OUTLINE

Traction has long been a mainstay for physical therapists when treating a variety of spinal problems. Many causes of spinal pain, as well as weakness, paresthesia, and pain referred from the spine, have traditionally been treated with traction techniques.

There have been mixed reviews from researchers regarding the actual physiologic effects of traction. The findings range from claims of profound changes in spinal occlusion[1,2] to studies showing no statistical differences between traction and bedrest.[3] The negative findings have largely been in studies of specific and dated methods such as bed traction.

Like most physical therapy treatments, the use of traction has been a subject of ongoing debate both with physical therapists and physicians. Controversy exists regarding optimal techniques, treatment times, positions, frequency, duration, force of pull, angle of pull, and overall efficacy of traction.

The scrutiny of research has helped drive the evolution of traction over the last several decades. Current use of polyaxial traction, inversion traction, home traction units, as well as the assortment of manual traction techniques has changed the perception of traction. The result of this controversy and change has been a seemingly endless variability of treatment techniques and protocols. In attempts to face this problem, several researchers have consolidated the quagmire of different protocols into useful information,[4–6] such as the general acceptance that supine is preferable to sitting when treating cervical disk lesions with traction.

Some therapists use traction liberally for a number of conditions such as herniated nucleus pulposus and lateral stenosis (a diminution of the intervertebral foramen). Some do not use traction at all. Although disagreement remains as to physiologic effects, traction has weathered the test of time as a useful treatment for many spinal problems.[1,2,7–11]

PRINCIPLES OF THERAPEUTIC APPLICATION

TERMINOLOGY AND DEFINITIONS

Traction

The word *traction* is derived from the Latin root "tractio," which means a process of drawing or pulling. By definition, this does not include a countertraction, which is necessary for separation of anatomic segments in the human body. The types of traction are listed in Table 7-1.

Distraction

With the addition of the prefix *dis*, which is from the Latin meaning "apart," the definition more accurately reflects the purpose of the treatment (to pull apart). Distraction is the separation of surfaces of a joint by extension without injury or dislocation of the parts.[12]

The Related Physics   A basic understanding of the physical principles of traction is necessary to understand the physiology of traction. Principles to be discussed include definition of force and friction as they pertain to traction.

A force, in the simplest sense, is a push or a pull. Its source may be gravitational, mechanical, electrical, magnetic, or generated from muscles (physiologic). A force is anything that can accelerate an object. In the case of traction, it is generated either by the therapist (physiologic), by a machine (mechanical), or by weight (gravitational). If a therapist places a 100-pound weight on a string and attaches it by way of a strap onto a patient, a traction force of 100 pounds is incident upon the patient (Fig. 7–1).

Friction is the resistive force that arises to oppose the motion or attempted motion of an object past another with which it is in contact.[13] It results from mutual contact of irregularities in the surfaces. The direction of frictional force is always parallel to the surfaces in contact and in the direction opposing motion (Fig. 7–2).

There are known constants of frictional forces between surfaces, the so-called coefficient of friction. The force of friction is dependent on the coefficient of friction between the two objects and the magnitude of the force compressing the two objects together (the greater the weight of the body part being pulled, the greater the friction). In the example of the 100 pounds of pull placed on the patient in Fig. 7–2, the traction force on the patient is therefore not 100 pounds. There is a force of friction that opposes the pull between the table and the patient. The net force is defined as the sum of the forces on an object (patient). The net force would be the 100 pounds of pull minus the friction (see Fig. 7–2). The coefficient of friction between the table and the patient has been calculated at approximately 0.5.[14] This means that, in the case of a 160-pound man, a force of one half the weight of the

TABLE 7–1.   **Traction Methods**

Type of Traction	Features	Advantages/Disadvantages
Autotraction	Involves the patient using his/her own muscle strength as the distraction source. This can be done in different ways, the use of a three-dimensional autotraction table (see Fig. 7–13) has gained popularity in Europe and is becoming more commonly used in the U.S. In addition, several home lumbar traction units utilize this method (see Fig. 7–16).	**Advantage:** Patient can control parameters such as position and amount of force. Some forms can be done at home. **Disadvantages:** Three-dimensional tables are expensive, have been shown to increase intradiskal pressure.
Cervical traction	Traction applied to the cervical spine by applying a force to move the heat superiorly, or mobilization technique used to distract the individual cervical vertebra. This can be done manually, with halters, or through Crutchfield tongs which are inserted directly into the skull.	
Continuous (bed) traction	Traction that is administered for several days to weeks. The traction force is often minimal because of the duration of the treatment. This form of traction has fallen into disuse because of studies indicating that the results are consistent with bedrest alone.	**Advantages:** Can be done at home, inexpensively. **Disadvantages:** Efficacy is questionable.
Elastic traction	Traction by use of elastic devices such as rubber bands.	
Gravity-assisted traction	Utilizes gravity to facilitate localized traction of target issue. This differs from inversion traction in that the body is not suspended in the air.	**Advantages:** Can be done at home, inexpensively. Does not require healthy cardiopulmonary systems as does inversion traction. **Disadvantages:** Traction force is limited by body weight.
Head traction	Traction applied to the head in the presence of injury to the cervical vertebra.	

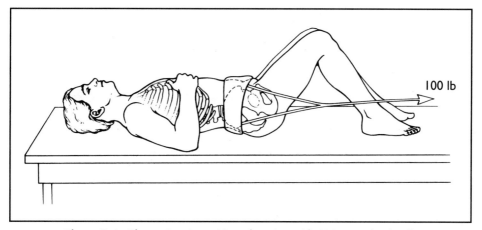

Figure 7–1. The patient is positioned supine with 100 pounds of pull.

body, or 80 pounds, is needed to overcome friction and move the body horizontally. In the example, then, if the body parts to undergo traction are the legs and pelvis (weighing usually about half body weight, or in this case, 80 pounds), then one half of 80 pounds (40 pounds) would be necessary to overcome the force of friction and the traction force on the patient would be 60 pounds; 100 pounds (traction force) − 40 pounds (frictional forces) = 60 pounds (Fig. 7–3). Notice that the total frictional force of 40 pounds was equal to one fourth the total body weight of 160 pounds (weight of legs and pelvis = 0.5 body weight × 0.5 [coefficient of friction] = 0.25). It takes a traction force of approximately one fourth of the body weight to overcome frictional forces when applying lumbar traction.

There are ways to reduce the coefficient of friction between surfaces. One way is to reduce the amount of "roughness" between the two surfaces. In the above example, then, if a smooth surface is placed between the patient and the table, the coefficient of friction could be reduced to perhaps 0.4. Then the net force of traction on the patient would be 100 − 32 = 68 pounds; 0.4 (coefficient of friction) × 80 (weight of legs and pelvis) = 32.

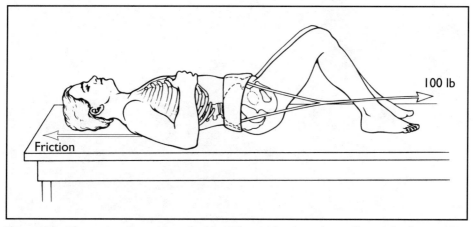

Figure 7–2. The patient is positioned with 100 pounds of traction pull, and the force of friction is depicted.

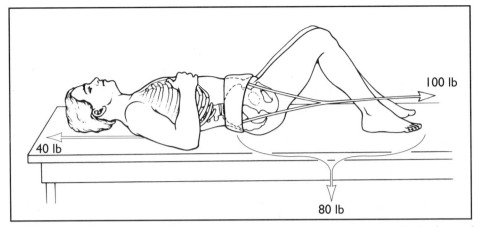

Figure 7–3. The patient is positioned supine with 100 pounds of traction pull; the force of friction is indicated. The resultant pull is equivalent to 60 pounds once the coefficient of friction is calculated into the formula. The weight of the individual was 160 pounds, and 50% of the weight of the individual (80 pounds) was distributed between the legs and pelvis. The coefficient of friction was 50%. Summary: 160-pound patient (80 pounds below the waist), coefficient of friction = 50% or 40 pounds to move the pelvis and legs. Traction force applied = 100 pounds − 40 pounds for the pelvis and legs = 60 pounds of traction force.

There is another and better way to reduce the amount of friction when performing traction. The use of a "split traction table" that separates at the point of distraction essentially eliminates movement of one surface (the patient) from the other (the table) (Fig. 7–4). This equipment is necessary only with lumbar traction.

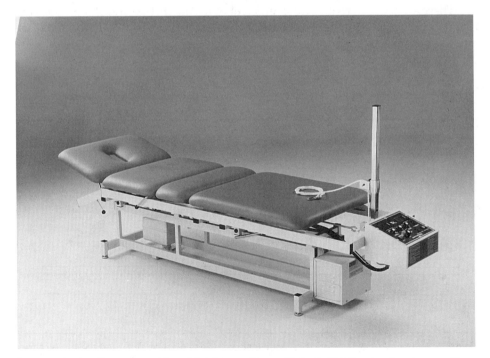

Figure 7–4. A split traction table, which lowers the coefficient of friction to close to zero. Traction force to cause movement or separation is greatly reduced through the use of a split table.

With cervical traction, the weight of the head does not offer enough friction to reduce the pulling force significantly.

THEORY OF APPLICATION

BRIEF HISTORICAL PERSPECTIVE

Traction has been a popular treatment for low back pain long before scientific method could test its efficacy. The use of traction may well have dated back to the time of the Egyptians and is documented at least to the times of Hippocrates (460–376 BC). The Hippocratic method was used by Galen (130–200 AD) and others (Fig. 7–5). The Turks have used a traction device for over 500 years, and the Italians used a traction table in the mid-sixteenth century that was based on the Hippocratic model.[15] Traction fell from grace based in part by studies challenging its efficacy. This, in addition to bad results (probably because of the rote manner in which physicians were prescribing and therapists were applying traction), convinced many therapists to abandon it as a therapy choice. Traction is a modality that makes such physiologic sense that it was never fully disregarded.

Traction enjoyed a renaissance starting with Cyriax in the 1950s and others who developed new and creative approaches to traction treatment. This spurred new research that verified some physiologic effects such as vertebral separation and reversal of spinal nerve root impingement.[11]

Current Trends and Research

Modern research involving traction has been going on since at least the 1950s and involves studies of the physical and physiologic effects and efficacy of traction as well as comparing different protocols of traction such as optimal patient positioning, intermittent versus continuous pull, angle of pull, and time and frequency of application. Some of the problems that arise when researching traction (and many other modalities) are (1) conclusively diagnosing the population base; (2) objectively measuring variables, that is, pain levels; and (3) eliminating unwanted variables.[16] It is probable that the future of traction research will be enhanced by better imaging equipment such as magnetic resonance imaging (MRI) and computerized axial tomography (CAT) scans. This will allow researchers to better categorize their diagnostic groups and better assess physiologic changes.

GENERAL TREATMENT GOALS FOR TRACTION

Goals of traction include reduction of radicular signs and symptoms associated with conditions such as disk protrusion, lateral stenosis, degenerative disk disease, and subluxations (i.e., spondylolisthesis). Other goals of traction include reduction of muscle guarding/spasm via prolonged stretch; reduction of joint pain via neurophysiologic pathways (gating mechanism); and increasing range of motion (ROM) via distraction/mobilization of joint surfaces. Traction has also been used for fracture immobilization. Examples include immobilization of cervical spine fracture via Crutchfield or Burton tongs and immobilization of lower-extremity long bones via skeletal or skin traction, that is, Buck's traction or Russell's traction. Further discussion of traction for fracture immobilization is beyond the scope of this book. The remainder of this chapter will address the issues of lumbar and cervical traction methods.

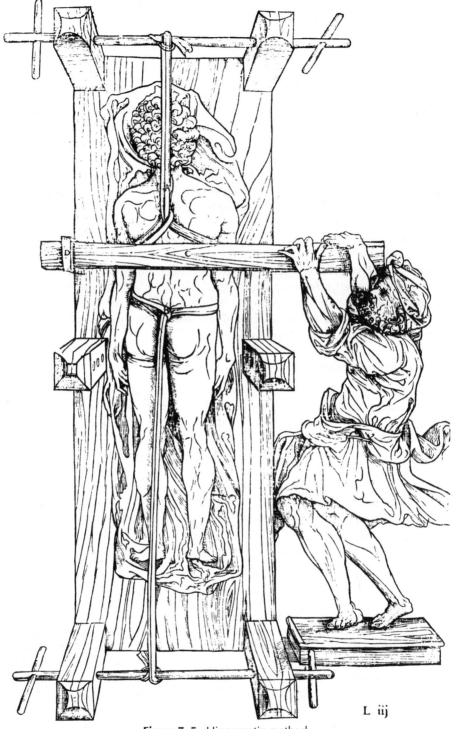

L iij

Figure 7–5. Hippocratic method.

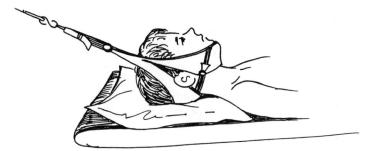

Figure 7–6. A traditional halter that pulls from both the occiput and the mandible.

CERVICAL TRACTION

MECHANICAL TECHNIQUES

Mechanical traction is the use of free weights and traction machines to create a pulling force. Programmable traction units are primarily used because of their versatility. Traditional halters pull from both the occiput and the mandible (Fig. 7–6). There is evidence that mandibular pull can create and aggravate temporomandibular problems.[17] Occipital halters have largely replaced traditional halters (Fig. 7–7). They have no mandibular strap and pull exclusively from the occiput. In addition, some models are capable of pulling the head into side flexion and rotation.

Position

Supine position has been shown to be preferable to sitting for most treatments.[21] There are those that prefer prone as a position of choice in cases of low back pain involvement.[22]

Poundage

The head weighs approximately 14 pounds. The poundage used for cervical traction varies according to the source, but it is generally accepted that to produce elongation of the spine, 25 to 30 pounds (11.25 to 13.5 kg) is necessary.[6] Greater amounts

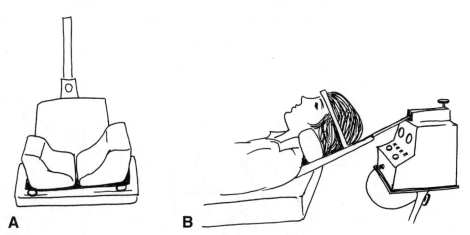

A   **B**

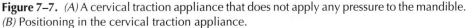

Figure 7–7. *(A)* A cervical traction appliance that does not apply any pressure to the mandible. *(B)* Positioning in the cervical traction appliance.

produce greater separation only to a point, and excessive traction may produce muscle guarding that can overcome up to 55 pounds of traction force.[11] It appears that the upper cervical spine requires less traction force to cause separation than does the lower cervical spine.[5] Weight approaching 120 pounds was necessary to cause a disk rupture at the C-5, C-6 level.[18] Some studies indicate that application of cervical traction can produce low back radiculopathy in some patients,[23] so care should be taken to use the least amount of force that is clinically effective.

Angle of Pull

The angle of pull varies according to target tissue. For maximal perpendicular facet separation, the angle would be zero degrees at the atlanto-occipital (A/O) joint and increasing amounts of extension to C-6, C-7 (Fig. 7–8). For increasing the intervertebral space, it is generally accepted that about 25° of flexion is optimal.[19] Too much flexion has been shown to actually decrease intervertebral space because of encroachment of the ligamentum flavum on the intervertebral foramen.[4,20] For some disk problems, a neutral spine is indicated because it causes the ligaments to be lax and the traction can be transmitted more completely to the disk. Three-dimensional or polyaxial traction is becoming more popular because of its ability to maximally gap vertebral segments unilaterally (Fig. 7–9).

Static Versus Intermittent

There is little agreement on one over the other, but intermittent traction seems to be more comfortable for most patients. The shorter the time of pull, the more poundage can generally be tolerated. Facet problems seem to respond better to shorter and equal on time versus off time (10 seconds/10 seconds), and herniated disk problems to longer on-off times with approximately 1:3 ratios (20 seconds/60 seconds), and sustained pulls.

Treatment Time

The optimal amount of time that traction is administered ranges from 2 minutes[24] to 24 hours.[25] One study showed that maximal vertebral separation per pull phase occurs after 7 seconds with intermittent traction.[26] Treatment time for cervical degenerative joint disease (DJD) should be approximately 25 minutes, for disk

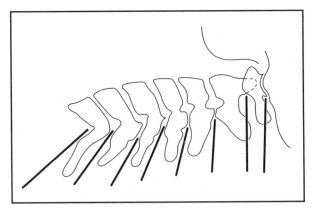

Figure 7–8. The cervical spine.

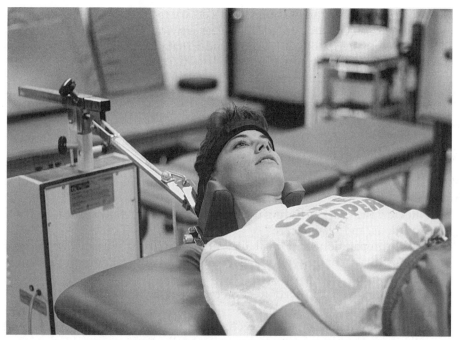

Figure 7–9. A polyaxial traction unit.

protrusion no more than 8 minutes. Traction for longer than 8 minutes with disk protrusions can cause the disk to imbibe excess fluid and increase intradiscal pressure.[5] No significant muscular relation was found on electromyography (EMG) after 10 minutes of traction.[27] The minimum amount of time that traction should be applied to allow full muscular relaxation is 20 to 25 minutes.[6]

Frequency of Treatment

The number of times per week the patient is treated is dependent on type and severity of the problem and duration of relief from traction. The frequency should generally be greater when the problem is more acute, as in the presence of neurologic findings.

Other Equipment for Traction of the Cervical Spine

Autotraction   Autotraction of the cervical spine has become more popular recently. The traction force is controlled by the patient through a footboard or other device. This allows constant adjustments to be possible at the patient's discretion and creates an active role of the patient in therapy. The Goodley polyaxial cervical traction unit (E-Z-Em, Westbury, NY) has the advantage of allowing the therapist to administer the line of force through three dimensions. Results using this method have been promising.[7]

Home Units   The use of the "over-the-door" variety of home units has endured in spite of the necessity to perform the traction sitting. The maximal weight of these units is 20 pounds. When considering the weight of the head at 14 pounds, this means the maximum force on the cervical spine can be only 6 pounds. It has already been established that 25 pounds is necessary to create a significant distraction of the cervical vertebra. In addition, less cervical muscle activity occurs in supine position than in sitting.[27] It is no wonder that patients usually do not show marked change with these units.

Other home units are available that allow the patient to be treated in the recumbent position and can deliver traction forces sufficient to allow vertebral separation (Fig. 7–10). Traction forces can be generated by gravity assistance and springs.

Procedure for Mechanical Cervical Traction

Before starting a mechanical cervical traction treatment, the following should be done:

1. Review the chart including diagnosis, indications, contraindications, precautions, and plan of care.
2. Table preparation including halter, pillows, draping sheets, call bell, timer.
3. Preset treatment time, poundage, time on and off, and duration and angle of pull as per plan of care.
4. Explain fully the effects of traction to the patient and answer all questions and concerns the patient has.
5. Use a mouthpiece or soft insert between the teeth if no occipital halter is available to reduce compression forces on the temporomandibular joint.
6. Position patient according to desired effect, that is, supine with 25° of cervical flexion in the case of intervertebral foraminal separation. Provide pillows for support and comfort.
7. Adjust the halter according to desired effect. Traditional halters should be positioned so that the patient feels the majority of the pull from the occiput. The posterior (occipital) part of the halter should cradle the occiput at the

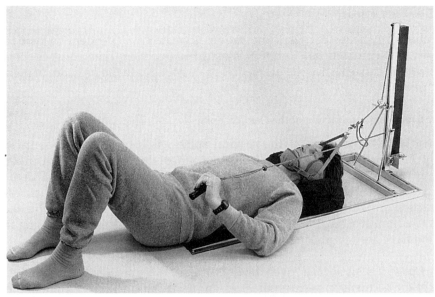

Figure 7–10. A home traction unit. (*Courtesy of C-Tract, Granberg International, Richmond, CA.*)

level of the inferior nuchal line to both mastoid processes. Place a tissue between the anterior (chin) pad and the chin. If properly applied, the anterior pad should cradle the mandible and be snug to patient's tolerance.

8. Attach halter to spreader bar and remove all slack from the rope.
9. Double check all settings.
10. Turn on machine and stay with patient at least through one entire cycle to ensure proper setup.
11. Explain use of call bell or safety switch before leaving.

MANUAL TRACTION

Therapists are using manual traction techniques in greater numbers. Techniques ranging from simple occipital distraction (Fig. 7–11) to various segmental locking techniques in unison with three-dimensional distraction to isolate specific vertebral levels are commonly applied. Specific techniques of manual traction are beyond the scope of this text.

POSITIONAL TRACTION

Positional distraction techniques are inviting because the patient can perform them at home with little to no equipment. The general principle is to place the neck in positions that either enhance limited ROM or maximize intervertebral foraminal space to release impinged tissues. Caution should always be taken to avoid prolonged positions that would place the facet joints in a closed-packed attitude.

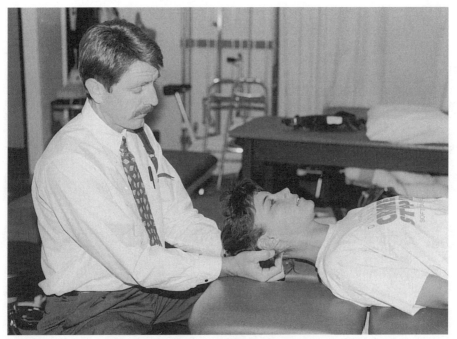

Figure 7–11. Proper positioning of both the patient and the clinician for manual cervical traction. Great care must be taken to assure an appropriate line of pull.

LUMBAR TRACTION

MECHANICAL TECHNIQUES

Mechanical traction using a traction machine is the most frequently used method. Free weights have largely been abandoned due to the large amount of weight needed.

Equipment

A programmable traction unit is generally used because of its versatility (Fig. 7–12).

Position

Lumbar traction has traditionally been performed with the patient in supine with knees and hips flexed to varying degrees. Approximately 45° to 60° of hip flexion will cause laxity at the L-5, S-1 level, 60° to 75° at the L-4, L-5 level, and 75° to 90° at the L-3, L-4 level. The point of laxity of the joint represents the neutral position for that joint and, theoretically, the position of maximal joint separation. As with the cervical spine, excessive lumbar flexion can decrease intervertebral foraminal space because of encroachment of the ligamentum flavum on the intervertebral foramen.[4,20]

Current trends include positioning the patient in supine with hips and knees extended, and prone, depending on the target tissue and desired effect. Prone has the advantage of accessing the back for modalities to be performed concurrently.

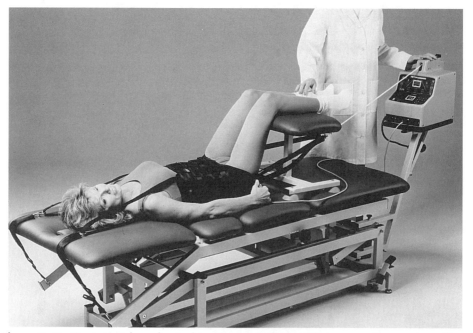

Figure 7–12. Commercial mechanical traction unit. *(From Chattanooga Corporation, Chattanooga, TN, with permission.)*

Poundage

As described under physics of traction, the poundage necessary to overcome the frictional forces of the lower body (in the absence of a split traction table) is one fourth body weight. When using a split traction table, the frictional force is negligible. The protocol for optimal tractional force varies according to source, ranging from 300 pounds[9] to the minimum one fourth body weight.[4] Maximal tolerance of the T-11, T-12 disks was found to be 440 pounds,[18] although estimates for the lumbar spine are considerably higher than that.

Angle of Pull

The angle of the traction force on the pelvis can ultimately determine the low back position during traction and can actually be more important than patient position.[19] With use of modern harnesses (Fig. 7–13), the differential pull can position the lumbar spine into lordosis in the case of an anterior pull, or into kyphosis in the case of a posterior pull. Therefore, supine with knees and hips straight with an anterior pull would maximize lordosis and might be indicated in cases of a disk protrusion, while prone with table flexed and a posterior pull would maximize kyphosis and might be indicated in the case of lateral stenosis secondary to spondylosis. Unilateral traction has the advantage of allowing side flexion and rotational forces to occur. This can be of use in cases of lateral disk protrusion or unilateral foraminal stenosis, to name a few. Unilateral traction can be performed by either positioning the patient askew to the line of force or by applying the traction pull on one side without the use of a spreader bar (Fig. 7–14).

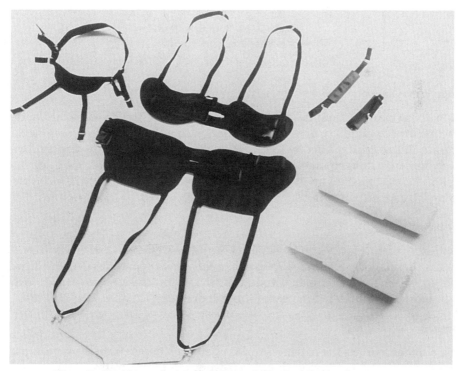

Figure 7–13. The typical components of a harness for lumbar traction.

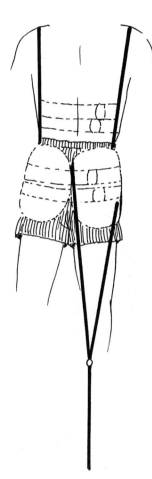

Figure 7–14. A unilateral pull of lumbar traction force.

Static Versus Intermittent

As with cervical traction, the physiologic difference of static versus intermittent traction force is poorly understood, although intermittent traction allows the therapist to utilize greater traction forces. Facet problems empirically respond better to shorter and equal on time and off time (10 seconds/10 seconds), and herniated disk problems to longer on-off times with approximately 1:3 ratios (20 seconds/60 seconds), and sustained pulls.

Treatment Time

The length of time for treatment depends on the desired effect and tends to shorter for disk herniations (8 minutes or less), and longer for spondylosis (about 25 minutes). Traction for longer than 8 minutes with disk protrusions can cause the disk to imbibe excess fluid and increase intradisk pressure.[5]

Frequency of Treatment

The number of times the patient is treated per week depends on the type of problem and severity. Generally, the more severe the problem, the greater the frequency.

Other Equipment for Traction of the Lumbar Spine

Autotraction   Lumbar autotraction has gained strong support in parts of Europe and the United States. Use of an autotraction table when performing this technique allows the therapist to control the three-dimensional pull on the patient accurately (Fig. 7–15) and allows the patient to control the amount of traction force. In one study, the use of autotraction compared to sustained mechanical traction showed significantly better results.[28] Another study comparing autotraction to manual traction showed them to be equally successful.[29] These studies sound favorable; however, the use of autotraction has been shown to increase intradiskal pressure, probably because of contraction of spinal and other muscles.[30]

Home Units   Many of the home units for lumbar traction use the patient's own muscle strength as a traction force and therefore would be considered autotraction. In addition, various gravity-assisted traction units have been developed as well as hydraulic and spring-loaded models.

Procedure for Lumbar Traction

Before initiating lumbar traction, the following should be done:
1. Review the chart including diagnosis, indications, contraindications, precautions, and plan of care.
2. Table preparation including harnesses, pillows, draping sheets, call bell, and timer. Always use a split traction table if available.
3. Preset treatment time, poundage, time on and off, duration, and angle of pull as per plan of care.

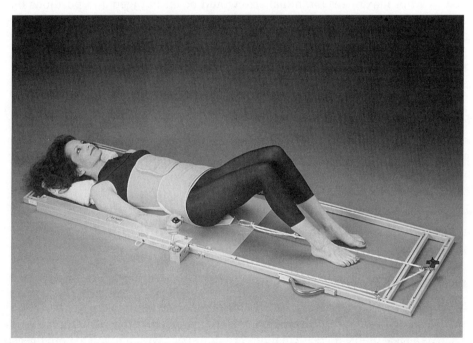

Figure 7–15. An "E-Z track" traction unit. *(Courtesy of Granberg International, Richmond, CA.)*

4. Explain the effects of traction to the patient and answer questions and concerns the patient has.
5. Remove clothing from around belt sites, drape patient appropriately. Position patient according to desired effect, that is, supine with knees and hips flexed to 45°. Provide pillows for support and comfort.
6. Adjust harnesses according to desired effect. Place a folded towel between patient's abdomen and traction harness. Attach traction (pelvic) harness first, the superior part should be in line with the umbilicus. The counter-traction (thoracic) harness should then be positioned so that the superior part fits snugly around ribs 8, 9, and 10. If properly applied, the two belts should overlap slightly and be snug to patient's tolerance.
7. Attach harness to spreader bar and remove all slack from the rope.
8. Double check all settings.
9. Turn on machine and wait for one complete cycle so that all of the slack is taken up; release catch of split table (during off cycle if using intermittent traction).
10. Explain use of call bell or safety switch before leaving.

MANUAL AND POSITIONAL TRACTION

Manual traction techniques can be as simple as providing a simple longitudinal traction force (Fig. 7–16) to locking techniques used in unison with three-dimensional pulls to create joint-specific traction in any desired direction.

Positional traction is used frequently in the lumbar area by therapists because it can be done at home and requires little or no equipment. The forces can be three-dimensional, and can be significant, because the weight of the legs can be used as the traction force. As with the cervical spine, the position that either enhances limited ROM or maximizes foraminal size would be encouraged and positions that create a closed-packed position over a prolonged period of time should be avoided.

Inversion Traction

The weight of the suspended body, either fully or from the waist down, is used as a tractive force. Both techniques create a lumbar traction force of about 40% of body weight. This method of traction is acceptable in patients without cardiopulmonary or cardiovascular compromise or hypertension, because it has been shown to raise both systolic and diastolic blood pressure significantly and to increase oxygen uptake.[31,32]

CLINICAL USES AND SAFETY CONSIDERATIONS

INDICATIONS AND EFFECTS

Herniation of Disk Material

Traction has been a treatment for impingement or irritation of nerves secondary to a variety of causes, including disk material contacting the spinal nerve roots. There is a measurable increase in intervertebral space with traction to both the cer-

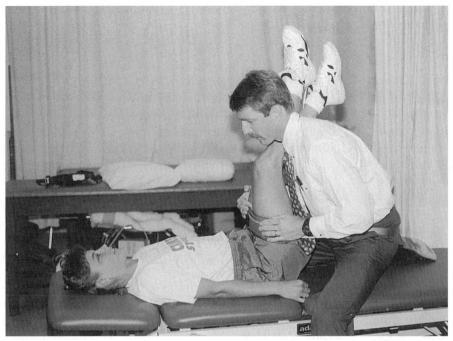

Figure 7–16. The effects on the lumbar vertebrae with an applied traction force sufficient to cause lumbar distraction.

vical and lumbar spine.[1,9,10,16,26,33] The debate to date revolves around how much separation occurs with specific distractive forces. There are studies that seem to indicate that the application of traction can reverse spinal obstruction secondary to disk protrusion.[1,2,34] It has been proposed that in the presence of increased volume of the disk, that intradiskal pressure would be lessened. In other words, the negative pressure that should accompany the increased volume should "suck" the disk material back into the disk.[9,34,35] This is generally accepted, although one study found that intradiskal pressure either stays the same or actually increases during application of different forms of traction.[30] Although the precise mechanisms of action are unclear, however, traction has been found to be effective in treatment of herniated disks.[1,9,10,16,26,33–35]

Degenerative Joint Disease

With degenerative joint disease (DJD) of the spine, there are at least two clinically significant occurrences: (1) a decrease of intervertebral space with an associated decrease of the intervertebral foraminal space, and (2) osteophyte production into the intervertebral space coming from the facet joint and the vertebral body (see Fig. 7–10). Collectively, this progression leads to lateral stenosis, which is a reduction of the intervertebral foraminal size. As mentioned before, traction has been shown to increase intervertebral space, and with it, the size of the intervertebral foramen. Although the increase in foraminal size seen with traction should return to pretreatment size after the treatment is over, the decrease in pain can last for a prolonged time. Once the nerve is decompressed, perhaps the swelling in the nerve subsides and the existing foraminal size is sufficient to accommodate the smaller-diameter nerve. Traction has been shown to be an effective treatment for impingement of the spinal nerve secondary to spinal stenosis.[4–6,8,9,15]

Muscle Spasm or Guarding

In the presence of spinal pain, be it cervical, thoracic, or lumbar secondary to muscle spasm or guarding, traction can be of use to cause a slow, prolonged stretch of the muscles. Although some sources state that prolonged stretch via traction can cause a reflex inhibition of the muscle,[25] others disagree.[27] Possible explanations include golgi tendon organ involvement, a "resetting" of the muscle spindle to a longer length, and relaxation of nociceptive reflexes.

Joint Hypomobility

In the presence of generalized decreased spinal ROM, spinal traction will mobilize the joint by moving the articular surfaces on each other as well as distract the surfaces and decreasing pressure. In addition, intermittent traction should have the effect of increasing synovial fluid production and thus nutrifying the cartilage as well as firing mechanoreceptors to "gate" the pain transmission. Treating patients with specific areas of hypomobility would be difficult with generalized traction; however, manual traction and mobilization or three-dimensional traction might be indicated in this case.

Facet Impingement

The facet joints have a capsule that can theoretically become impinged within the joint space.[36] Traction techniques, especially in combination with positions that maximize specific joint separation, will cause a decompression of the facet joints and thus could be of some use in treating impingements. Although standard mechanical traction could be used for this condition, polyaxial autotraction, positional traction, and manual traction would be the preferred methods because of their ability to isolate specific joints.

Contraindications

The following are potential contraindications to the use of traction:
1. Spinal infections (i.e., spinal meningitis, arachnoiditis) that could be spread by the use of traction.
2. Rheumatoid arthritis (RA) or other acute inflammatory disorders affecting the joints. Ligaments, such as the transverse ligament of the atlantoaxial joint, are particularly vulnerable with RA.
3. Osteoporosis. Traction may exceed the tolerance of the structurally compromised bone.
4. Spinal cancers. Traction may increase the chance of metastasis of cancer cells.
5. Spinal cord pressure. In the presence of impingement directly on the spinal cord secondary to a central disk herniation or spinal tumor, traction has not been shown to be effective and may aggravate the condition.[37]

Precautions

The following are precautions to the use of traction:

1. Joint hypermobility. In the presence of hypermobile joints, traction could aggravate the condition.
2. Acute inflammation. In almost all cases traction could aggravate the condition.
3. Claustrophobia or other anxiety associated with traction. If the patient is not relaxed, muscle guarding can overcome strong traction forces.
4. Cardiac or respiratory insufficiency with inversion traction.
5. Pregnancy. Due to constriction of the abdomen as well as joint laxity secondary to endogenous production of relaxin.
6. Patients whose symptoms increase with traction. For example, with cervical traction, pre-existing lumbar radiculopathy that was aggravated by traction.
7. With cervical traction, temperomandibular joint (TMJ) dysfunction when using a chin strap.

PATIENT EDUCATION

As with all treatments, the patient should be as completely informed as possible regarding the effects and goals of traction treatment. Patient compliance strongly correlates to an understanding of the treatment they are to receive. The use of a spinal model with spinal nerves and drawings of the physical effects are useful tools for traction education. For example, the therapist, upon explaining the effects of cervical traction to treat lateral stenosis, might use a finger to represent a nerve and form an "O" with the finger and thumb of the other hand to represent the foramen, then pass the "nerve" through the "foramen" demonstrating the normal relationship. By reducing the size of the "foramen," impingement is represented. Next, the therapist might show on a spinal model how distraction can increase the size of the foramen to allow the nerve unimpeded passage.

If the patient is to be given a home traction device or technique to perform, the therapist should demonstrate the use of it and have the patient demonstrate the use to the therapist. Have the patient bring the device in the next treatment (or use a similar model available in the clinic) and demonstrate the proper use again. These "pop quizzes" will give the therapist valuable information regarding compliance and will alert one to improper use of the modality. Improper use of traction units and improper positional traction positioning can aggravate many conditions.

CLINICAL DECISION MAKING

During the patient's treatments, certain questions can help prevent problems from arising. The following is an example of some of the questions to ask patients that could yield valuable information.

Questions to rule out contraindications and precautions include:

1. Is your pain in both legs (arms)? Contraindication—spinal tumor or central spinal cord impingement.
2. Are you having problems going to the bathroom? Contraindication—spinal cord tumor or central spinal cord impingement.

3. Have you had any swelling or pain in other joints for no reason (without a traumatic event)? Contraindication—Rheumatoid or other systemic inflammatory disorders.
4. Tell me about any bones that you have broken. Contraindication—osteoporosis.
5. Have you had a fever or sweating and unusual tiredness as of late? Contraindication—spinal infection.
6. Is your pain worse at night, any changes in your appetite, sleep patterns, etc.? Contraindication—spinal tumor.
7. When did you last injure your back or neck? Precaution—acute inflammation, avoid excessive forces in traction.
8. Does all movement hurt your back or neck or specific movements and do you experience any excessive popping, clicking, or other noises with movement? Precaution—hypermobility, avoid excessive forces in traction.
9. Do you get short of breath easily? Precaution—respiratory insufficiency, avoid inversion traction.
10. Do you have high blood pressure? Precaution—cardiac insufficiency, avoid inversion traction.
11. Do you have popping or clicking in your jaw, jaw pain or frequent headaches? Precaution—TMJ dysfunction.
12. Have you ever received traction before, and if so, did it aggravate your condition? Contraindication/Precaution—all of the above.

PATIENT POSITIONING AND DRAPING CONSIDERATIONS

Patient positioning is especially important when dealing with problems for which traction is indicated.

Although there remains controversy about extension versus flexion when treating spine patients, patient comfort is paramount. As mentioned earlier, if the patient is in an uncomfortable position and is in spasm, the strength of the spinal muscles will overcome any desired physiologic effects of traction. Because patient position greatly affects intradiskal pressure,[38] it is of particular importance for patients with disk herniations.

Lumbar Spine

Prone positions tend to increase lumbar extension (lordosis) of the spine with a relative anterior wedging of the disk, decreased intervertebral foraminal space, and increased weight-bearing forces on the facets. Prone positioning might be indicated with disk bulges without total dissociation of the nuclear material. It would be contraindicated with severe osteoarthritis with lateral stenosis.

The supine position without leg support can also create lumbar extension (lordosis), which has the same effects as above. Supine with knees and hips flexed creates flexion of the lumbar spine and produces a relative posterior wedging of the disk, increased intervertebral foraminal space, and decreased weight-bearing forces on the facets. Excessive lumbar flexion has actually been shown to decrease intervertebral space, probably because of the movement of the ligamentum flavum into the foraminal space.

Cervical Traction

When performing cervical traction, positioning is usually performed either sitting or supine. As mentioned earlier, there is less muscle activity in the paraspinals when supine compared to sitting, and therefore this appears to be the position of choice if the patient can tolerate it. Prone positioning creates an extension bias and should be avoided unless the therapist can create a neutral spine with supports. The supine position maintains an approximately neutral cervical spine in patients with normal thoracic kyphosis. Patients with excessive kyphosis or a dowager's hump are apt to experience a position of excessive cervical lordosis when supine without at least one pillow for support. A position of slight hip and knee flexion during cervical traction prevents lumbar lordosis in persons with tight hip flexors and can relax the patient to ensure greater efficacy.

Patient draping should be consistent with room temperature and patient modesty and expose only the skin necessary to perform techniques effectively.

SUMMARY

In summary, traction has endured as a treatment technique for hundreds of years because of its ease of application and versatility. Although not a panacea, traction can be an effective treatment technique for a variety of spinal disorders, and can be utilized with a modicum of equipment both in the clinic and in the home setting. Although there is a plethora of research that substantiates the efficacy of certain traction methods, more research needs to be done to validate (or invalidate) specific methods of traction treatment in all of its applications.

DISCUSSION QUESTIONS

1. Why would position make a difference in the treatment outcome when utilizing either cervical or lumbar traction?
2. Of what significance is the presence of a lordosis in the lumbar spine if lumbar traction is utilized?
3. How does knowledge of the coefficient of friction influence your decision regarding the amount of traction required to cause distraction of the joint surfaces?
4. How would you explain the purpose of cervical traction to a patient who was referred for treatment with a diagnosis of a cervical strain with radiating pain and paresthesia in the right upper extremity following an automobile accident?
5. Describe the differences between the use of an occipital pull harness and a typical head halter for cervical traction.

REFERENCES

1. Mathews, J: Dynamic discography: A study of lumbar traction. Ann Phys Med 9:275, 1968.

2. Gupta, R and Ramarao, S: Epidurography in reduction of lumbar disc prolapse by traction. Arch Phys Med Rehabil 59:322, 1978.

3. Pal, B, et al: A controlled trial of continuous lumbar traction in the treatment of back pain and sciatica. Br J Rheumatol 25:181, 1986.

4. Saunders, H: Lumbar traction. J Orthop Sports Phys Ther 1:36, 1979.

5. Saunders, H: The use of spinal traction in the treatment of neck and back conditions. Clin Orthop Rel Res 179:31, 1983.

6. Harris, P: Cervical traction: Review of literature and treatment guidelines. Phys Ther 57:910, 1977.

7. Walker, G: Goodley polyaxial cervical traction: A new approach to a traditional treatment. Phys Ther 66:1255, 1986.

8. Larsson, U, et al: Auto-traction for treatment of lumbago-sciatica. Acta Orthop Scand 51:791, 1980.

9. Cyriax, J: The treatment of lumbar disk lesions. Br Med J 2:1434, 1950.

10. Judovich, B: Herniated cervical disc. Am J Surg 84:649, 1952.

11. Bard, G and Jones, M: Cineradiographic recording of traction of the cervical spine. Arch Phys Med Rehabil Aug:403, 1964.

12. Taber's Cyclopedic Medical Dictionary, ed 17. FA Davis, Philadelphia, 1993.

13. Hewitt, P: Conceptual Physics, ed 6. HarperCollins, New York, 1989.

14. Judovich, BD: Lumbar traction therapy—elimination of physical factors that prevent lumbar stretch. JAMA 159:549, 1955.

15. Natchev E: A manual of auto-traction treatment for low back pain. Folksam, Stockholm, Sweden, 1984.

16. Goldie, I and Reichmann, S: The biomechanical influence of traction on the cervical spine. Scand J Rehabil Med 9:31 1977.

17. Shore, A, et al: Cervical traction and temporomandibular joint dysfunction: Report of case. J Am Dental Assoc 68:4, 1964.

18. DeSeze, S and Levernieux, J: Les traction vertebrales. Semin Hip Paris 27:2075, 1951.

19. Saunders, H: Evaluation, treatment, and prevention of musculoskeletal disorders, ed 3. WB Saunders, Philadelphia, 1993.

20. Maslow, G and Rothman, R: The facet joints, another look. Bull NY Acad Med 51:1294, 1975.

21. Deets, D, et al: Cervical traction: A comparison of sitting and supine positions. Phys Ther 57:255, 1977.

22. Sood, N: Prone cervical traction. Clin Manag 7:37, 1987.

23. LaBan, M, et al: Intermittent cervical traction: A progenitor of lumbar radicular pain. Arch Phys Med Rehabil 73:295, 1992.

24. Frazer, H: The use of traction in backache. Med J Australia 2:694, 1954.

25. Crue, BL and Todd, EM: The importance of flexion in cervical halter traction. Bull Los Angeles Neurol Soc 30:95, 1965.

26. Colachis, SC and Strom, BR: Cervical traction: Relationship of traction time to varied tractive force with constant angle of pull. Arch Phys Med Rehabil 46:815, 1965.

27. Murphy, M: Effects of cervical traction on muscle activity. J Orthop Sports Phys Ther 13:220, 1991.

28. Tesio, L and Merlo, A: Autotraction versus passive traction: An open controlled study in lumbar disc herniation. Arch Phys Med Rehabil 74:871, 1992.

29. Ljunggren, A, et al: Autotraction versus manual traction in patients with prolapsed lumbar intervertebral discs. Scand J Rehabil Med 16:117, 1984.

30. Andersson, G, et al: Intervertebral disc pressures during traction. Scand J Rehabil Med 9:88, 1983.

31. Ballantyne, B, et al: The effects of inversion traction on spinal column configuration, heart rate, blood pressure, and perceived discomfort. J Orthop Sports Phys Ther 7:254, 1986.

32. LeMarr, J, et al: Cardiorespiratory responses to inversion. Phys Sport Med 11:51, 1983.

33. Mathews, W, et al: Manipulation and traction for lumbago sciatica: Physiotherapeutic techniques used in two controlled trials. Physiother Pract 4:201, 1988.

34. Onel, D, et al: Computed tomographic investigation of the effect of traction on lumbar disk herniations. Spine 14:82, 1989.

35. Goldish G: Lumbar traction. In CD Tollison and M Kriegel (eds): Interdisciplinary Rehabilitation of Low Back Pain. Williams & Wilkins, Baltimore, 1989.

36. Paris, S: The Spine: Etiology and treatment of dysfunction including joint manipulation. Course notes, 1979.

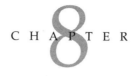
Passive Motion Devices for Soft Tissue Management: Continuous Passive Motion

Gisele Larose, OTR, CHT

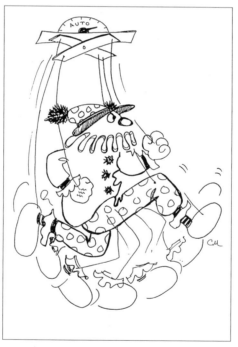

CHAPTER OBJECTIVES

- Define continuous passive motion (CPM).
- Describe the benefits of using CPM for recovery from joint immobilization and in the presence of pain.
- Describe the contraindications and precautions for use of CPM.
- Describe safety issues inherent in the use of CPM.
- List items to be included when documenting a treatment session with CPM.
- Provide CPM treatment guidelines.

CHAPTER OUTLINE

Continuous passive motion (CPM) is a form of passive motion delivered via a motorized device. CPM has been suggested following open reduction, internal fixation (ORIF) of an intra-articular fracture when fracture fragments are stable. Other uses include postdiaphyseal and metaphyseal fractures, capsulotomy and arthrolysis, arthroplasty, ligament reconstruction, synovectomy, arthrotomy, and drainage of acute specific arthritis (after incision and drainage and pharmaceutical management), tendon reconstruction, and burns. There is a biologic significance to what occurs in the healing process with longer doses of passive motion. Adhesion formation is consequential to all injury or surgery. CPM can reduce adhesion formation or promote healing with less fibrous tissue. This chapter is designed to provide the reader with an understanding of CPM as a method of moving a limb or joint to benefit from biologic changes of passive motion. CPM will stimulate an improved biologic healing response of articular cartilage, tendon, ligament, skin, and periarticular tissue when applied within the first postoperative week and continued for 24 hours per day for a period of at least 3 weeks.[1] Parameters of motion, protective precautions, and continuation of CPM beyond 3 weeks will vary according to the patient's diagnosis.

CPM is based on the efficacy of clinically applied small-dose, passive range of motion (PROM). Through empiric success, a spectrum of passive motion techniques have been utilized by clinicians. Passive motion can include joint manipulation (controlled accessory motion) or joint mobilization (slow, repetitious accessory movements).[2] Many variables, such as range, speed, force, and the addition of compressive forces, are important to result in a therapeutic benefit. This motion is provided by a machine. Intermittent passive motion is defined as motion applied by an external source at intermittent intervals within a 24-hour period, and is applied by a person or a machine.

THEORY OF APPLICATION

The early documented biological benefits of CPM are the hallmark work of Robert Salter, MD. His basic premise is that: "Joints are meant to move and last a lifetime."[3] Articular cartilage is the protective lining of every synovial joint in the body. This cartilage supports joint loading and unloading capabilities that contribute to functional joint motion. Salter published extensive research findings using an animal experimental model to document the biomechanical and biochemical changes that occur under the influence of CPM. In 1970, he proposed CPM as a means of stimulating the healing and regeneration of articular cartilage[4] (Fig. 8–1). A cartilage defect created in the femoral condyles of a rabbit's knee was managed by immobilization, by intermittent active motion (rabbits moved actively limited only by pain), or by continuous passive motion. Salter hypothesized that due to the fatiguability of skeletal muscle, longer doses of movement would have to be passive. Continuous motion was chosen because the animals ate well and were calmer when the units continued without start and stop periods. Table 8–1 represents a summation of numerous animal experimental investigations.[3,5–17] CPM utilization prevented complications of immobilization and stimulated the healing of articular tissue defects. The healed tissue resembles hyaline cartilage morphologically and histochemically.[1]

The biochemical changes to the fibrous connective tissue matrix resulting from stress deprivation include (1) decreased water content, (2) decreased total glycosaminoglycans (GAGS), (3) decreased collagen mass, (4) increased collagen turnover with increases of both synthesis and degradation, and (5) parallel increases in certain types of collagen cross-linking associated with increased syn-

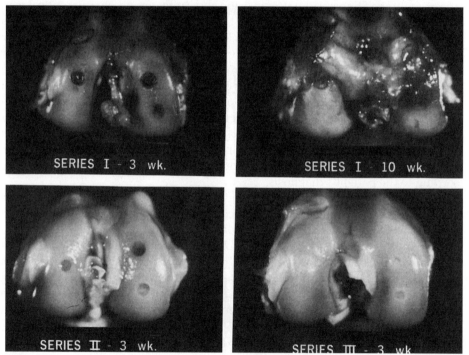

Figure 8–1. Gross appearance of typical defects in the three series of experiments (adolescent rabbits). Series Ia (immobilization for 3 weeks): Note the granulation-like tissue in the defects. Series Ib (immobilization for 10 weeks): Note the numerous extensive intra-articular synovial adhesions in the region of each of three defects in the femoral condyles; there are no adhesions in the region of the defect in the patellar groove. Series II (intermittent active motion for 3 weeks): Healing of the defects is somewhat better in this series than in Series Ia at 3 weeks, but healing is still incomplete. Series III (CPM for 3 weeks): Healing of the defects is by tissue grossly resembling articular cartilage. Healing in this series is considerably more complete than in either Series I or Series II. *(From: Continuous Passive Motion: Full Thickness Defects. William & Wilkins, Baltimore, 1993, p. 55, with permission.)*

Table 8–1   Summation of Findings on Effects of CPM in Animal Models

CPM Animal Investigations	Findings
Intra-articular fractures[3]	Healing articular cartilage replaced with tissue resembling hyaline cartilage.
Full-thickness defects[4]	CPM group healed with new hyaline cartilage (chondrogenesis) in more than half the defects within four weeks compared to control group.
Prevention of arthritis[5]	Motion may prevent iatrogenic damage to articular cartilage.
Partial-thickness patella tendon lacerations[6]	CPM animals had significantly thicker tendon callous formation and a greater mean breaking strength.
Semitendinosus tenodesis[7]	Semitendinosus tenodesis combined with CPM decreased atrophy changes associated with immobilization and significantly increased the strength of the repair at 6 and 12 weeks.
Effect of CPM on intra-articular pressure[8]	CPM produces sinusoidal oscillation in intra-articular pressure.
Analysis method for type I and type II collagen[9]	An accurate and reliable method is demonstrated to determine percentage of type II collagen in small samples of articular cartilage.
Major defects repaired with autogenous grafts and CPM[10]	Major osteochondral defects repaired with autogenous osteoperiosteal grafts and CPM will produce new chondrocytes, a phenomenon of "biological resurfacing."
Acute septic arthritis[11]	Knee joints treated with CPM showed fewer X-ray abnormalities, erosion and fewer adhesions.
Clearance of hemarthrosis[12]	CPM was shown to accelerate the clearance of hemarthrosis.
Free periosteal autografts[13]	Free avascular periosteal grafts survive and grow when transplanted into rabbit synovial joints. CPM stimulates cartilage growth.
Chondrogenic potential of free autogenous periosteal grafts[14]	Free autogenous periosteal grafts and CPM can repair a large full-thickness defect with tissue that resembles articular cartilage grossly, histologically, biochemically, and contains predominantly type II collagen.

Continued

Table 8–1 **Summation of Findings on Effects of CPM in Animal Models (Continued)**

The fate of allogeneic periosteum[15]	Periosteal allografts are immunologically compatible. Also, if an allograft is used instead of an autograft, a harvest incision is avoided.
Cryopreservation of periosteum[16]	This study verifies that the cryopreserved periosteum is viable and retains the ability to undergo neochondrogenesis.
Durability of regenerated articular cartilage[17]	Hyaline cartilage produced by free periosteal grafts in full-thickness defects is capable of withstanding a full year of articular function without marked deterioration.

thesis.[14] "Physical forces provide important stimuli to tissues for the development and maintenance of homeostasis."[18] *Stress deprivation* refers to the changes that occur at a cellular level in soft tissue when a limb is immobilized. The negative effects of stress deprivation or immobilization on connective tissue appear to be common to all synovial joints studied. Most researchers identify peak collagen synthesis to occur in the early postoperative period of 5 to 7 days postinjury or surgery. In order for CPM to influence an improved biologic healing response, it should be applied in that same postoperative period for improved tissue healing.

Continuous motion has been shown to favorably influence the cellular, biochemical, and biomechanical processes of healing in connective tissue. Not only are tissues "stressed" and "lubricated" by repeated motion, but metabolic activities are enhanced with longer doses of motion. Hypothetically, changes might result from a "direct" translation of stress or motion, such as pressure, vibration, electric potentials, or local chemical differences (sensed directly, in some way, by the cells). Another theory suggests that cellular changes may result from "indirect" translation of stress or motion, such as secondary changes in vascularity or diffusion and, therefore, regional difference in nutrition, metabolism, or waste removal.[2]

The advantages of early motion programs in rehabilitation will continue to be researched in animal and clinical models. The current use of CPM devices requires a good understanding of the specific events occurring in the initial stages of wound healing, the effects of passive motion, and the benefits of longer durations of motion via a CPM device. (The reader should review principles of tissue healing outlined in Chapter 1.) The first 3 weeks after injury or surgery offer a window of time when CPM will favorably influence biologic tissue healing. Table 8–2 is a guide to prescribe CPM according to the type of connective tissue damaged and precautions specific to certain diagnoses. The clinician must combine his or her understanding of the biologic benefits that CPM offers with the rehabilitation goals specific to each diagnosis. For example, a patient who has undergone a tenolysis of the digital flexor tendons will benefit from improved nutrition during healing (Fig. 8–2). As a result of adding CPM to the postoperative

Table 8–2 **Clinical Guidelines for CPM Applications***

Tissue / Diagnosis	Dosage / Duration	Rationale / Benefit
Cartilage • ORIF intra-articular fracture (stable) • Hemarthrosis • Joint infection	Post-op 24 hr/day max, 8–10 hr/day min, 0–3 wks min or until Ac = Pas max	Regnerative hyalinelike cartilage Prevent adhesions Maintain joint ROM
Tendon • Rotator cuff repair • Flexor tendon repair • Tenolysis	Post-op 24 hr/day max, 8–10 hr/day min, 0–3 wks min or until OK'd for AROM Protective ranges are indicated	Improved nutrition facilitating intrinsic healing response Greater tensile strength Improved tendon gliding
Ligament • ACL repair	Post-op 24 hr/day max, 8–10 hr/day min, 0–3 wks min or until OK'd for AROM Protective ranges are indicated	Maintain collagen matrix organization Normalize collagen concentration and maintain tissue strength
Periarticular tissue • Shoulder joint manipulation • Total knee replacement	Post-op 24 hr/day max, 8–10 hr/day min, 0–3 wks min or until OK'd for AROM Protective ranges may be indicated	Maintain collage matrix organization Normalize collage concentration and maintain tissue strength
Skin • Burn	Post-op 24 hr/day max, 8–10 hr/day min, 0—3 wks min or until Ac = Pas max Protective ranges may be indicated	Improved biologic healing response Maintain collagen tissue constituents Maintain ROM without pain

*Guidelines for CPM prescriptions are specific to the damaged connective tissue. Precautions are specific to the patient's diagnosis. Note the diagnoses listed are just a few examples; this table does not include all potential diagnoses.

management, an intrinsic healing response is enhanced, perhaps resulting in less adhesion formation. The rehabilitation goal for the care following tenolysis is active motion. The patient removes the CPM device for active exercise every hour during his or her 8- to 24-hour wearing schedule. The added benefit of decreasing pain as a result of continuous movement can increase the patient's compliance in performing active tendon excursion exercise. Future clinical studies on large patient populations will advance our understanding of CPM on specific diagnoses.

Animal studies have demonstrated the following findings: healing of cartilage defects with tissue that resembles hyaline cartilage,[1] prevention of adhesions,[1] an in-

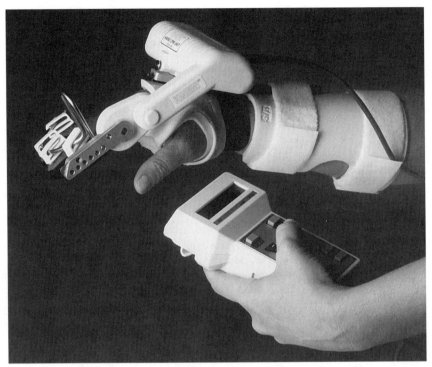

Figure 8–2. The CPM device is one of several hand models typically used in a postoperative tenolysis application. Attachments can be made for a single or multiple digit application. *(From Smith-Nephew Richards, with permission.)*

trinsic healing response within tendons,[19] and a greater tendon tensile strength.[19] Homeostasis of collagen tissue constituents can enhance collagen fiber alignment.[20]

TREATMENT GOALS

A clinician has two treatment goals in the application of CPM. The first goal is to maximize the biologic benefits stimulated through continuous motion. A period of at least 8 to 24 hours for a minimum of 3 weeks is suggested by this author. The second goal is to evaluate the clinical benefits associated with those biologic changes. A multitude of experiments have led to the use of CPM devices in the postoperative management of skeletal and soft tissue disorders. Clinical applications of CPM have demonstrated a decrease in pain, swelling, and stiffness. To understand the biologic rationale for prescribing CPM, the clinician must recognize which type of connective tissue was damaged based on the patient's diagnosis and history of injury. For example, an intra-articular fracture of the proximal phalanx of the finger will result in cartilage damage. CPM offers an adjunctive treatment technique to regenerate hyalinelike articular cartilage. In the example of rotator cuff tear, tendon is damaged and CPM offers a treatment adjunct to promote an intrinsic healing response in tendon and decrease adhesion formation (Fig. 8–3). CPM is rarely a standalone treatment choice. Therapy paradigms unique to each condition are implemented in addition to CPM.

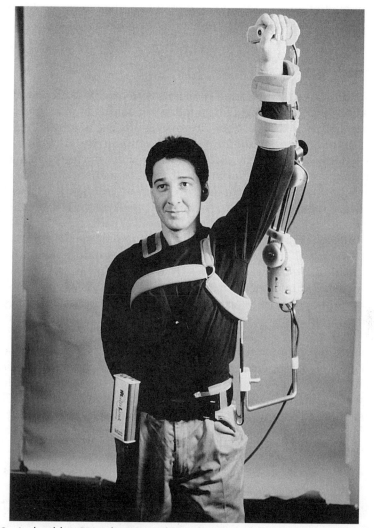

Figure 8–3. A shoulder CPM device is often selected for a postoperative application in a shoulder reconstructive procedure. Initial fitting is conducted in the hospital and again at home once the patient is discharged. *(From U.S. Orthopedics/Toronto Medical, Inc., with permission.)*

The physiologic changes that occur with longer doses of passive motion are unique to each kind of connective tissue. Therefore, treatment goals will be identified according to connective tissue types, that is, cartilage, tendon, ligament, and skin.

ARTICULAR CARTILAGE

Articular cartilage is avascular, relying on synovial fluid diffusion for its nutrition. It has a limited ability to repair itself. Local destruction of articular cartilage, such as injury or infection, represent irreparable lesions. CPM promotes healing of articular cartilage defects with tissue that is comparable to hyaline cartilage, or with a smaller amount of fibrous adhesions compared to the defects healed under the influence of small doses of active motion or immobilization.

TENDON AND LIGAMENT

Research models have not provided clinicians with precise clinical guidelines for the application of CPM in management following tendon repair. Tendon loading achieved through early motion does improve tendon excursion and tensile properties when compared to immobilization. The optimum duration and frequency is yet to be determined. Synovial diffusion can enhance intrinsic healing (healing within), which is proposed to diminish adhesion formation. Once adhesion formation is minimized, tendon excursion should improve. Ligaments, like tendons, consist of dense regular connective tissue. Noyes's[20] work on ligaments has led numerous investigators to address the question, "What is the effect of immobility on the functional properties of ligaments or the permanency of such alterations once they exist?" His work has demonstrated significant alterations in ligament mechanical properties resulting from long-term immobilization. Early motion has been documented to maintain collagen matrix organization during healing, normalize collagen concentration, and maintain tissue strength.[20] The most common CPM application after ligament repair is anterior cruciate reconstruction (Fig. 8–4).

Epithelium depends on the underlying skin connective tissue for all of its nutrients and most of its oxygen. In serious skin wounds, such as massive burns, the cells (fibroblasts) from the underlying connective tissue (epidermis) proliferate to repair the wound. In the animal model, wounds under the influence of CPM for 3 weeks are significantly stronger, stiffer, and tougher than those in the cast group.[21] Histologically, the structural organization of the collagen fibers was superior in the scars treated with CPM.

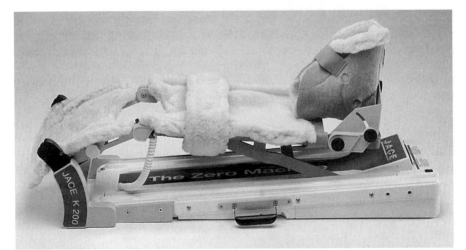

Figure 8–4. Numerous knee models for orthopedic applications are available. Some CPM knee devices have been tailored to meet the postoperative needs of the patient has undergone an anterior cruciate ligament repair. (*From Thera- Kinetics, Inc., with permission.*)

CONTRAINDICATIONS AND PRECAUTIONS

Tissue damage from CPM can result from a combination of improper methods used in incorrect situations. Most trauma from improper manual passive motion is a direct mechanical irritation or injury, with significant effects from excessive bleeding or swelling. Therefore, precaution must include precise ranges of protected motion, proper positioning, and proper monitoring to avoid mechanical irritation or injury. These same precautions exist for longer duration of passive motion when applied via a CPM machine. CPM is most effective when applied postoperatively; particular care must be exercised not to irritate or injure newly repaired or reconstructed tissues. Additional precautions would include monitoring any vascular and/or sensory impairment that may be present. The clinician should provide written instructions for the patient to monitor changes in color and/or sensitivity.

Surgical procedures for the release of joint contractures require special consideration for the nearby neurovascular structures. The clinician and patient will upgrade the range on a CPM device within tolerable levels that do not place the neurovascular structures under unnecessary levels of tension. Each patient's diagnosis and subsequent rehabilitation carries precautions specific to the diagnosis and operative findings. For example, manual passive motion begun post rotator cuff repair begins within protective ranges based on the surgical repair performed. The application of CPM would include the same precautions and protective ranges. Specific contraindications to CPM include an unstable fracture or active infection.

TREATMENT WITH CONTINUOUS PASSIVE MOTION

The therapist and physician must collaborate on a case-by-case basis to determine an adequate prescription for motion in the postoperative case. Similar to a pharmacologic prescription, a prescription for motion must encompass amount, frequency, and duration. Research in precise prescriptions for clinical applications of CPM is ongoing. Currently clinical reasoning for CPM applications must rely on information from animal experimental models combined with the preliminary findings from recent clinical research. Additionally, the purpose of motion, precautions, contraindications, and protective ranges must all be well defined before determining the CPM prescription.

Evidence seems to suggest that "more is better" in terms of certain healing effects. The application of longer duration of motion via CPM devices offers practitioners one alternative to increasing the dose-response benefits of motion to healing connective tissue. Until additional diagnosis-specific research is conducted, it is our obligation to determine a tailored prescription on a case-by-case basis. A thorough understanding of the principles of passive motion, the timetable of wound healing, and diagnosis-specific precautions will promote adequate clinical reasoning.[21] Optimum use of CPM devices requires close scrutiny, since the minimum duration with maximum effect would be superior in terms of conservation of time and cost, as well as achieving patient compliance.[2]

SAFETY CONSIDERATIONS

The clinician should provide written CPM instructions to the patient and a family caretaker whenever possible. A brief verbal explanation on the purpose of using CPM is beneficial. The clinician provides instructions on all setting indicators on the device. A thorough demonstration and explanation on proper limb positioning and limb relaxation in the device is provided. Written instructions for nursing personnel and for family members are included to avoid excessive pressure and circulation or nerve irritation problems (tingling). The patient must be cautioned not to change CPM limits unless instructed to do so by a physician or therapist. The CPM speed is set to patient comfort. Most units are equipped with a safety "kill" switch in the event a sudden device stop is required. Additional safety measures may be specific to the patient's condition. Provide the patient with instructions to check power source and a technical service number in the event of equipment failure. Most CPM distributors have technical support phone numbers for assistance once the patient leaves the hospital or clinic.

Positioning in most devices will change depending on whether the patient will lie supine or sit during CPM use. Clinicians must familiarize themselves with device adjustments and whether or not the device requires soft goods for attachment and positioning of the limb. A set of replacement straps to stabilize the unit and pads should accompany rental units.

CLINICAL APPLICATION AND DECISION MAKING

Ideally, CPM is begun immediately after surgery in the recovery room or preferably within the first postoperative week. The benefit of starting motion in the recovery room is to avoid the pain associated with the initial fitting. If the patient can wake up with the operated limb already moving, the initial pain response that occurs with starting and stopping the device can be eliminated. Motion is continued on a 24-hour basis (minimum 8 hours), for a period of 1 to 3 weeks (this may extend to 6 weeks in some cases). Early application of CPM must be well controlled and monitored at regular intervals to enhance healing as opposed to interrupting newly repaired tissue. The CPM device often requires programming within protective ranges. The patient and all parties involved in the patient's care must understand the merits of CPM to achieve patient compliance in the optimum wearing schedule.

Efficacious results of CPM are dependent on good clinical reasoning and compliance on time and duration schedules. One-week delay in the application of CPM in an articular cartilage defect model was not as effective as placing the CPM device on the injured joint immediately.[22] On the other hand, CPM for about 8 hours per day was as effective as 24 hours per day in the articular cartilage model. The CPM application for 2 hours a day did not demonstrate the same beneficial effects.[23] Clinically, one criterion for the amount of CPM is patient comfort. Pain relief occurs when motion is constant, gradual, and predictable. A slow rate of motion appears superior to a faster rate (45 seconds per cycle).

CPM seems to have its greatest effect during the first postoperative week.[1] Regarding the optimum duration, as a general rule, improved biologic healing has peaked within the first 3 weeks of CPM application.[4,17] Thereafter, the patient may be weaned from the CPM and active exercise encouraged. Each case will have specific precautions regarding when a patient may begin active motion. Once active motion maintains the patient's maximum available passive motion, CPM utilization can be weaned or discontinued.

PAIN

Beyond the physiologic benefits, which are tissue-specific, clinical benefits of decreased pain, swelling, and stiffness are consistently documented with the use of CPM devices when applied immediately post-operatively.

In Salter's early work with clinical applications, the reported patients are more comfortable when the involved limb is attached to the CPM device and is only interrupted for periods of bathing or other activities of daily living.[24] In the majority of CPM applications, CPM had a favorable effect of reducing pain (in a series of 128 patients with various upper extremity injuries).[25] Only 28% of the patients required an analgesic 8 hours following surgery. Theoretically, this finding is consistent with the gate control hypothesis, proposed by Melzack and Wall,[26] which states that the perceived intensity of pain is the result of a balance of input from myelinated and unmyelinated fibers.[27] The myelinated afferent nerve fibers are proposed to excite the inhibitory interneuron, consequently inhibiting pain. The large myelineated primary afferent nerve fibers, the muscle proprioceptors, and joint mechanoreceptors are excited by mild mechanical stimuli, that is, the passive motion that a CPM provides.

Weekly assessment of pain, swelling, and mobility will assist clinicians in their clinical decision making for determining the optimum CPM duration.

EDEMA

CPM can assist in edema control postoperatively. In a reported series of upper-extremity injuries, volumetric and circumferential measurements decreased during the first 2 weeks of CPM utilization.[25] Abramson, in 1965, proposed the theory that limb elevation permits gravity to increase the rate of venous lymphatic flow from the extremity.[28] Active and passive motion has been reported clinically and experimentally to compress adjacent veins and lymphatic vessels, thereby creating a pumping action that may enhance venous and lymphatic flow. Giudice demonstrated results where 30 minutes of intermittent passive motion (via a CPM device) of the digits in the combination with limb elevation resulted in significantly greater reduction of hand edema than 30 minutes of limb elevation alone.[28] An additional finding demonstrated a positive relationship between outcome to amount of pretreatment edema (the greater the amount of pretreatment edema, the greater the treatment effect) for hand volume and finger circumference following CPM with elevation. There was no relationship for these same measures following elevation alone.

MOTION

Optimum mobility is easily achieved in postoperative CPM applications if the patient remains compliant in the wearing schedule. The use of CPM devices after cast immobilization, for intermittent periods, in the treatment of joint stiffness has not been well documented. Osterman[29] shared his clinical impression: "In a small controlled series of patients with wrist fractures, we have used continuous passive motion to improve both rotation and flexion-extension during the early weeks following cast removal. Thus far, the series indicate that motion is re-established much sooner." The effectiveness of low-load prolonged stretch splinting for the management of existing joint stiffness has been documented.[30] CPM devices may be another technique besides splinting for long-lived stress delivery (resulting in biologic remodeling) to shortened connective tissue.[31] Patients may not tolerate an adequate dosage of low-load prolonged stretch through traditional techniques of splinting, serial casting, and traction because of pain responses. Patients may tolerate a therapeutic dose of total end-range time better with a CPM device initially, then convert to splinting.

If the patient is using a CPM device to increase end range of motion (ROM) of a stiff joint after cast removal, a wearing schedule should be determined on a "trial-and-error" basis, much like a splint-wearing schedule is determined. The clinician will set the device parameter within a pain-free range of motion.

POSTTREATMENT ASSESSMENT AND DOCUMENTATION

A biopsy is the only current accurate means of assessing induced biologic changes in connective tissue with the use of CPM. Of course, this is neither practical nor likely to occur in a clinical setting. Therefore, clinicians rely on subsequent objective clinical outcomes such as ROM, edema reduction, and subjective decreases in pain perception to measure the effectiveness of CPM. ROM measures, both active and passive, should be performed weekly in a postoperative application. Circumferential or volumetric readings can be used to determine changes in edema. The visual analogue scale, although subjective, can ascertain the patient's perception of his or her pain level from day to day or week to week. Additional documentation should include the number of hours a day the patient is using the CPM device, if the patient can sleep in the device (if needed), and current parameters of movement and range that the patient tolerates.

SUMMARY

Therapists strive to shorten recovery time and enhance the healing process in orthopedic management. The timetable of wound healing, principles of passive range of motion, and diagnosis-specific precautions will allow clinicians to make adequate decisions for the use of CPM as one alternative versus complete immobilization versus intermittent active motion. Trends and paradigms for individual diagnoses are being researched for determining the optimum CPM frequency and duration. Current research indicates an improved connective tissue healing response is achieved using an immediate postoperative application, an 8- to 24-hour dosage within pain-free and protective range of motion for an average of 1 to 3 weeks' duration.

DISCUSSION QUESTIONS

1. Are the concepts related to early motion following orthopedic injury or surgery more beneficial than immobilization? If so, what duration of passive motion gives the most benefit? Is longer better?

2. Specific to a cartilage defect, CPM may prevent development of degenerative joint disease. Biologic changes appear to be tissue-specific. Do these same concepts for healing of articular cartilage apply to tendon, periarticular tissue, ligament, and skin? Will ROM reflect those biologic changes?

3. How do these biologic changes translate to clinical benefits? Do these biologic events continue once the stimulus of motion is removed?

4. The ROM is likely to be the same a year later in CPM patients, yet the healing of connective tissue occurs faster with CPM patients and results in a stronger connective tissue. Does this translate to faster return to function?

REFERENCES

1. Salter, RB: The biological concept of continuous passive motion of synovial joints. The first 18 years of basic research and its clinical application. Clin Orthop 42:12, 1989.

2. Frank, C, et al: Physiology and therapeutic value of passive joint motion. Clin Orthop 185:113, 1984.

3. Salter, RB and Harris, DJ: The healing of intra-articular fractures with continuous passive motion. Am Acad Orthop Surg Lecture Series 6:28:102, 1979.

4. Salter, RB, et al: The biological effect of continuous passive motion on the healing of full-thickness defects in articular cartilage: An experimental investigation in the rabbit. J Bone Joint Surg 62A:1232, 1980.

5. Salter, RB: The prevention of arthritis through the preservation of cartilage. Royal College Lecture, J Radiol 32:5, 1981.

6. Salter, RB and Bell, RS: The effect of continuous passive motion on the healing of partial thickness lacerations of the patellar tendon in the rabbit (abstract). Ann Royal Coll Phys Surg Can 14:3:109, 1981.

7. Salter, RB and Minster, RR: The effect of continuous passive motion on a semi-tendinosus tenodesis in the rabbit knee (abstract). Orthop Trans (Orthop Res Soc) 6:292, 1982.

8. O'Driscoll, SW, Kumar, A, and Salter, RB: The effect of the volume of effusion, joint position and continuous passive motion on intra-articular pressure in the rabbit knee. J Rheum 10:3:60, 1983.

9. O'Driscoll, SW, Salter, RB, and Keeley, FW: A method for quantitative analysis of ratios of types I and II collagen in small samples of articular cartilage. Analyt Biochem 145:227, 1985.

10. O'Driscoll, SW and Salter, RB: The repair of major osteochondral defects in joint surfaces by neochondrogeneis with autogenous osteoperiosteal grafts stimulated by continuous passive motion. An experimental investigation in the rabbit. Clin Orthop 208:131, 1986.

11. Salter, RB, Bell, RS, and Keeley, F: The protective effect of continuous passive motion on living articular cartilage in acute septic arthritis: An experimental investigation in the rabbit. Clin Orthop 159:223, 1981.

12. O'Driscoll, SW, Kimar, A, and Salter, RB: The effect of continuous passive motion on the clearance of a hemarthrosis from a synovial joint. Clin Orthop 76:305, 1983.

13. O'Driscoll, SW and Salter, RB: The induction of neochondrogenesis in free periosteal autografts under the influence of continuous passive motion. J Bone Joint Surg 66A:1248, 1984.

14.   O'Driscoll, SW, Keeley, FW, and Salter, RB: The chondrogenic potential of free autogenous periosteal grafts for biological resurfacing of major full-thickness defects in joint surfaces under the influence of continuous passive motion. J Bone Joint Surg 68A:8:1017, 1986.

15.   Salter, RB, et al: The fate of allogeneic periosteum transplanted into an osteochondral defect and subject to continuous passive motion. An experimental investigation in the rabbit (abstract). Clin Invest Med (Suppl) 10:4:B127, 1987.

16.   Kreder, HJ, Salter, RB, and Keeley, FW: Cryopreservation of rabbit periosteum for transplantation (abstract). Trans 34th Annual Meeting Orthop Res Soc 113:113, 1988.

17.   O'Driscoll, SW: Durability of regenerated articular cartilage produced by free autogenous periosteal grafts in major full thickness defects. J Bone Joint Surg 70A:4, 1988.

18.   Akeson, WH, et al: Effects of immobilization on joints. Clin Orthop Rel Res 219: 1987.

19.   Gelberman, RH, et al: Flexor tendon healing: A prospective clinical trail evaluating controlled passive motion rehabilitation. Abstract presented at ASSH 44th Annual Meeting. Seattle, Washington, September 1989.

20.   Noyes, FR: The functional properties of knee ligaments and alterations induced by immobilization. A correlative biomechanical and histological study in primates. Clin Orthop 123:21, 1977.

21.   Vay Royen, BJ, et al: A comparison of the effects of immobilization and continuous passive motion on surgical wound healing in mature rabbits. Plast Reconstr Surg 78:3, 1986.

22.   Dimick, MP: Continuous passive motion for the upper extremity. In Hunter, JM, Schneider, L, Mackin, E, and Callahan, A (eds): Rehabilitation of the Hand, ed 3. CV Mosby, St Louis, 1990, p 1140.

23.   Shimizu, T, et al: Experimental study on the repair of full thickness articular cartilage defects: The effects of varying periods of continuous passive motion, age, activity and immobilization. J Orthop Res 5:2, 1987.

24.   Salter, RB, et al: Clinical application of basic research on continuous passive motion for disorders and injuries of synovial joints. A preliminary report of a feasibility study. J Orthop Res 3:325, 1983.

25.   Osterman, AL, Bora, FW, and Skirven, T: The use of continuous passive motion in hand rehabilitation. Presented at Am Soc Surg Hand 42nd Annual Meeting, San Antonio, TX 1987.

26.   Melzack, R and Wall, PD: Pain mechanism: a new theory. Science 150:971, 1965.

27.   Fields, HL: Pain. McGraw-Hill, New York 1987, p 137.

28.   Giudice, ML: Effects of continuous passive motion and elevation on hand edema. Am J Occup Ther 44:10, 1990.

29.   Coutts, RD, et al: Symposium: The use of continuous passive motion in the rehabilitation of orthopedic problems. Contemp Orthop 16:3, 1988.

30.   Light K, et al: Low-load prolonged stretch vs. high load brief stretch in treating knee contractures. Phys Ther 64:330, 1984.

31.   Flowers, K and Michlovitz, S: Assessment and management of loss of motion in orthopedic dysfunction. Postgrad Advances Phys Ther, APTA (Vols. II–VII of independent study course), 1988.

32.   McCarthy, MR, et al: The clinical uses of continuous passive motion in physical therapy. J Orthop Sports Phys Ther 15:3, 1992.

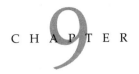

Edema Management: Intermittent Compression as a Therapeutic Modality

Joyce L. Adcock, MA, PT

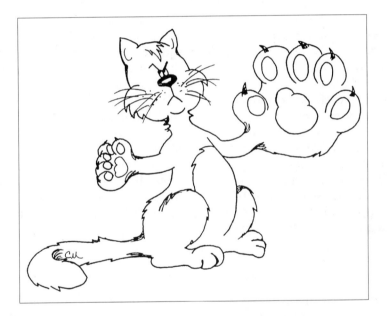

CHAPTER OBJECTIVES

- Define the types of edema.
- Describe the causes for the different types of edema.
- Outline the medical precautions when treating a patient with edema.
- Discuss the signs of edema and infection.
- Discuss the assessment of edema.
- Outline the available compression options and the rationale for their selection.
- Discuss the options and potential benefits of those options on compression devices.

Management of edema or swelling is a difficult medical problem with a multiplicity of causes and varied distribution throughout the body. The individual with edema can have a host of functional and cosmetic problems. Treatment may include interventions such as ice, exercise, and elevation or massage techniques such as retrograde massage or manual lymph drainage. Manual and/or mechanical compression techniques can also be used to facilitate the return of venous or lymphatic fluids. Techniques may include bandaging, elastic stockinette, and intermittent compression via a pump with an appliance. The appliance or sleeve may consist of one or several chambers (nonsequential and sequential, respectively). These appliances provide compression with the use of air or a combination of water and antifreeze. When indicated, custom compression garments or stockings are measured for each patient individually and fabricated to meet their specific needs.

Selection of appropriate treatment interventions is dependent on findings from a detailed patient history, an understanding of the basic pathology and physiology of edema, careful patient assessment, and clinical experience. Much of the material presented in this chapter is based on empirical data obtained through valuable feedback and participation by hundreds of patients. These individuals have generously shared their self-discoveries, small successes, and experiences, and have guided this author in developing a variety of protocols to provide patients with useful treatment options.

THEORY AND RESEARCH

In the mid-1600s, anatomists and physiologists recognized the role of the lymphatic and venous systems regarding fluid transport in the body. Thomas Wharton and Niels Steensen[1] addressed the lymphatics, while William Harvey more clearly defined the venous system. In the early 1900s, Henry Gray described these systems and their function in detail.[2] The current understanding of fluid dynamics and the regulation of fluid in the body, the relationship of the lymphatic and venous system, and the causes of edema are well described in the basic physiology texts.

How to successfully manage edema has not received the same attention or interest. As early as 1867, there were advertisements for compression stockings in the Vienna Medical Weekly.[3] Definitive treatment interventions proposed by Emil Vodder[4] and Leo Clodius[5] offer conservative, symptomatic management to a variety of surgical interventions. This work has long been confined to the European medical community.

In the United States, much of the research and development of treatment interventions for edema have been confined to patients with congenital edemas or edemas secondary to cancer and its treatment. Other types of edema tend to be transient, as in trauma. Traumatic edema is mainly a vascular phenomenon. The edema is a reaction of the vascular and supporting elements of the tissue to injury.[6] Individuals experiencing problems with edema have been seeking a well-regimented, conservative approach to managing their problem, as evidenced by anecdotal experiences exploring traditional and nontraditional medicines for treatment and relief.

PATHOPHYSIOLOGY OF EDEMA

Edema is an accumulation of excess fluids in the spaces between the cells of tissues, known as *interstitial space*. It can be classified into two types: lymphatic edema, in which plasma proteins in the tissues stagnate owing to mechanical insufficiency of lymph drainage, and venous edema, which results from increased capillary pressure and venous obstruction. When the lymphatic system is incompetent, obstructed, or surgically obliterated, proteins and their products accumulate in the tissue space. Edema occurs when there is an imbalance of the affected pressures across the capillary membrane or when there is obstruction to the venous or lymphatic flow. Thus, the tissue has abnormally large quantities of fluid in the intercellular spaces.[7]

In order for the body to maintain a homeostasis, there is movement of water and diffusible solutes from the vascular space at the arteriolar end of the microcirculation into the interstitial space. Fluid is returned from the interstitial space into the vascular system by way of the lymphatics, and unless these channels are obstructed, lymph flow tends to increase if there is a net movement of fluid from the vascular compartment to the interstitium.[8]

Edema may be localized or generalized. Localized edema is usually caused by venous or lymphatic obstruction or to increased vascular permeability as seen in post-traumatic edema. Localized edema tends to be limited to one area of the body, but it can be seen in bilateral extremities. This edema can be the result of trauma, infection, or obstruction. Generalized edema is a systemic process that occurs with chronic illnesses such as advanced cardiac disease, kidney failure, or liver disease. These types of edema usually are apparent in both lower extremities, the groin, and abdominal areas, but some patients exhibit a more generalized appearance of "whole body edema." The management of localized edema will be the focus of this chapter.

CAUSES OF EDEMA

Edema is usually a symptom of a disease process or injury rather than a disease itself. Many times, treating the underlying cause can alleviate the problem. Some causes include: malnutrition and toxicity; cardiac, kidney, and liver disease for generalized edema; trauma, lymphatic, or venous compromise for localized edema.

One of the most common causes of edema is trauma. This is an acute inflammatory edema in which there is damage to the capillary wall. The permeability is increased, allowing fluid containing more protein into the interstitial space.[9] Common causes of trauma are blows, strains and sprains, burns, and fractures. This edema has clearly identifiable characteristics, which include inflammation, a nonpitting edema, redness, warmth, and local tenderness. Traumatic edema is usually acute and resolves with conservative treatment. Depending on the severity of the injury, resolution may require as little as 6 weeks to as long as a year.

A frequent cause of edema is lymphatic and/or venous compromise. Much of this chapter will be devoted to the specific treatment interventions of these problems. It is important to note that we are discussing two distinct but interrelated types of edema. It is a misnomer to refer to any swelling as lymphedema, and this labeling demonstrates an incomplete understanding of the pathophysiologic process. The lymphatic system removes excess proteins that have escaped from blood vessels. It then returns it to the blood via the main lymph ducts. If the lymphatic system is compromised, proteins will progressively accumulate in the interstitial fluid causing an imbalance in capillary dynamics resulting in edema.[11] Lymphatic edema is typically characterized by a pitting quality, that is, pressure on the edematous area leaves a depression, or "pit," because of fluid translocation. Within 30 seconds this fluid will flow back into the area and the depression disappears. Lymphatic edema is also a local process and its turgor can be soft or hard. As plasma proteins are laid down in the tissue over time, this stagnation tends to result in a much harder edema, which can contribute to loss of joint motion, sensory impairment, and pain. Venous edema results from a rise in venous pressure with a concomitant increase in capillary pressure. Unique characteristics of venous edema are that it is generally a soft pitting edema, it has a tendency to pool in the distal extremities, and the skin has a glossy, tight appearance.

Other causes of edema include malnutrition and toxicity. Nutritional or famine edema may be related to hypoalbuminemia (loss of protein in the blood) or perhaps loss of fat, which is replaced by loose connective tissue in which fluid can accumulate.[12] This type of edema is usually localized in the lower extremities. Toxicity or exposure to a poison is usually a transient local response that follows the insult. This can include toxins such as snake venom, insect bites, chemotherapy, and allergic responses. These insults cause the capillaries to dilate and increase in permeability causing a local swelling, redness, and pain.

As discussed previously, advanced cardiac and kidney disease and liver failure can result in generalized edema. The individual with congestive heart failure retains both sodium and water. This edema is first noticed in the distal lower extremities and can spread proximally. Edema acts as a safety valve allowing fluid to be displaced into the tissues to prevent overloading of the heart.[13] The individual with renal disease has edema because of fluid and salt retention, resulting in increased capillary pressure causing fluid to accumulate in the interstitial spaces.[14] A more critical problem occurs when the patient loses protein into the urine and salt and water do not remain in the vascular compartment. Individuals with liver disease will first develop edema in their abdomen because of obstruction of hepatic portal drainage. This pressure in the abdomen can obstruct venous return from the lower extremities, causing bilateral lower-extremity edema.

SIGNS AND SYMPTOMS OF EDEMA

There are clear visible and palpable signs and symptoms that accompany an edematous process (Table 9–1). These include the distribution, color, sensitivity, tissue changes, temperature, and overall quality of the edema. Recognition of the dis-

Table 9–1 **Summary of Edemas**

Causes	Signs and Symptoms
Traumatic	Redness Warmth Local tenderness Generally nonpitting Can spread proximal and distal to sight of injury
Malnutrition	Weight loss Skin rashes Abdominal filling Bilateral lower extremity edema
Toxins	Redness Rashes Itching Local pain Nonpitting
Organ failure (heart, kidney, liver)	Weight gain Abdominal ascites Lower-extremity swelling Migrating edema Can become generalized Generally pitting
Lymphatic	Can be pitting or nonpitting Can be soft or hard Can pocket, particularly below elbow and below knee Local tenderness along lymph channels
Venous	Distal swelling of extremities Pitting Skin is thin Skin loses natural creases, texture, and tone

tribution of the edema pattern can provide the health care provider with clues as to the cause of edema. Traumatic edema is always localized about the area of injury, with regional swelling, including distal and proximal, to the site of the injury. In the case of venous or lymphatic obstruction, edema is often confined to a single extremity or part of an extremity, although bilateral involvement can be seen. Typically, this edema is better in the morning and increases as the day proceeds, with activity and gravitational forces. Edema related to nutritional deficits is often seen in the legs, but with progressive loss of protein there can be soft edema about the eyes and face in the morning. The pattern seen with traumatic edema is also typically seen with toxic edema, but depending on the sensitivity of the patient can be more widespread and even life threatening.

Systemic edemas are often confined to the legs and abdomen. They may have a hard texture and increase with vertical posturing. Skin color can vary greatly among individuals with edema. Most frequently, acute edemas have a pink or red color similar to that of a mild sunburn. Sometimes with venous obstruction the skin is cyanotic, or bluish. Longstanding edema may cause significant tissue discoloration, which is patchy in nature and variegated in color.

Not all individuals with edema have pain, but many complain of an exquisite sensitivity that is increased with palpation. It is not surprising to find the individual with traumatic edema to have pain and sensitivity at the site of injury. Gross edema can impinge on nerve tissue, and those patients with gross or longstanding edema may complain of neuropathic pain, burning or electric shock sensation, heaviness, and pain in attempting normal joint motion. Patients with true lymphatic edema often have exquisite tenderness along the lymph channels on palpation and complain of an unremitting aching or tenderness.

With edema there is change in the texture and health of the tissue. With persistent chronic edema, brawny induration is clearly evident. The tissue has a hard, ungiving turgor and lacks normal definition. There may be changes in hair growth patterns (generally loss of hair), normal skin creases, and tissue elasticity.

Tissue temperature is a significant sign and symptom of edema and a critically important element in patient evaluation. This will be discussed in the next section. It is important to note that with most inflammatory processes one will observe warmth or an increase in tissue temperature. Depending on degree, this could be a sign of infection. Decreased skin temperature is also commonly seen and may be an indication of infection or significant vascular compromise.

Quality of edema refers to whether the edema is pitting or nonpitting, the general health of the tissue, and overall assessment. It is an overall view of both the patient and the body part.

ASSESSMENT OF THE PATIENT WITH EDEMA

In order to select the most appropriate treatment interventions, one must be able to evaluate each patient, attending to detail in the physical exam and listening carefully to the information the patient is providing. This information will help to elucidate the cause of the edema, the current status, and the available treatment options for the individual (Table 9–2).

One of the common causes for venous or lymphatic edema is infection. The main function of the lymphatic system is to remove waste excreted from body tissue. The fluid that it carries contains phagocytes, which digest bacteria, and lymphocytes, which trap and destroy invading cells. If the immune system is compromised, those vital functions do not occur, which makes the patient susceptible to infection. It is important to point out that these patients are vulnerable to any type of infection. Systemic infection can precipitate edema. The patient does not have to sustain direct insult to the body part. Past experience indicates that spontaneous edema (i.e., edema without an identifiable cause) is extremely rare.[14] Consequently, this is one of the first things to assess. This can be done by taking the patient's temperature to see if he or she is febrile. In addition, skin temperatures must also be taken. A superficial probe connected to an electronic or battery-operated monitor is relatively inexpensive and not difficult to use. Temperatures must be taken throughout the extremity and compared to the unaffected extrem-

Table 9–2   **Key Components of Edema Evaluation**

1. Infection
   Assess with a skin thermometer
   Compares affected and unaffected sides
   Be sure patient has been in environment at least 20 minutes with body part uncovered
   Note pre-existing conditions that may skew skin temperature

2. Circumferential measurements
   Must be taken at designated landmarks
   Take at same time of day, same tool, same person
   Compare affected and unaffected sides if possible

3. Range of motion and muscle testing
   Assess baseline function of involved body part
   Note if limitations are due to pre-existing conditions
   Note if limitations are due to excessive weight or swelling of body part

4. Neurologic assessment
   Assess sensation including: hot/cold, sharp/dull localization and light touch
   Check reflexes
   Look for muscle wasting, changes in hair growth patterns and skin texture

5. Assess tissue quality
   Check skin for color, temperature, wounds, rashes, and texture changes
   Palpate for sensitive area, changes in muscle bulk, tissue resistance, temperature changes

6. Photograph
   Take pretreatment photographs of affected and unaffected body parts

ity if possible. They can be recorded on measurement forms (Figs. 9–1 and 9–2). Skin temperature will naturally decrease as one moves distally along the extremity because of the distance from the heart, narrowing of vessels and capillaries, and decreased fat content of the tissue. The range of differentiation of temperature varies with the age, general health, and vascular status of the individual. If comparing affected and nonaffected sides at the same landmark, one finds a 2 to 3°F increase in skin temperature, this may be indicative of a superficial infection and antibiotic therapy may be indicated. If one finds a 2 to 3°F decrease in skin temperature, this is also a sign of infection. We speculate that this is a much deeper longstanding infection in which heat is actually drawn away from the superficial tissue, thus yielding a decrease in skin temperature. This is clearly an indication for antibiotic therapy and should be discussed with the patient's physician. Signs of infection include change in color, texture, temperature, and size (Fig. 9–3).

Accurate baseline and follow-up girth measurements are critical in evaluating the patient with edema. Forms are used to record measurements to ensure consistency (see Figs. 9–1 and 9–2). The unaffected extremity is measured, first noting the date and time of day. The affected extremity is then measured and the two sets of measurements are compared. The literature substantiates the accuracy of volumetric measurements.[15] These may be best used for edema localized to the hand or foot. Circumferential measurements are recommended because they require no specific

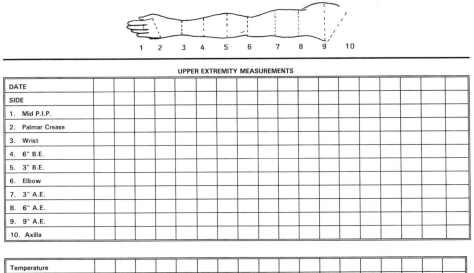

UPPER EXTREMITY MEASUREMENTS

DATE																			
SIDE																			
1. Mid P.I.P.																			
2. Palmar Crease																			
3. Wrist																			
4. 6" B.E.																			
5. 3" B.E.																			
6. Elbow																			
7. 3" A.E.																			
8. 6" A.E.																			
9. 9" A.E.																			
10. Axilla																			

Temperature																			
1. Hand																			
2. Forearm																			
3. Upper Arm																			

JLA/bm

Figure 9–1. Upper-extremity measurement and temperature form.

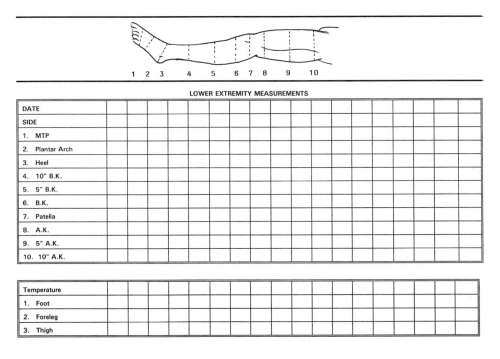

LOWER EXTREMITY MEASUREMENTS

DATE																			
SIDE																			
1. MTP																			
2. Plantar Arch																			
3. Heel																			
4. 10" B.K.																			
5. 5" B.K.																			
6. B.K.																			
7. Patella																			
8. A.K.																			
9. 5" A.K.																			
10. 10" A.K.																			

Temperature																			
1. Foot																			
2. Foreleg																			
3. Thigh																			

JLA/bm

Figure 9–2. Lower-extremity measurement and temperature form.

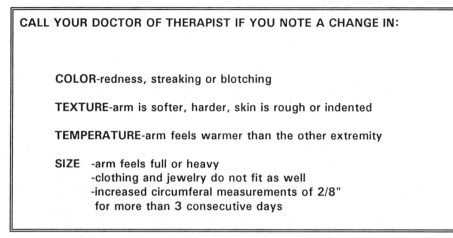

Figure 9–3. Possible signs of infection.

setup and they will enable one to clearly localize areas of edema. There are, however, very specific guidelines to ensure accurate and consistent measurements (Table 9–3). First, the same landmarks must be used with every measurement. Depending on the site of the edema, one may have to establish one's own landmarks and document them clearly. Second, the same person should measure the patient every time. Studies have shown that there is consistency in the manner that one individual measures, but this cannot be demonstrated among a variety of individuals, regardless of the tool.[16] Third, measurements must be taken at the same time of day. There is evidence that as one proceeds through the day in an upright posture, an increase in capillary permeability occurs, increasing girth and weight.[17] If this is the case, one's measurements could be skewed by varying the time of day. Fourth, one must use the same tool. An inexpensive fiberglass tape measure that does not stretch with repeated use and can be wiped down with alcohol between patients is suggested.

Table 9–3   Guidelines for Consistent Circumferential Measurements

1. Use the same tool every time a measurement is taken.

2. The same individual should measure the patient every time.

3. Measurements should be taken at approximately the same time of day.

4. Measure both unaffected and affected body parts if possible.

5. Landmarks must be easy to identify and used consistently.

6. Measure directly over the landmark.

7. All measurements should be documented, preferably on a form, to provide comparative data.

8. Conditions that may skew measurements should be noted, e.g., use of a diuretic, 10-pound weight gain or loss, additional medical problems, change in treatment regimen.

Muscle strength and range of motion must also be assessed, with particular note in limitations caused by edema. Some patients will exhibit loss of power simply from the weight of the extremity. Others will have limitation in joint motion, particularly flexion, because of the bulk of their edema. In addition, if movement is difficult or uncomfortable, patients tend to use the body part less, creating the perfect scenario for an adhesive capsuilitis or other fibrotic processes about the joint.

A thorough neurologic assessment is another critical element of the evaluation. Individuals with edema can experience neuropathic changes that can include pain, hyperesthesia, paresthesia, weakness, and trophic changes. Nerve entrapments related to edema in breast cancer patients have been well documented.[18] A sensory evaluation must include hot/cold, sharp/dull, localization, and light touch. Check reflexes and position sense. Muscle wasting may be a sign of disuse or nerve compression. One must also note any changes in skin texture and hair growth patterns that can be indicative of neurologic involvement.

Throughout the course of the evaluation, make observations about the quality of the patient's skin. The importance of noting temperature, texture, color, wounds, and open areas have been previously mentioned. All of these observations can provide clues as to the severity and duration of the edema, the exact type of edema, and guidelines for treatment intervention.

If available, it is always helpful to document edema with photographs. At one time a sophisticated 35-mm camera with a special lens had to be used. Now there are instant cameras on the market with easily attachable magnifying lenses and grid film that do an excellent job providing immediate documentation in an economical manner. The Briggs new Polaroid HealthCam System (Cambridge, MA) utilizes a Spectra camera, close-up lens, and grid film. As in all assessments, the affected and unaffected sides should be compared.

Besides these specific assessment tools, a good clinical evaluation also includes a detailed medical and social history, medication regimen, vital signs, functional assessment, previous treatment interventions and the patient's goals. Any evaluation is only as good as the eyes, the ears, and the hands of the evaluator.

TREATMENT

Regardless of the choice of patient treatment, success is dependent upon the patient having a complete understanding of the treatment goals and how they will be achieved. For lymphatic and/or venous edema treatment can be arduous and take several months to a year with continual follow-up. Both parties must clearly understand the time commitment and need for patience and persistence. Ideally, the best program starts with education and prevention, but if intervention is required, the sooner the better. For those individuals who know they are at risk for the development of edema, some preventive measures can be offered. These include instruction in monitoring circumferential measurements at least once a week, distributing and reviewing with the patient a hand and arm care sheet (Fig. 9–4), instructing the patient in signs of infection, and ensuring that he or she clearly understands the risks and are able to intervene early and appropriately. Patients must be told that once they have developed a problem with edema they are more susceptible to another incidence. Most importantly it must be conveyed to the pa-

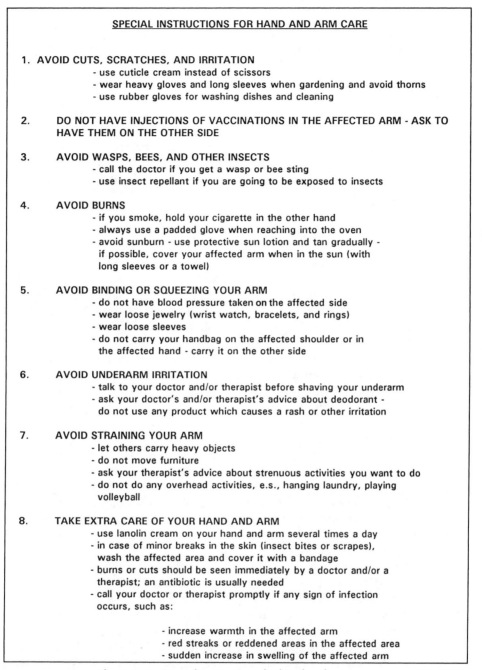

SPECIAL INSTRUCTIONS FOR HAND AND ARM CARE

1. AVOID CUTS, SCRATCHES, AND IRRITATION
   - use cuticle cream instead of scissors
   - wear heavy gloves and long sleeves when gardening and avoid thorns
   - use rubber gloves for washing dishes and cleaning

2. DO NOT HAVE INJECTIONS OF VACCINATIONS IN THE AFFECTED ARM - ASK TO HAVE THEM ON THE OTHER SIDE

3. AVOID WASPS, BEES, AND OTHER INSECTS
   - call the doctor if you get a wasp or bee sting
   - use insect repellant if you are going to be exposed to insects

4. AVOID BURNS
   - if you smoke, hold your cigarette in the other hand
   - always use a padded glove when reaching into the oven
   - avoid sunburn - use protective sun lotion and tan gradually - if possible, cover your affected arm when in the sun (with long sleeves or a towel)

5. AVOID BINDING OR SQUEEZING YOUR ARM
   - do not have blood pressure taken on the affected side
   - wear loose jewelry (wrist watch, bracelets, and rings)
   - wear loose sleeves
   - do not carry your handbag on the affected shoulder or in the affected hand - carry it on the other side

6. AVOID UNDERARM IRRITATION
   - talk to your doctor and/or therapist before shaving your underarm
   - ask your doctor's and/or therapist's advice about deodorant - do not use any product which causes a rash or other irritation

7. AVOID STRAINING YOUR ARM
   - let others carry heavy objects
   - do not move furniture
   - ask your therapist's advice about strenuous activities you want to do
   - do not do any overhead activities, e.s., hanging laundry, playing volleyball

8. TAKE EXTRA CARE OF YOUR HAND AND ARM
   - use lanolin cream on your hand and arm several times a day
   - in case of minor breaks in the skin (insect bites or scrapes), wash the affected area and cover it with a bandage
   - burns or cuts should be seen immediately by a doctor and/or a therapist; an antibiotic is usually needed
   - call your doctor or therapist promptly if any sign of infection occurs, such as:

     - increase warmth in the affected arm
     - red streaks or reddened areas in the affected area
     - sudden increase in swelling of the affected arm

Figure 9–4. Special instructions for hand and arm care.

tient that edema management is not a passive activity but one that requires a high level of compliance. For many patients, their edema is so distressing, particularly from a cosmetic and functional perspective, and they have sought out many resources with poor success that they are willing to attempt any program which may offer even a modicum of success.

ELEVATION

One of the most simple interventions, which requires little expertise, is elevation. Elevation of the affected extremity lowers the hydrostatic pressure exerted by the blood against the capillary walls by counteracting the force produced by the heart with the force of gravity.[19] The patient must be instructed to avoid extremes of elevation in order not to compress the axillary or groin areas. Advise the patient to elevate the extremity just enough so that if a drop of water were placed on his or her hand or foot, it would slide toward the shoulder or hip. Elevation can be accomplished with a bed pillow, foam wedge, inverted quadriceps exercise board, or a towel sling attached to a mobile intravenous (IV) pole. Patients should be instructed to elevate their extremity whenever possible, and particularly when at rest.

THERMAL AGENTS AND ELECTROTHERAPY

There have been many papers written on the use of modalities for the reduction of edema, including the use of heat, cold, ultrasound, electrical stimulation, and intermittent compression. Many of the patients may have some sensory impairment which could predispose them to a burn, affording the perfect opportunity for infection. The use of any type of thermal agent should be carefully monitored with these patients. If edema is the result of an inflammatory process, such as in acute edema relative to trauma or venom, heat will only exacerbate the inflammation, causing more edema. Further, when heat increases local blood flow, but the system is incompetent to return fluids, one may get pooling without a mechanism to clear the accumulation of fluids.

The use of ice or cold for acute edema has been a long accepted form of management. This modality is usually readily available, inexpensive, and easy to use. Cold has been shown to decrease blood flow in superficial tissue and increase capillary permeability, thus decreasing inflammation and pain. Cold can be used with patients who have infection and, if monitored, with patients with impaired sensation. In order to counteract the effect of vasodilation with prolonged application of cold, it is recommended that treatment not exceed 12 minutes. Prolonged cold can produce vasodilation. This allows escape of fluid from the vascular to extravascular space resulting in edema.

Ultrasound has never been well substantiated as a technique for management of lymphedema. Further, because many edemas are a direct result of a cancer and/or its treatment, a conservative approach is not to use ultrasound even if the patient is clinically disease free. If one agrees that micrometastasis (the spread of cancer cells to distant sites where they form microscopic secondary tumors) can be freely circulating in the lymph and venous system,[20] the use of ultrasound is definitely contraindicated. Physiologically on acute edema, ultrasound may be helpful in that it increases the permeability of the cell membrane, increases movement and dispersement of fluids, and increases absorption of interstitial fluid.[21]

Electrical stimulation to activate a muscle pump mechanism is one method to assist in fluid return. Individuals with persistent hand edema and loss of function who cannot volitionally activate the muscle pump, are good candidates for this approach. Using continuous high-voltage pulsed current with the hands submerged in water, in the least-dependent position, has been a comfortable setup for our patients. One recommended protocol includes a frequency of 2 to 8 pulses per second, negative polarity, with an intensity set to accomplish a minimal muscle contraction, with 10 seconds on and 40 to 50 seconds off for 20 to 30 minutes.[22]

MASSAGE

The healing effects of massage and laying on of hands is probably the oldest method of practicing "the art of medicine." Besides the psychologic effects, massage also has a well-founded therapeutic value of mechanically assisting in venous and lymphatic flow.[23]

Massage is not indicated for all edemas. In acute traumatic injuries with hematoma, massage to the area could contribute to further internal bleeding and more edema. In cases of infection, active malignancy, pleural effusion, liver disease, kidney disease, and congestive heart failure massage is contraindicated. Massage, however, is an effective adjunctive treatment for those individuals with venous and lymphatic edema because it naturally enhances the movement of fluid. It also aids in improving skin integrity and can help to desensitize tissue and improve mobility.

Traditionally, retrograde massage has been used in this country. More recently, manual lymph drainage has been gaining popularity in the United States. The basic principle behind massage is to mechanically restore or assist normal venous and lymphatic flow. It is essential to understand that the lymphatics are fragile and vigorous methods of massage could be traumatic to this system.[24] Both Vodder and Clodius[25] recommend pressures of 20 to 30 mm Hg because more aggressive pressures close the lymphatic valves and obstruct the intercellular junctions blocking the lymphatic flow.[25] Among the various schools of thought there is agreement that all strokes should be light, should follow the course of the lymphatics, and should not be painful, but rather should be soothing to the patient. Proximal areas need to be cleared before distal areas.

Massage alone, without other complementary treatment, is time-consuming. Obviously, this is one-on-one, uninterrupted treatment. In our current health care environment with an emphasis on cost containment, we will be faced with difficult decisions administering a treatment with clear therapeutic value but lacking in cost efficiency. One may be forced to choose alternatives that are economically more efficient but may not be optimal therapeutically.

EXERCISE

Exercise complemented with elevation is another simple intervention. Patients can be instructed in active exercise via isometric or concentric contraction to help activate the muscle pump and assist to move fluids proximally. For the upper extremities, the use of a R-Lite Foam Block (Smith & Nephew Roylan, Inc., Germantown, WI) cube is very effective. This is an open-cell foam that when compressed slowly returns to its original shape. Each cube is $1\frac{3}{4} \times 1\frac{3}{4} \times 3$ inches and comes in three resistances. The patient must compress the cube and hold for a count of 5. Because the R-Lite Foam takes about 20 seconds to resume its normal shape, it paces the patient, controlling his or her exercise regime. Caution the patient to avoid any stretching exercises in the extreme ranges or activities that would compress the axillary or groin lymph nodes. A walking program is recommended for outpatients, both for the cardiovascular benefits and as a method to stimulate the muscle pump to assist in resolving lower-extremity edema. In order to avoid pooling, short walks for 7 to 12 minutes at a time are suggested, based on patient feedback. This can be done several times a day, however. In hot, humid weather, walking in an indoor mall or other climate-controlled environment is recommended. Brisk walking in an outside pool in water at least chest high is an excellent form of compression as well as exercise therapy. Many indoor pool facilities are environmentally counterproductive to patients because of high humidity in the pool room as well as higher water temperatures.

NONMECHANICAL COMPRESSION

Nonmechanical compression techniques range from something as simple as the use of a disposable latex surgical glove to a custom measured and manufactured support garment. There is general agreement in the literature that regardless of what technique is used to manage edema, some type of compression is required to sustain or maintain any edema reduction achieved. Compression dressings exert pressure on the limb, providing support and facilitating the muscle pump in doing its job.[26]

There are many products available today, some of which are inexpensive and easy to use. Common compression dressings include elastic bandages, elastic stockinette, prefabricated garments, and custom garments. Bandaging and stockinette are good models to test a patient's response to compression before investing the time and expense involved in a custom garment.

The problem with use of bandaging such as Ace wraps or Coban (3M Corporation, St. Paul, MN) is that consistent pressure and proper technique require skill and practice. Figures 9–5 through 9–10 are examples of this skill with excellent results (Fig. 9–11). A "figure-of-eight" wrap is recommended to prevent a tourniquet effect and avoid any bulging of the tissue. The advantage to Coban is that it adheres to itself and remains fixed on the tissue, but it is only designed for one-time use and one must use new material with each wrapping.

Elastic stockinette comes in a wide variety of sizes, giving the user many options. It is reusable, relatively inexpensive, washable and does not require special skill by the patient. One can use more layers distally to provide progressive compression or can use layers of smaller circumference distally for the same effect. These products provide a more consistent pressure and patients generally do not require help doffing and donning them. For those patients who may not be candidates for a custom garment, elastic stockinette is often a good alternative. There are prefabricated garments on the market from gloves to panty hose with varying compressions from 4 to 35 mm Hg. Most of these are for the lower extremities and are a good option for some patients. Often, they are cosmetically acceptable, easy to doff and don, and cost efficient. For most upper-extremity edemas and moderate to severe lower-extremity edemas, a custom-made support is indicated. These come in a variety of styles with many options (Fig. 9–12). Measuring a patient takes some experience both in technique and in selecting the most appropriate garment for the patient. All of the companies now have customer service representatives available by telephone and some have local representatives who will see patients in the home or the treating facility.

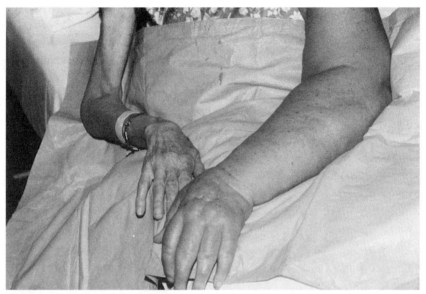

Figure 9–5. An example of a patient who has combined lymphedema in the upper extremity with classic venous edema in the hand.

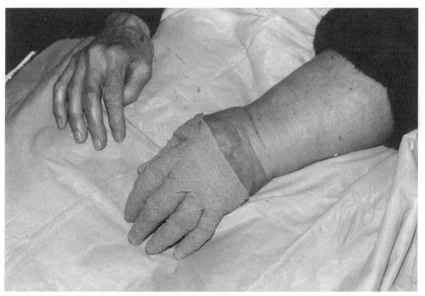

Figure 9–6. Each digit is individually wrapped with ½-inch Coban.

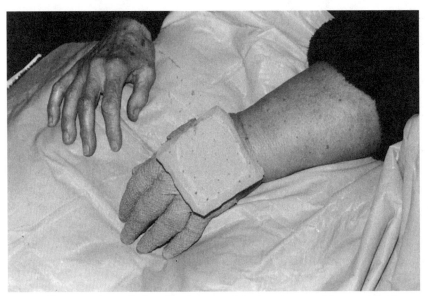

Figure 9–7. Plastazote is applied to the dorsum of the hand to provide more rigid compression.

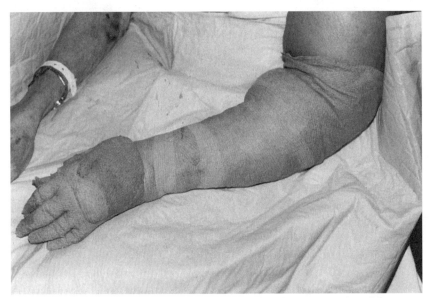

Figure 9–8. Three-inch Coban is used to wrap over the Plastazote and up the extremity.

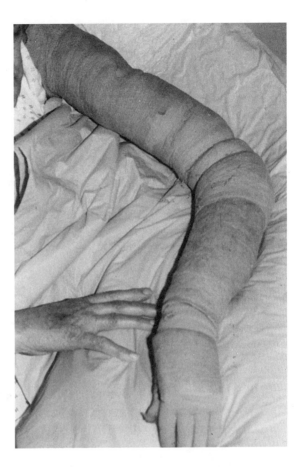

Figure 9–9. Arm is completely wrapped with Coban with a shoulder cap.

MECHANICAL COMPRESSION DEVICES

Another tool available to treat edema is the mechanical compression extremity pump, which consists of a pneumatic pump and a variety of appliances to fit extremities (see Fig. 9–13). Some of these pumps are nonsequential in that the appliance is a single chamber that fills with air. There are also nonsequential pumps in which the chamber fills with water and antifreeze to provide cold compression. Sequential appliances have a series of bladders that fill with air starting distal to proximal. Manufacturers have done their own studies to substantiate the value of sequential or nonsequential pumps to promote their product. To the knowledge of the author, no truly independent study has been performed to date.

Guidelines for equipment selection take into account: (1) the type and number of patients in a facility who will require this equipment, (2) cost of the pump and appliances themselves, (3) ease of operation of the pump, (4) noise generated by the pump, (5) maintenance, (6) available options such as ability to set inflation and deflation pressures and variable timing cycles, and (7) patient comfort while wearing the appliance.

In purchasing a mechanical compression pump, one should explore the following options: (1) whether the appliances for that pump are washable, (2) whether the appliances have a soft fabric liner, or (3) whether the appliance has an insert to provide more sizing options. In addition the pump should be relatively quiet, should

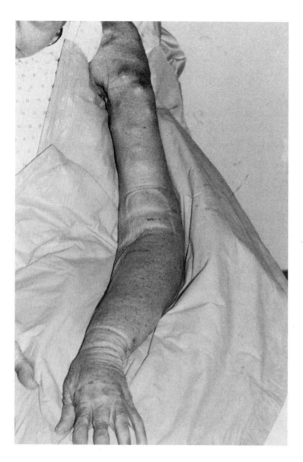

Figure 9–10. Appearance of upper extremity after several days of continuous wrapping.

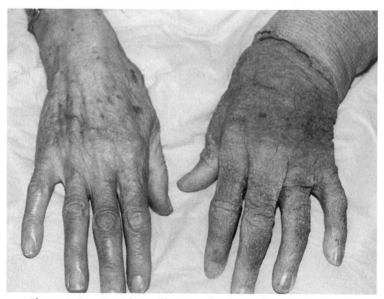

Figure 9–11. Complete reduction of venous edema in the hand.

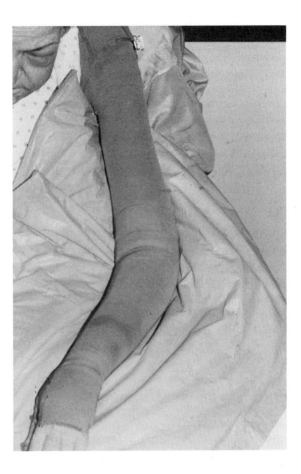

Figure 9–12. Patient fitted with a custom-made compression garment with a shoulder cap and attached gauntlet.

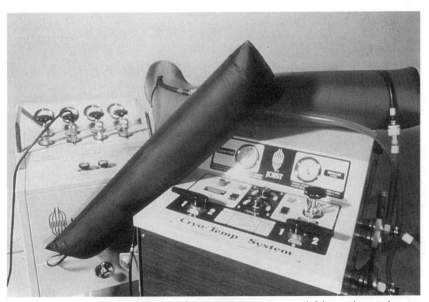

Figure 9–13. A few examples of compression units available on the market.

allow setting of both the ON and OFF timing cycles, and should allow inflation and deflation pressures to be set independently. (This feature would allow for a static compression with an intermittent compression superimposed upon, it preventing refilling of the extremity.) (Fig. 9–14).

Intermittent compression can facilitate edema reduction, normalize tissue texture, and increase patient comfort. It is important that the patient understand the rationale for treatment and that the program be as time efficient as possible to ensure compliance. Each individual patient will require a program unique to his or her problem; there are no concrete protocols but there are some general guidelines that will contribute to patient safety and success. These guidelines are outlined in Table 9–4.

Orthopedic or elastic stockinette should be applied to the extremity inside of the appliance to absorb perspiration and help keep the appliance clean. The treated extremity should be slightly elevated during compression (Fig. 9–6). Patients should be instructed to relax their fingers and toes before beginning the compression. They should also be advised that they may notice some parethesias that should resolve if they move their hand or foot during the OFF cycle. They should be told they may need to urinate frequently and that this is to be expected and that treatment may be terminated at their request.

When starting a new patient, he or she should be monitored every half hour. This includes taking the extremity out of the appliance and checking it for edema, treatment, sensation, and unusual markings. If time permits, measurements should be taken again. The opportunity for the patient to provide feedback, use the bathroom, and stretch should also be provided on a regular basis.

If use of a mechanical compression pump is the best option for the patient, the program should be aggressive. This includes 1 to 5 days of daily pumping for 8 to 10 hours per day. The actual number of days is determined by the rate and quantity of edema reduction. If the patient shows no reduction in edema by day 3, the pumping is discontinued. If the reduction has not leveled off by day 3, add another day or two of pumping. Home pumping is typically not recommended because of

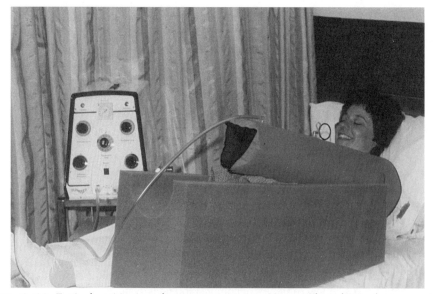

Figure 9–14. Typical positioning of patient to initiate treatment of mechanical compression.

Table 9–4   Guidelines for Safety and Success with Intermittent Compression

1. Monitor and record blood pressure, heart rate circumferential measurement. (This will enable you to monitor patient response to treatment.)

2. The environment must be conducive to patient comfort.

3. The area should be quiet and private with lighting control and music.

4. The patient should be in a recumbent position and be warm.

5. Some type of a call bell should be readily accessible.

6. Each patient must be provided with fluids, and the opportunity to use the bathroom as well as scheduled rest periods.

poor patient compliance and the inability to monitor the patient. In addition, home units are expensive, poorly calibrated, and offer fewer options. If a facility is unable to offer this service, they have the option of recommending another facility.

In terms of parameters for treatment, again this is highly individualized. Lower pressures (20 to 50 mm Hg) for the upper extremity as opposed to 30 to 70 mm Hg for the lower extremity are suggested. These are comfortable for the patient and less traumatic, inhibiting any type of rebound phenomenon. A very short timing cycle with 15 to 20 seconds on and 3 to 6 seconds off is preferred. This cycle again promotes patient comfort and tolerance and does not permit any reflux. It is a personal preference to use a combination of static and intermittent compression, the static component being about 30% of the total pressure. For example, the static, or constant, compression could be 10 mm Hg with an intermittent component of 30 mm Hg. This static component diminishes tissue refilling during the rest phase.

Patients who have infection; longstanding hard, unremitting edema; cardiac disease; altered cognitive status; and active malignancies are not candidates for any type of mechanical compression.

Intermittent compression without follow-through is of little value. In between treatment sessions, elastic stockinette is used to maintain reduction in edema. Mechanical compression is usually followed by fitting the patient with a custom compression garment to maintain the reduction. This is then followed by a serial sleeve program, fitting the patient with progressively smaller garments every 4 to 6 weeks. Ordering the sleeve 1 to 2 mm smaller than the actual measurements is recommended.

If a patient elects not to use a pump because of his or her life-style, personal wishes, or poor response, one can go directly to a serial sleeve program. The patient must understand that this may require more time in the long run to achieve the desired results. It is, however, a very effective option.

Once a patient's initial course of treatment is completed, he or she is monitored monthly for at least 3 months. If their course is uneventful, the time between visits can be extended to 3 months and then eventually to 6 months. The majority of patients with lymphatic and/or venous edema, even well controlled, will require lifelong monitoring, and they may always have to use a compression garment on a regular basis. A small percentage, in my experience, 10% to 15%, can be weaned from the garment in about 12 to 18 months. They still require constant checkups, care of the extremity, and early intervention in the event of a problem. Once again, patient education is the main component to the success of the program. For most individuals, any reduction in edema increases their mobility, softens the tissue, improves skin integrity, and generally makes them feel more comfortable.

In most cases, third-party payers will reimburse for an edema management program, including compression garments. They will require documentation on a case-by-case basis. One must be able to explain the rationale behind the program, predict expected outcome, provide a time frame, and demonstrate improvement. This can be time consuming, but the goal is to meet the needs of the patients. Clinicians are the best advocates for patients. If these programs are well documented via patient outcome, third-party payers will be less resistant to the inclusion of this program on their payment schedules.

SUMMARY

The individual caring for the patient with edema has a variety of available treatment options that can be used individually or in conjunction with one another. There is no one right way to manage every edema problem and an understanding of its etiology and physiology is necessary to make good clinical decisions. The patient is an active participant in most of these interventions and, therefore, patient education and compliancy are critical elements of any successful program. Good edema management takes practice and our patients are our best teachers.

DISCUSSION QUESTIONS

1. Edema is a complex condition that requires management both in the clinic and in the home. Prepare an explanation for a patient to cover the importance of their participation in the management of their edema, using terminology that they will understand.

2. Describe how cardiac disease, kidney disease, and liver failure would adversely influence the reduction of edema.

3. Prepare an explanation for a patient describing the visible signs of edema and some simple remedies that they can perform until they are able to be assessed in the clinic.

4. The successful application of intermittent compression devices stresses the importance of making sure that a patient has access to both fluids and a restroom. Why?

5. Describe the potential options that are available to patients for the management of chronic edema. (Give at least three options with both advantages and disadvantages to each option selected.)

REFERENCES

1. Lyons, AS and Petrucelli, RJ: Medicine: An Illustrated History. Harry N Abram, New York, 1987, pp 433, 439.

2. Gray, H: 1901 Edition Anatomy, Descriptive and Surgical. Running Press, Philadelphia, 1974, p 1082, 1130.

3. Hohlbaum, GG, et al: The Medical Compression Stocking. Schattauer, New York, 1989, p 109.

4. Wittlinger, B and Wittlinger, H: Introduction to Dr. Vodder's Manual Lymph Drainage, Vol. 1, Haug Publishers, Heidelberg, 1982.

5. Clodius, L (ed): Lymphedema. Georg Thieme, Stuttgart, 1977.

6. Walter, JB: An Introduction to the Principles of Disease, ed 3. WB Saunders, Philadelphia, 1992, p 64.

7. Adcock, JL: Rehabilitation of the breast cancer patient. In McGarvey, CL (ed): Physical Therapy for the Cancer Patient. Churchill Livingstone, New York, 1990, p 80.

8. Wilson, JD, et al (eds): Harrison's Principles of Internal Medicine, ed 12. McGraw-Hill, New York, 1991, p 167.

9. Wilson, JD, (ed) et al: Harrison's Principles of Internal Medicine, ed 12. McGraw-Hill, New York, 1991, p 167.

10. Guyton, AC: Basic Human Physiology: Normal Function and Mechanisms of Disease. WB Saunders, Philadelphia, 1971, p 189.

11. Walter, JB: An Introduction to the Principles of Disease, ed 3. WB Saunders, Philadelphia, 1992, p 19.

12. Hohlbaum, GG, et al: The Medical Compression Stocking. Schattauer, Stuttgart, 1989, p 38.

13. Guyton, AC: Basic Human Physiology: Normal Function and Mechanisms of Disease. WB Saunders, Philadelphia, 1971, p 193.

14. Adcock, JL: Rehabilitation of the breast cancer patient. In McGarvey, CL (ed): Physical Therapy for the Cancer Patient. Churchill Livingston, New York, 1990, p 80.

15. Michlovitz, S and Firuta, H: Peripheral Edema: Pathophysiology, Evaluation and Management. Alexandria, VA APTA, 1987, p 8.

16. Adcock, JL: Unpublished material. 1982.

17. Wilson, JD, et al (eds): Harrison's Principles of Internal Medicine, ed 12. McGraw-Hill, New York, 1991, p 170.

18. Ganel, A, et al: Nerve entrapments associated with post mastectomy lymphedema. Cancer, 44:2254, 1979.

19. Hargens, AR: Tissue Fluid Pressure and Composition. Williams & Wilkins, Baltimore, 1981, p 2.

20. Scanlon, EF: The process of metastasis. Cancer, 55:1163, 1985.

21. Mullins, T: Use of therapeutic modalities in upper extremity rehabilitation. In Hunter, JM (ed): Rehabilitation of the Hand. CV Mosby, Philadelphia, 1990, p 202.

22. Ibid, p 215.

23. Tappan, FM: Healing Massage Techniques Holistic, Classic, and Emerging Methods. Appleton & Lange, Norwalk, 1988, p 23.

24. Casley-Smith, JR: The structural basis for the conservative treatment of lymphedema. In Clodius, L (ed): Lymphedema. Georg Thieme, Stuttgart, 1977, p 22.

25. Stijns, HJ and Leduc, A: The contribution of physical therapy in the treatment of lymphedema. In Clodius, L (ed): Lymphedema. Georg Thieme, Stuttgart, 1977, p 27.

26. Hohlbaum, GG: The Medical Compression Stocking. Schattauer, Stuttgart, 1989, p 30.

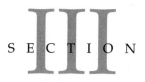

SECTION

III

Electrical Stimulation

Foundations for Electrical Stimulation

Cheryl A. Gillespie, MA, PT

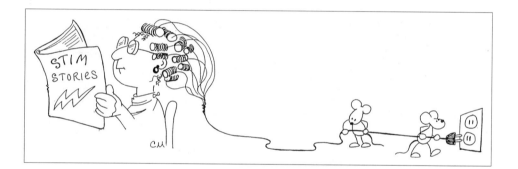

CHAPTER OBJECTIVES

- Introduce the physical concepts and terminology of electricity.
- Describe and differentiate among appropriate electrical parameters.
- Describe current and waveform characteristics as they relate to the delivery of electrical stimulation.
- Describe the present utilization of electrical stimulation with patient populations.
- Outline clinical treatment decisions regarding the use of electrical stimulation to maintain a safe treatment environment.

Every beat of the heart, every twitch of a muscle, every stage of secretion of a gland is associated in some way with electrical changes."[1]

In July 1986, the section on Clinical Electrophysiology of the American Physical Therapy Association published a booklet defining and standardizing electrotherapeutic terminology.[2] Clinicians, researchers, and manufacturers were not communicating with the same terms. The clinician must be familiar with this terminology to select and communicate the electrical parameters of treatment. This chapter explains electrotherapeutic terminology; presents general guidelines for the safe application of electricity; and discusses the rationale, indications, and therapeutic goals of electrical stimulation.

APPLICATION OF ELECTRICAL STIMULATION: YESTERDAY AND TODAY

The history of electricity and electrotherapeutics is well documented by numerous authors.[3–7] Three fields emerged from early research and the use of electricity. *Electrotherapy* applies electricity to treat disease. *Electrodiagnosis* diagnoses disease by interpreting the response of nerves and muscles to electrical stimulation. *Electromyography (EMG)* records the electrical activity of motor units.

Physicists, physiologists, and physicians developed the concepts and the practical application of electricity. Treatment progressed from general body stimulation with electrostatic air baths and electric water baths to more selective stimulation with electrodes. *Static, galvanic,* and *faradic* currents were three forms of electricity dominating the early years. Static and galvanic electricity generated a twitch response from the body. Faradic electricity produced a tetanic or holding response. A historical view of these currents and their application is presented in Table 10–1.

Electricity today continues to be a viable modality to treat dysfunction. Static and faradic currents are obsolete. The introduction of newer pulsatile waveforms has improved comfort levels of treatment.

The fields of electrodiagnosis and electromyography have merged to become

Table 10–1   History of Electricity Related to Electrotherapeutics

400 BC	Greeks recognize electrical qualities in *elektron*, the name for amber.
46 AD	Pain treated with electrical discharges from the torpedo fish, an electric ray.
1744	First recorded treatment with *static electricity* to contract muscle.
1791	Galvanic defines *animal electricity* generated within the body. He touches metal to a frog nerve and muscle, causes a contraction, and describes the release of internal electricity through the metal.
1796	Volta constructs the *voltaic pile*, the forerunner to the battery. The current is named galvanic or *direct current*, marking the beginning of therapeutic *galvanism*.
1823	Galvanic current is introduced through needle electrodes. Concept of electropuncture for pain management.
1831	Faraday's discovery of electromagnetic induction leads to the development of inductoriums that produce a new current called *faradic current*. The asymmetrical alternating pulses of short duration are capable of tetanizing muscle. Therapeutic *faradism* is born.
1833	Duchenne designs the first surface electrodes, which are cloth-covered and moist.
1840	Observation that paralyzed muscles respond to galvanic and not faradic current. Beginnings of electrodiagnosis.
1864	Zeimssen charts the motor points of muscles.
1905	Lapicque develops the "law of excitation" relating intensity and duration of the stimulus. The *strength duration curve* illustrates this concept.
1916	Adrian defines the strength duration curve for healthy and diseased muscle.
1920	Introduction of coaxial needle electrodes to pick up muscle potentials developed by one fiber.
1928	Beginning of clinical electromyography.
1965	Melzak and Wall describe gate control theory of pain perception, providing a scientific basis for use of electrical stimulation for neuromodulation.

the field of *electroneuromyography (ENMG)*. ENMG combines the diagnostic procedures of nerve conduction studies and electromyography. The older forms of electrical testing to determine the integrity of peripheral nerve, such as reaction of degeneration (RD), strength duration (SD), and chronaxie, have been mostly abandoned.

A flourishing area of electrical stimulation is the field of biomedical technology. Manufacturers are developing more highly technical and versitile stimulator units. Small portable stimulators have augmented electrical stimulation for home use, initially for pain management, later for many conditions requiring neuromuscular stimulation. The development and improvement of neural prostheses for implantation is expanding to the blind, deaf, and spinal cord injured.

THERAPEUTIC GOALS

The goals and applications of electrical stimulation are popularly communicated by acronyms. Electrical muscle stimulation (**EMS**) is stimulating denervated muscle to maintain muscle viability. Electrical stimulation for tissue repair (**ESTR**) uses electrical stimulation for edema reduction, enhancement of circulation, and wound management. Neuromuscular electrical stimulation (**NMES**) is stimulation of innervated muscle to restore muscle function and includes muscle strengthening, spasm reduction, atrophy prevention, and muscle re-education. Functional electrical stimulation (**FES**) activates muscles with electrical stimulation to perform functional activities. NMES and FES are often used interchangeably. Neural implants include cardiac pacemakers,[8] electrophrenic respirators,[9] dorsal column stimulators,[9–11] and visual and auditory implants.[9] Neural implants are also used for voiding bladders,[9] managing urinary and anal incontinence,[9,12,13] orthotic substitution,[9] and cerebellum stimulation for convulsions.[9,11] Trancutaneous electrical nerve stimulation (**TENS**) has become synonymous with stimulation for pain management and also refers to a group of portable electrical stimulators developed specifically to achieve this goal. TENS is any application of electrical stimulation to the skin inducing nerve stimulation. All stimulators with appropriate electrical features can be used for pain management.

ELECTROPHYSICS: ELECTRICITY BASICS

CHARACTERISTICS OF MATTER

Atoms are electrically neutral. The positive charge of the proton in the nucleus is equally balanced by the negatively charged electrons surrounding the nucleus. Electrons move in imaginary spherical spaces called electron shells. The atom is charged and becomes an *ion* when proton and electron numbers are not equal. Charging of a body is the removal or addition of electrons. Negative ions are always trying to lose electrons and positive ions are trying to gain electrons to attain a neutral state. Electrons that are loosely attached to atoms are *free electrons* and are capable of moving from one atom to another.

Matter, including biological tissues, is composed of atoms, ions, and free electrons. The charged particles move and produce a current flow because of a concentration difference or electrical potential. The reactivity of atoms determines how well the charged particles move and depends on the number of electrons in the outer shell.[14] An atom is stable and less reactive when the outer shell of electrons is full and electrons are tightly bound.

Conductors of electric current are materials composed of very reactive atoms with freely moving and loosely bound electrons in the outer orbit. Nerves and muscles are examples of biological conductors, while metal is an example of a non-biological conductor. *Insulators* are materials whose electrons are tightly bound in the outer shell. Skin, adipose tissue, and bone function more like insulators. The conductivity of most tissues really falls somewhere between conductor and insulator. The electrons of these *semiconductors* can be displaced but with difficulty.

CHARACTERISTICS OF ELECTRICITY

"Electricity is a form of energy which, when in motion, exhibits magnetic, chemical, mechanical and thermal effects and when at rest or in motion exerts force on other electricity."[1]

Static electricity is produced by friction. It is present when electrons are in a state of tension on an insulated conductor and ready to flow.[1] Electric current is the actual flow of electrons in a conductor. Electrons flowing continuously in one direction is called *direct current (DC)*. The periodic reversal of electron flow is called *alternating current (AC)*.

Electricity is most often described by its strength, rate of flow, driving force, and opposition. These characteristics are popularly compared with similar features of water (Table 10–2).

Charge

Charge is the number of free electrons flowing. It represents the *quantity* of electricity and is measured in coulombs (C). One coulomb equals 6.26×10^{18} electrons.[14] Therapeutic currents are measured in microcoulombs or one millionth of

Table 10–2 Comparison of the Characteristics of Electricity and Water

Electricity	Water
Electron	Water drop
Coulomb	Gallon of water
Current	Water flow
Voltage	Water pressure
	Low voltage: in old house
	High voltage: Water Pik
Resistance (impedance)	Water pipe: Narrow pipe
	Hair clog

a coulomb. Charge can be stored or it can be moved. Stored charge or voltage has the potential to do work by providing a driving force or electrical potential.[15] The movement of charge is current.

Current

Current (I) is how fast free electrons flow. The ampere (A) is the unit measuring the *rate* of flow. One ampere equals the flow of one coulomb per second.[14] Therapeutic current flow is measured in milliamps (mA) and microamps (μA).

Voltage

Voltage (V) is the electromotive *force* (EMF) produced by an electrical potential. Two regions have electrical potential when there is a difference in electron charge between them. The difference in potential creates a force that pushes the charge, causing the flow of electricity from one place to another. Electrons move from an area of high concentration (more negativity) to an area of low concentration (less negativity). Electron flow is from negative to positive. The EMF pushes electrons until the two electrical potentials are equal. Volt (V) is the unit of electrical potential. Therapeutic ranges are in millivolts and volts. The voltmeter is an instrument calibrated to measure potential differences.

Resistance

Resistance (R) determines the ease or difficulty of current moving through substances. Conductance is the ease of movement. A good conductor has low resistance and an insulator has high resistance. All materials offer some opposition to current flow but the amount depends on the material's composition, dimensions, and temperature. Resistance is inversely proportional to the substance's free electron number and cross-sectional area. It is directly proportional to the length and temperature of the material. The ohm is the unit of electrical resistance. One ohm will limit current flow to one ampere when there is a voltage of one volt.[16] Resistors are organized in an electric circuit. The arrangement may be parallel or in series. There is only one pathway for electricity to flow when resistors are in series and that is through each resistor in turn. When resistors are in parallel, the current has a choice of pathways and will always flow through the path of least resistance.

The term *resistance* is electrically used to describe the circuit's opposition to the flow of direct current (DC).

Impedance

Impedance (Z) is the opposition of electrical circuits to the flow of alternating current (AC). The opposition to current flow in biologic tissues is more accurately described by impedance than the term resistance. Ohm is the electrical unit for both resistance and impedance.

Impedance combines the properties of resistance and reactance. Capacitance and inductance are two types of reactance. The body's tissues have capacitive reactance but do not possess significant inductive reactance.[17] The opposition to current flow in the body essentially results from the resistive and capacitive reactance properties of tissue.

Capacitance

Capacitance is the ability to store charge in an electric field and oppose change in current flow. Capacitance is expressed in microfarads. A capacitor is simply two conductors separated by an insulator. Nerve and muscle membranes function as capacitors. When delivering electrical stimulation, the electrode and the nerve-muscle complex function as the conductors. The intervening skin and adipose tissue act as the insulator.

Body tissues can function as resistors in an electrical circuit. Skin and adipose tissue function as resistors in series, whereas muscle, blood, tendon, and bone act like resistors in parallel.[18] Electric current takes the path of least resistance once skin and subcutaneous tissues have been penetrated.

Tissue impedance varies throughout the body. Conductivity depends on the water content of tissue. High water content decreases impedance and improves conductance; thus current flows more easily. Bone, fat, tendons, and fascia are poor conductors with low water contents of 20% to 30%.[19] The intracellular components of nerve and muscle have high water contents of 70% to 75%,[19] but their membranes have a high capacitive reactance. Moist skin will conduct better than dry skin. Healthy skin contains a thin layer of water containing salt, yet it offers one of the highest impedances (1000+ Ω)[14] to current flow because the outer layer of the epidermis contains little fluid. The amount of moisture in the deeper layers is determined by age and the number of sweat glands. Skin resistance is also inversely proportional to its temperature.[20] Heat increases moisture and surface salt content, which promotes conductivity.

Impedance changes in the presence of injury and disease. It increases with edema, ischemia, atherosclerosis, scarring, and denervation and decreases in open wounds and abrasions.[20]

Ohm's Law

The relationship between current, voltage, and resistance (impedance) is defined by Ohm's law and is illustrated in Figure 10–1. Current flow is directly proportional to voltage. An increase in voltage with constant resistance increases current. Current flow is inversely proportional to resistance. An increase in resistance

$$Current = \frac{Voltage}{Resistance}$$

$$\frac{Voltage}{Resistance} = Current$$

$$\frac{Voltage}{Resistance} = Current$$

Figure 10–1. The relationships of Ohm's law.

(impedance) with constant voltage decreases current. The magnitude of current therefore increases with higher voltages and less resistance. High skin impedance requires high voltages to produce necessary current flow in the tissues below.[21]

CHARACTERISTICS OF CURRENT FLOW

Current will flow under two conditions. There must be a source of energy creating a difference in electrical potential and there must be a conducting pathway between the potentials.

Electron flow needs to be distinguished from conventional current flow. Electron flow is described by the movement of the negative charge (electron) from negative to positive. Conventional current flow is described by the movement of positive charge.[14] This concept took root before electron theory was known and has never been abandoned. The current flow is arbitrarily viewed as flowing from positive to negative, even though this actually never happens. It is based on the concept that current leaves the positive terminal of the battery and flows through the circuit to the negative terminal.[17]

The type of current flow changes and a charge transfer occurs between the electrical generator and the biologic tissue at the electrode interface.[22] The current that has been conducted through the wires as *electron flow* converts in the body to *ionic flow*.[15] Ions, such as sodium chloride (NaCl), are charge carriers in the body.

Conventional current flow is used to describe current flow from the electrical generator to the body. Positive ions are driven into the tissues beneath the positive pole (electrode), flow through the tissues to the negative pole (electrode) and then back to the electrical stimulation unit.[23] The ions actually move in two directions under the electrodes. Negative ions move in the same direction as electrons, from negative to positive.[17] Positive ions move in the same direction as conventional current, from positive to negative.[17] These concepts of current flow are illustrated in Figure 10–2.

Ionic flow occurs because of the elementary law underlying electrophysics. This law states *like charges repel, unlike charges attract*.[1] The ions move toward their respective poles to give up or gain electrons. The positive ions (cations) migrate toward the negative electrode (cathode) and the negative ions (anions) migrate toward the positive electrode (anode). Chemical reactions occur at the interface between electrode and tissue during the transfer of charge.[17] The description of the body as a "bag of skin holding a salt solution (NaCl)"[24] is appropriate for explaining these reactions. The positive sodium ions (Na^+) migrate to the negative pole and combine with water, forming the base sodium hydroxide (NaOH). This chemical reaction increases the alkalinity of the area and promotes liquefaction of proteins and the softening of tissues.[18] The negative chloride ions (Cl^-) migrate to the positive pole and combine with water, forming hydrochloric acid (HCl). This chemical reaction increases the acidity of the area, thus promoting coagulation of proteins and the hardening of tissues.[18] Circulation is enhanced as the body attempts to neutralize the changes in the pH.[21] The magnitude of the chemical reaction depends on how long the current flows and how much current flows per square centimeter of surface area. Large charge accumulations occurring when the current is too strong can potentially cause tissue damage such as burns. Small

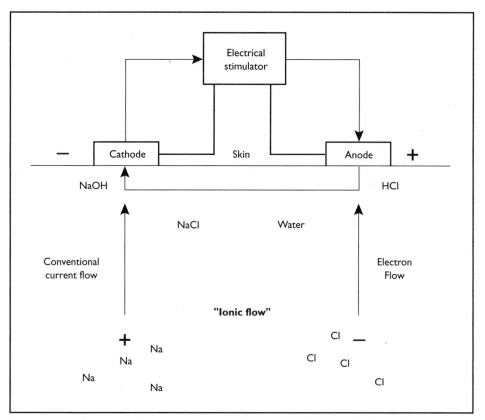

Figure 10–2. Concepts of current and ionic flow with application of electrical stimulation. Current flow through the electrodes and the ionic flow of sodium (Na^+) is portrayed as following the direction of conventional current flow, while the ionic flow of the chloride (Cl^-) ions follows the direction of electron flow.

charge accumulations are advantageous to certain electrical stimulation treatments such as wound and fracture healing.

STIMULATOR OUTPUTS

The output of the electrical generator classifies the unit as either a *constant- (regulated) current* or a *constant- (regulated) voltage* stimulator. Some units are capable of delivering both outputs.

The stimulators only function within a set resistance (impedance) range. The current or voltage cannot increase beyond a fixed limit set by the machine. This safety feature prevents excessive voltage or current outputs when large changes in resistance occur.

Electrical stimulators in the clinic may be of the constant-current or constant-voltage output type. The selection of constant-current or -voltage equipment for treatment depends on which is available for use, and if both are, then the clinician's preference or therapeutic goal determines the choice. There are advantages and disadvantages to both types of output.

CONSTANT-CURRENT STIMULATORS

A constant-current stimulator produces a current that does not vary and is independent of resistance (impedance). This generator maintains the same current output regardless of changes in resistance. The voltage output increases or decreases to maintain constant current flow. The mechanism is similar to cruise control in a car. The car speed (current) is preset and the accelerator (voltage) maintains this constant speed even when the car is going up and down hills (resistance).

The advantage of stimulation with constant current output is consistency of the physiologic response. It is the level of current that determines the physiologic effect of electrical stimulation. The quality of the muscle contraction, for example, remains the same throughout the treatment when current level is constant as long as treatment parameters are such that muscle fatigue is avoided or at least minimized.

The disadvantage of this output is the effect on the tissue when resistance changes. Impedance increases as electrode size decreases. Electrode size is decreased with loss of electrode contact or electrode drying. This changes conductivity and increases impedance. The voltage increases to maintain the same level of current flow, which is now focused in a smaller area. The result can be pain with potential for tissue damage.

Electrical stimulation units producing AC and DC are generally constant current. Some TENS and neuromuscular units are also constant current output. Clinicians can easily determine *on themselves* if a machine has a constant-current or constant-voltage output by slowly peeling the electrode away from the skin surface. The machine is a constant-current stimulator if the current sharpens and starts to bite. The machine's output is constant voltage if the current lessens when the electrode is peeled away from the skin.

CONSTANT-VOLTAGE STIMULATORS

A constant-voltage machine produces voltage that does not vary. The current output increases or decreases depending on changes in resistance. This mechanism is similar to conditions of normal driving. The car will decrease speed (current) as it negotiates a steep hill (resistance) or increase speed going down the hill if the same amount of pressure is maintained on the accelerator (voltage).

A constant-voltage stimulator has the advantage of decreased current levels with increased resistance preventing discomfort or damage.

The disadvantage of this output is that the quality of the response, such as muscle contraction, will change with resistance. Constant voltage can be a problem if there are large decreases in resistance. The current could increase to levels causing injury to tissue.

High-voltage pulsatile units, some TENS units, and some neuromuscular units are constant-voltage stimulators.

CURRENT CLASSIFICATION

A clinically popular, but inappropriate and often confusing practice, is communicating the types of current by their *commercial* or *trade* names. These names stem from the manufacturer and not from the current output of the unit. Commercial generators include low-volt, high-volt, interferential (IFC), Russian, neuromuscular, TENS, and microelectrical nerve stimulators (MENS).

The recognized *generic* forms of current are *direct current* (DC), *alternating current* (AC), and *pulsatile* (pulsed) *current* (Fig. 10–3). The current output of all generators can be classified as one of these three forms.

DIRECT CURRENT

Direct current (old term, *galvanic current*) is a continuous unidirectional flow of charged particles with a duration of at least one second. One electrode is always positive and one electrode is always negative for the period of stimulation. One

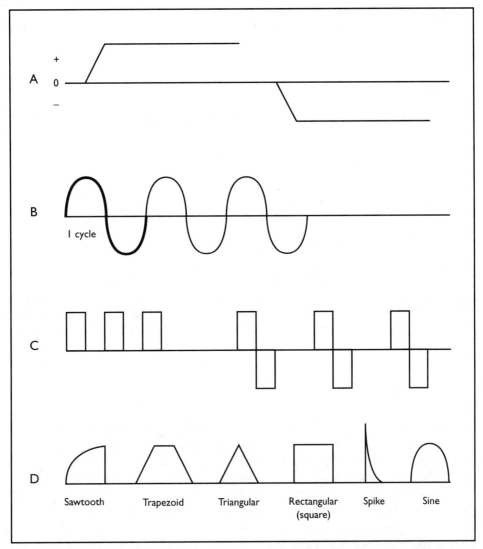

Figure 10–3. Types of current. *(A)* Direct current. *(B)* Alternating current. *(C)* Pulsatile current. Common classifiers used to describe the shape of either the interrupted direct current, one phase of AC, or one phase of a pulse is depicted in *(D)*.

electrode always receives current from the machine and current is returned to the machine by the other electrode. Direction of current flow in any given electrode is determined by the polarity selected on the electrical stimulation unit. The unidirectional property of DC produces residual charges in the tissues under the respective electrodes. DC has a chemical effect.

Direct current can be delivered continuously to promote absorption of medication through the skin (iontophoresis) or it can be interrupted and used to stimulate denervated muscle. DC is the only current form capable of these two treatments.

ALTERNATING CURRENT

Alternating current is an uninterrupted bidirectional flow of charged particles changing direction at least once a second. Alternating current can also be delivered in an interrupted form, sometimes referred to as bursts. Each electrode becomes positive for one phase of the cycle and then negative as the current reverses. Charges do not build up in the tissues and chemical effects are negligible since each electrode continually changes polarity.

AC is no longer used to directly stimulate tissue. Several commercial stimulators, including interferential and Russian, use an alternating current as the base or carrier current which is then modified in the machine and delivered to the patient in the form of *beats* or *bursts*, respectively.

PULSATILE CURRENT

Pulsed or pulsatile current is the unidirectional *or* bidirectional flow of charged particles periodically ceasing for a period of less than one second (milliseconds or microseconds) before the next electrical event. The current is comprised of individual pulses of short duration. Each individual pulse is comprised of one or more phases. A continuous series of individual pulses delivered over time is a *pulse train.*

Electrochemical reaction in the tissue depends on whether the pulse is unidirectional like DC or bidirectional like AC. A cathodal *or* anodal effect will occur under each electrode when the pulse is unidirectional. When the pulse is bidirectional, one phase of the pulse has anodal characteristics and one phase of the pulse has cathodal characteristics.

ELECTRICAL PARAMETERS

Pulsatile current is the most commonly generated and clinically used current form. This chapter section defines terminology primarily associated with this form of current. AC and pulsatile current share many similar properties, and some terms are applicable to both forms of current.

Although the description of the individual pulse and the pulse train is important, the physiologic effect depends predominantly on the parameters defining the single pulse. Table 10–3 lists the characteristics of the pulse and the pulse train.

DESCRIBING THE SINGLE PULSE

The pulse is described by time, amplitude and time/amplitude dependent characteristics.[2]

Table 10–3   **Characteristics Describing Pulsatile Current**

Single Pulse	Pulse Train
Waveform	Interpulse interval
Amplitude	Frequency
Rise time/decay time	Duty cycle
Intrapulse interval	On-off time
Duration	Ramp time
Charge	Total current

Waveform

Waveform is a visual representation of the pulse. It is a spatial drawing depicting the amplitude and duration of the pulse with respect to charge.

Pulses are classified as *monophasic* or *biphasic*. Some clinicians use a third classification, *polyphasic*. This waveform will be discussed briefly. Figure 10–4 summarizes waveform classification.

An additional description is often added to the waveform (see Fig. 10–3), such as *biphasic square wave* or *twin-spiked monophasic pulse*. The body does not distinguish between a square or trapezoid shape. It does respond to the amplitude and time characteristics of the waveform. The waveform classification with the specific electrical description suffices for communication.

Waveforms are diagrammatic only and rarely reflect what is actually going into the patient. Two factors influence the shape of the waveform and account for the difference between the illustrative waveform and the real. The first is the capacitive reactance property of tissue.[17] A load applied to a current, such as the resistance encountered in the body's tissues, will change the configuration of the waveform. The actual waveform that is delivered when a load (resistance) is applied can be visualized on an oscilloscope. The second factor that determines the actual shape of the waveform is whether the equipment has constant-current or constant-voltage output.

Monophasic Waveform   A *monophasic* pulse has only one phase. This pulse is always unidirectional from the baseline carrying a positive or negative charge. The

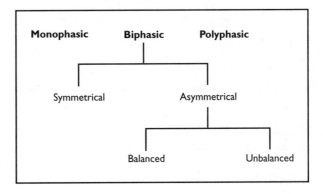

Figure 10–4. Classification of waveforms.

polarity effects are not of the magnitude of DC because pulsatile current flows for a shorter time period. The monophasic pulse is depicted in Figure 10–5.

There has been some confusion regarding the usage of the terms *interrupted DC* and *pulsed monophasic*. Interrupted DC is not the same as delivering monophasic pulses. Pulsed monophasic current, such as that delivered by the commercial high-voltage units, is often wrongly referred to as interrupted or pulsed DC. Monophasic pulsatile current and interrupted DC are different currents with different durations and physiologic effects. The terms are not interchangeable.

Biphasic Waveform   A *biphasic* pulse is bidirectional with two phases. One phase deviates from the baseline in a positive direction and the other phase deviates in a negative direction.

The variables of the two phases are identical and mirror one another in the *symmetrical biphasic* pulse (Fig. 10–5). The chemicals formed in one phase are neu-

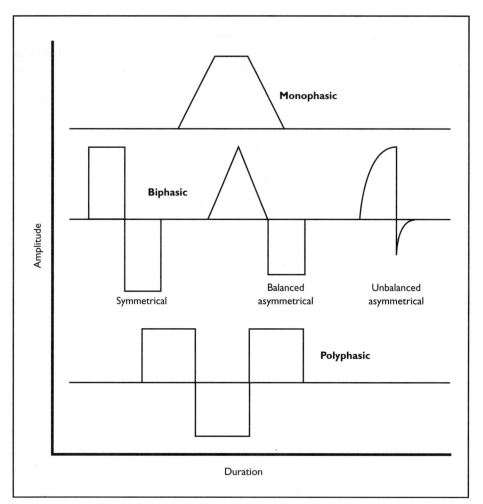

Figure 10–5. Classification of pulsatile waveforms into monophasic, biphasic, and polyphasic. Biphasic can be subdivided into symmetrical versus asymmetrical and balanced versus unbalanced.

tralized by the reversal of current in the second phase. The charges of the two phases cancel each other out and there is a zero net charge (ZNC) across the baseline. No accumulation of positive or negative charge occurs. Some neuromuscular units produce this waveform.

A pulse is *asymmetrical biphasic* when the variables of the two phases are not identical. When the charge of one phase is electrically equal to the charge of the other phase, the waveform is a *balanced asymmetrical biphasic* (Fig. 10–5). The equal charges cancel each other out and a ZNC still exists across the baseline. A pulse is an *unbalanced asymmetrical biphasic* when the electrical charge of one phase is greater than the electrical charge of the other phase (see Fig. 10–5). The old faradic current is an example of this waveform. The unbalanced asymmetrical biphasic pulse produces a net charge across the baseline with some residual charge in the tissues. This pulse is similar to the monophasic pulse because of the accumulation of charge, but the electrochemical reactions are much less because the pulse is biphasic.

Most commercial TENS units and some neuromuscular units produce both balanced and unbalanced asymmetrical biphasic waveforms.

A single cycle of AC is biphasic (Fig. 10–3). The two phases of the AC cycle can either be symmetrical or asymmetrical. The durations of interrupted AC and the biphasic pulse differ and the terms are not synonymous.

Polyphasic Waveform   A *burst* groups together a finite series of pulses and delivers them to the body as a single charge (Fig. 10–6). The single pulse is like the pull of a trigger on a gun. The burst is more like the pull of a trigger on a machine gun. A burst is perceived by the body as a single pulse. It behaves physiologically as a single pulse and has no physiologic advantage over the single pulse.[21] Packet, beat, and envelope are other terms sometimes used synonymously for burst.

The burst is also occasionally referred to as a polyphasic waveform. *Polyphasic* means three of more phases (see Fig. 10–5). Polyphasic pulses are all bursts, but

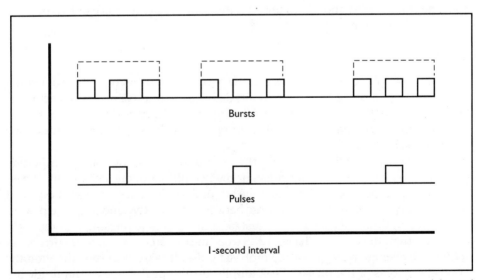

Figure 10–6. The burst and single pulse. Example of three bursts and three pulses delivered in a 1-second time interval. Each burst comprises three monophasic pulses in this illustration.

not all bursts are polyphasic. A burst can also be a group of monophasic or biphasic pulses delivered as a single charge.

The modified or bursted AC produced by the commercial interferential and Russian stimulators are examples of what may be referred to as a polyphasic pulse.

Phase Versus Pulse   The physiologic effect the pulse will have on tissue is determined by the phase not the pulse parameters. The monophasic pulse has only one phase. The phase characteristics therefore describe the whole pulse.

The biphasic pulse has two individual phases. The terms phase and pulse are not the same. The description of one phase is sufficient in the symmetrical biphasic pulse since the phases are equal. The characteristic of each phase needs to be identified in the asymmetrical biphasic pulse, especially the unbalanced where the charges are not equal.

Waveform Comfort   Several studies have investigated the comfort levels of different waveforms during electrical stimulation.[25-29] It is difficult to summarize from these studies what is the most comfortable waveform for clinical use because of the procedural variations. A single conclusion that may be drawn from all of these studies is that patients will perform best with the waveform they perceive as most comfortable. This varies not only from person to person but also between different muscle groups within the same person. The symmetrical biphasic waveform seemed to be preferred more often.

Waveform Selection   The choice of waveform for treatment depends on the available equipment in the clinic and the treatment goal. All waveforms are basically effective for most treatments but some techniques dictate the waveform selection. The requirement of specific electrochemical effects in treatment, as in wound healing, precludes the use of the biphasic waveforms. Patient preference best determines selection of waveform when treatment goal does not dictate the choice. Some neuromuscular and TENS units on the market offer a choice of two or more waveforms within the same unit.

Amplitude

Peak amplitude (old term, *peak current*) is the maximum current or voltage delivered in one phase of a pulse. It is the magnitude of the stimulus and is one factor determining strength of stimulation. Peak amplitude describes the maximum amplitude of the monophasic pulse but refers only to the maximum amplitude of one phase of the biphasic pulse.

Peak-to-peak amplitude denotes the maximum current or voltage amplitude over the two phases of biphasic pulses or the two phases of one cycle of AC. Peak-to-peak amplitude does not indicate the strength of the *pulse* because it does not reflect the difference in electrical charge between the positive and negative phases. The peak amplitude of each phase must be compared to determine differences in electrical strength between phases. RMS (root-mean-square) voltage or current describes the average strength of the biphasic pulse. It takes into consideration the opposite charges of the phases. Peak amplitude and peak-to-peak amplitude are shown in Figure 10–7.

Peak amplitude is measured in current (milliamperes or microamperes) or

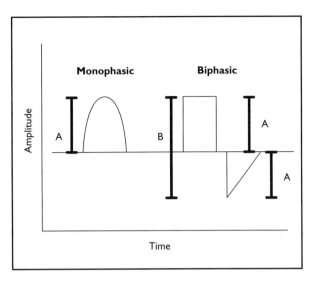

Figure 10–7. Characteristics describing the single pulse. *(A)* Peak amplitude. *(B)* Peak-to-peak amplitude.

voltage (volts) depending on the stimulator. The amplitude is read either on a milliammeter or a voltmeter. The amplitude control on stimulator units is labeled *intensity*. This term can be confusing because intensity usually refers to current flow.

Current and voltage are directly related as defined by Ohm's law. A machine with a high voltage output is capable of producing a high peak current.[21] Most commercial units are low-voltage (0 to 100 V), except for the high-voltage units, which have a maximum output of 500 V.

Peak amplitude is associated with depth of current penetration.[18] Higher peak amplitudes penetrate deeper into tissue. The electrical conductivity of the tissues under the electrode decides *how deep* this penetration will be. A high voltage output generating a high peak amplitude will have no more penetration than a low-voltage output if the tissues as adipose and bone are not good electrical conductors.

Electrical stimulation produces three excitatory responses which are sensory, motor, and pain.[30] Peak amplitude influences the response of tissue to electrical stimulation. Low peak amplitudes may fail to excite tissue, whereas high peak amplitudes may cause pain and not produce the intended response. The level of current necessary to excite a nerve fiber is inversely proportional to the fiber's diameter.[18] The larger-diameter nerve offers less resistance because of its greater cross-sectional area. The larger sensory fibers are recruited before small pain fibers in "ideal" conditions. The anatomic location of the nerve fiber to the electrode is a factor with electrical stimulation.[15] Sensory fibers will generally fire first with the sensation of tingling, prickling or pins and needles. Sensory fibers have a higher threshold than motor fibers but are usually more superfical and closer to the electrode. Selective discrimination of each excitatory response occurs as amplitude is increased slowly over time. When amplitude is increased rapidly, all nerve fibers meet threshold and are recruited simultaneously. The response is pain, usually described as a sharp burning.

Four clinical levels of stimulation are therefore possible with electrical stimulation. The amplitude of the stimulus can produce a subsensory, sensory, motor, and noxious response (Table 10–4). The strength of the stimulus needed for treatment depends on the problem, muscle group treated, type of electrodes used, in-

Table 10–4   **Clinical Levels of Stimulation**

Subsensory:	No nerve fiber activation
	No sensory awareness
Sensory:	Nonnoxious paresthesias
	Tingling, prickling, or pins and needles
	Cutaneous *A-beta* nerve fiber activation
Motor:	Strong paresthesias
	Muscle contraction
	A-alpha nerve fiber activation
Noxious	Strong, uncomfortable paresthesias
	Strong muscle contraction
	Sharp or burning pain sensation
	A-delta and *C-fiber* activation

tended goal, and patient tolerance. A training period may be necessary for the patient to achieve target stimulus strength.

Rise Time and Decay Time

Rise time is the time it takes for the amplitude to increase from zero to peak amplitude. The rate of rise directly affects the ability to excite nervous tissue.[18] Nerve membranes accommodate to slow introductions of current over time (slow rise time) with an automatic rise in threshold. The membrane has time to adjust to the voltage change and a greater stimulus is then needed to cause a response. Increasing amplitude can compensate for waveforms with slow rates of rise. Denervated muscle does not exhibit accommodation and can be selectively excited by current forms with slow rates of rise.[18]

Decay *time* is the time it takes for the peak amplitude to decrease back down to zero and defines the terminal end of the phase. Rise and decay times are fixed by the pulse shape. Figure 10–8 depicts these parameters.

Intrapulse Interval

The *intrapulse interval* (synonym, *interphase interval*) defines the time period between the end of one phase and the beginning of the second phase of one pulse (Fig. 10–9). It is measured in microseconds and usually fixed by the manufacturer. The monophasic pulse does not have an intrapulse interval.

It has been reported that when the anodal phase immediately follows the cathodal phase, the excitation caused by the stimulating cathode phase is depressed and may reverse.[31] Greater peak amplitude is then required for excitation. The introduction of an intrapulse interval abolishes this effect of the anodal phase and decreases the amount of amplitude needed to evoke excitation.[31] There is some discrepancy in the literature concerning the length of the intrapulse interval needed to abolish the anodal effect.[27,31]

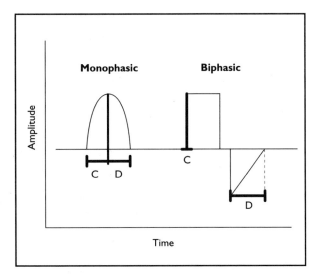

Figure 10–8. Characteristics describing the single pulse. *(C)* Rise time. *(D)* Decay time.

Duration

Phase duration (old term, *pulse width*) is the time period extending from the beginning to the end of one *phase* of a pulse. It also describes the time elapse of one cycle of alternating current. *Pulse duration* is the time interval between the beginning and end of all the phases of the *pulse,* including the intrapulse interval. The terms phase and pulse duration are synonymous in the monophasic pulse. The pulse duration of a biphasic pulse includes the *first-phase duration + intrapulse interval + second-phase duration.* Phase and pulse durations are measured in microseconds and are illustrated in Figure 10–10.

The strength and duration of current determines tissue excitability. This is the *law of excitation.*[4] The strength duration curve (SDC) demonstrates the inverse relationship between these two variables. As phase duration increases, less peak amplitude is required to achieve the desired physiologic response (Fig. 10–11). There is a minimum stimulus duration below which no magnitude of stimulus can cause

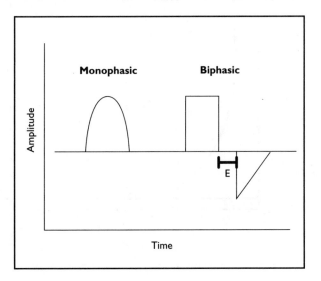

Figure 10–9. Characteristics describing the single pulse. *(E)* Intrapulse interval.

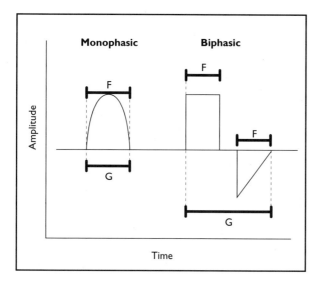

Figure 10–10. Characteristics describing the single pulse. *(F)* Phase duration. *(G)* Pulse duration.

excitation and a minimum amplitude below which no duration can cause excitation.[18] Nerve and muscle membranes function as capacitors. The membranes are capable of absorbing a certain amount of charge before reaching threshold. The minimum duration necessary to excite muscle is longer than that of a nerve because muscle membranes have greater capacitance than nerve membranes.[18]

Phase duration is also associated with discrimination between the excitatory responses. Each excitable tissue has its own SDC. Discrimination, therefore selectivity, is greatest between the different nerve fibers at the shortest durations. The ability to discriminate between the different fibers decreases as phase durations increase[18] as shown in Figure 10–12. Shorter durations excite the large sensory afferents, while the longer durations are necessary to excite the smaller A delta and

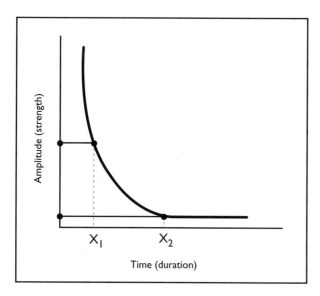

Figure 10–11. Relationship between peak amplitude and phase duration as defined by the strength duration curve (SDC). Note the different amplitude requirements at durations (X_1) and (X_2). Less current amplitude is required to achieve threshold as phase duration increases.

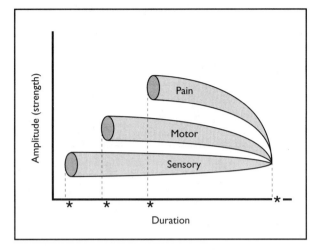

Figure 10–12. Discrimination of the excitatory responses in electrical stimulation. As the phase duration increases, the ability to selectively discriminate between the activation of sensory, motor, and pain nerve fibers decreases, and a point is reached where all the excitatory responses are evoked at the same time.

C fibers.[15,32,33] Stimulus durations between 20 and 200 μs are effective for discrimination.[21] Discrimination ability is lost at phase durations exceeding 1000 μs (1 ms).[34]

Phase duration affects comfort of stimulation. Comfort decreases as phase duration increases. No optimal phase duration has been defined for surface electrodes. Several studies have indicated that 50 to 1000 μs may be within an optimal range with 300 μs being the most comfortable duration when compared to 50- and 1000-μs duration.[25,27]

The magnitude of chemical changes in the tissue is directly proportional to the phase duration. Increased chemical effects occur as phase duration increases. The electrochemical effect is less with pulsatile currents than with DC but still appreciable in monophasic pulses and to a lesser extent in unbalanced asymmetrical biphasic pulses.

Short pulse and phase durations are associated with decreased impedance and better conductivity of current into the tissue.[21] Phase duration can be fixed by the manufacturer or a variable control on the stimulation device. A variable phase duration permits custom fitting of the strength and duration of the current to the patient. The phase duration is still labeled pulse width on some electrical stimulation devices. Other units use the label *pulse duration* when *phase duration* is meant. The manufacturer's specification sheet should be checked to clarify pulse characteristics.

Charge

Phase charge is the amount of electrical energy delivered to the tissue with each phase of each pulse (microcoulombs per second [μC/s]). It is quantity of charge defined by amplitude and duration. Charge is represented by the area of the phase. *Pulse charge* is the sum of all the phase charges in the pulse. The phase charge equals the pulse charge in a monophasic pulse. Phase charge is illustrated in Fig. 10–13.

Phase charge reflects the strength of the electrical stimulation unit. Machines are classified as weak, moderate, or powerful depending on the maximum phase charge that the unit is capable of producing. The phase charge of the unit may be

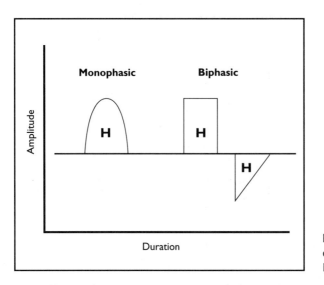

Figure 10–13. Characteristic describing the single pulse. *(H)* Phase Charge.

as weak as 12 μC or as powerful as 40 μC. Adequate phase charge determines tissue excitability. Excessive phase charge results in tissue damage.

The amount of charge necessary to evoke the three excitatory responses decreases as pulse and phase durations decrease.[30] This may be the result of reduced impedance at shorter pulse or phase durations lowering the charge needed for excitation.[21]

Some machines offer the feature of reading phase charge during treatment.

DESCRIBING THE PULSE TRAIN

All the parameters so far discussed describe the single pulse and are summarized in Figure 10–14. The parameters detailed in this section define the electrical characteristics of a *series of pulses* or the current as a whole.

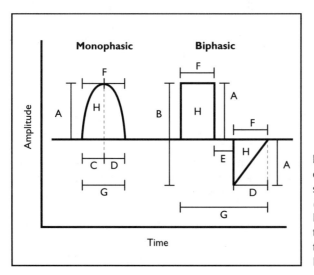

Figure 10–14. Summary of the characteristics describing the single pulse. *(A)* Peak amplitude. *(B)* Peak-to-peak amplitude. *(C)* Rise time. *(D)* Decay time. *(E)* Intrapulse interval. *(F)* Phase duration. *(G)* Pulse duration. *(H)* Phase charge.

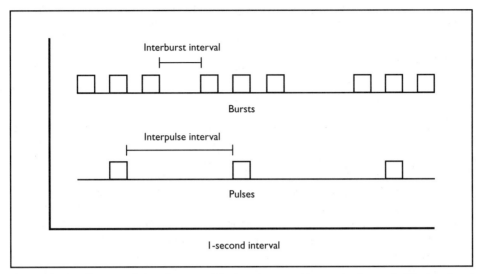

Figure 10–15. Characteristics of current. The interburst and interpulse intervals. The interburst interval is shorter because the duration of the burst is longer than that of the pulse.

Interpulse and Interburst Intervals

The *interpulse interval* is the time period extending from the end of one pulse to the beginning of the next pulse and is measured in milliseconds (Fig. 10–15). The interpulse interval decreases as phase or pulse durations increase (Fig. 10–16). Most stimulators produce relatively short pulse durations with long interpulse intervals. The interpulse interval interrupts current and results in less electrical stimulation fatigue, but is not a true interruption of current because relaxation does not occur.[34] Any parameter decreasing the interpulse interval will increase the time of current flow and increase fatigue to electrical stimulation.

Polarity effects are less with pulsatile current than with DC because the *intrapulse* and *interpulse* intervals shorten the period of time the current is on. The tis-

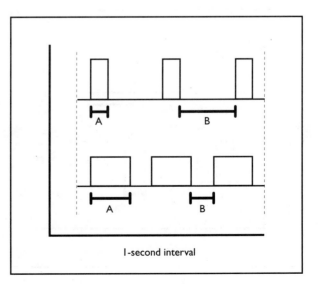

Figure 10–16. Relationship between *(A)* phase duration and *(B)* the interpulse interval. The interpulse interval shortens as phase duration increases.

sues have time to neutralize the chemical effects between phases or pulses and there is less residual electrical charge buildup in the tissues.

Bursts are separated by an *interburst interval.* The interburst interval is shorter than the interpulse interval because each burst contains more phases—therefore the pulse duration is longer (see Fig. 10–15).

Frequency

Pulse frequency, which often is referred to as pulses per second (pps) or pulse rate (Fig. 10–17), is the number of pulses delivered to the body in one second. The body responds to the *number of pulses* not the number of phases. A single monophasic, biphasic, or polyphasic pulse is "counted" as *one* by the body. *Carrier* frequency is the base frequency of the AC sine wave produced in a machine before it is modified and delivered to the patient at a different frequency. The frequency of AC is expressed in hertz (Hz) or cycles per second (cps). Burst frequency is the number of burst per second. Fatigue is greater at higher frequencies because the interpulse interval shortens (see Fig. 10–17).

Frequency defines the quality of the muscle response dictating a twitch or tetanic (holding) contraction. Muscle response changes from twitch to tetany as frequency increases. The importance of this concept will be discussed in Chapters 11 and 12.

Impedance is influenced by frequency. The capacitive reactance characteristic of tissue is inversely proportional to frequency.[35] Impedance will decrease as frequency increases.

Electrical stimulators are often referred to as low-, medium-, or high-frequency units, the low and medium frequencies having the ability to stimulate excitable tissue. Unfortunately, the classification of electrical stimulators into low and medium frequency has just resulted in confusion. Essentially all therapeutic electrical stimulation machines are low frequency. The "medium" frequency machines simply utilize a carrier frequency of AC that is delivered to the patient as a low-frequency current in the form of bursts. A carrier frequency of 2500 Hz has been found to be more comfortable than stimulation with 1000 or 5000 Hz.[26]

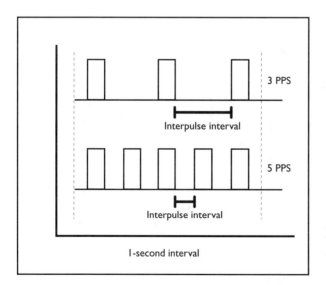

3 PPS

Interpulse interval

5 PPS

Interpulse interval

1-second interval

Figure 10–17. Characteristics of current. Pulse frequency. The length of the interpulse interval decreases as frequency increases.

Frequency is a variable control on electrical stimulators and is usually labeled pulse rate. A frequency range of 1 to 120 pps is sufficient for most therapeutic goals.[34] Smooth muscle contractions occur at frequencies from 15 to 50 pps.[23] Large-diameter nerves have higher firing rates than small-diameter nerves. Bioelectric investigations are providing some insight into the most appropriate frequency ranges for affecting both excitable and nonexcitable tissues. A frequency window has been postulated suggesting that cells may be receptive to certain frequencies and unresponsive to others,[36] an important concept for tissue and bone healing.

Duty Cycle

On time is the period of time the current is delivered to the patient. *Off time* is the period of time current flow stops. Both times are measured in seconds and are shown in Figure 10–18. The current must be on for at least one second and off for at least one second to be a true interruption of current with relaxation. Intrapulse, interpulse, and interburst intervals are much shorter than one second.

On time versus off time can be expressed as a ratio. If the current is on for 5 seconds and off for 20 seconds, the ratio is 1:4. *Duty cycle* is the percentage of total time that the current is actually on. It represents the *on time* divided by *the sum of on and off time* expressed as a percentage. The duty cycle must be known to calculate total stimulation time. A clinical example is given in Figure 10–19. Cycling is generally reported by use of the on and off times.

Muscle contractions generated by electrical stimulation are more fatiguing than those generated by the nervous system. The on-off time ratio plays an important role in circumventing muscle fatigue during stimulation. The longer the *off* time relative to the *on* time, the less the fatigue.

Ramp Time

Ramp time is the increase in amplitude to peak of the pulse train. It is how long it takes for the *current* to go from zero to peak amplitude and how long it takes for the current to go from peak amplitude back down to zero (Fig. 10–20). *Ramp time*

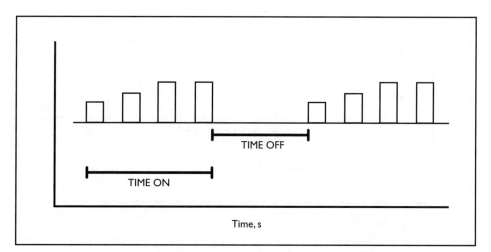

Figure 10–18. Characteristics of current. On time/off time.

PROBLEM: *The total stimulation time needed for a specific treatment protocol is 30 minutes. The stimulation time is 15 seconds and the on/off ratio is 1:4. How long would the total treatment time have to be?*

SOLUTION: $\dfrac{\text{on time}}{\text{on + off time}} = \dfrac{15}{15 + 60} = \dfrac{15}{75} = \dfrac{1}{5} \times 100 = 20\%$

Duty Cycle is 20%, therefore the current is only on for one fifth of the time.

The total treatment time would have to be 2 hours 30 minutes (150 minutes) to achieve 30 minutes of stimulation time.

Figure 10–19. Clinical implications of the duty cycle.

is not synonymous with rise time. Rise time describes the change in amplitude in a single pulse. Ramp time describes the change in amplitude of the pulse train or current over a specific time period of current flow. *Ramp up* is an increase in amplitude over time. *Ramp down* is a decrease in amplitude over time. Both ramp times are measured in seconds.

Ramp time may be fixed or variable, depending on the stimulator. There may be one ramp feature, usually ramp up, or none at all. When variable, the adjustable range is generally 1 to 8 seconds.

Ramp time is associated with the comfort of stimulation, and a 2-second ramp is often adequate.[23] The ramp-up feature allows for more normal motor recruitment and smoother muscle contraction with slow buildup of current to peak amplitude. The ramp-down feature can increase patient comfort. An 8- to 10-second ramp-up is recommended when applying electrical stimulation to the antagonist of a spastic muscle.[23] Quick stretch and activation of the 1A afferents in the spastic muscle is then avoided.

The ramp time must be added to the on time to assure contraction time is long

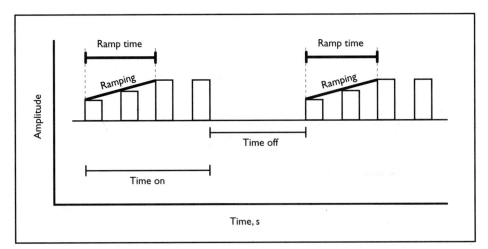

Figure 10–20. Characteristics of current. Ramp time.

enough. If a 10-second peak muscle contraction is desired with a 2-second ramp-up, the on time must be set at 12 seconds.

Total Current

Total current (synonym, *average current*) is the amount of current delivered to the tissue per second and is measured in milliamperes. Total current is very closely related to phase charge. *Total current equals phase charge times number of phases times pulses per second.*[21]

Total current determines safety of treatment and magnitude of the physiologic effect. Tissue damage is the result of thermal and electrochemical effects in the tissue and both are a function of total current.[37] Heat dissipation is generally not a problem with surface stimulation.[37] The tissues can be harmed if the total current is excessive or there will be no physiologic response if total current is too low. Most machines function within safe limits, but there are several commercial units with excessively high total current outputs.

Any parameter increasing the strength of the current stimulus or decreasing the length of the interpulse interval will increase the total amount of current to the patient. *Peak amplitude, pulse frequency,* and *phase duration* are all directly proportional to total current, as shown in Figure 10–21. Changes in peak amplitude and

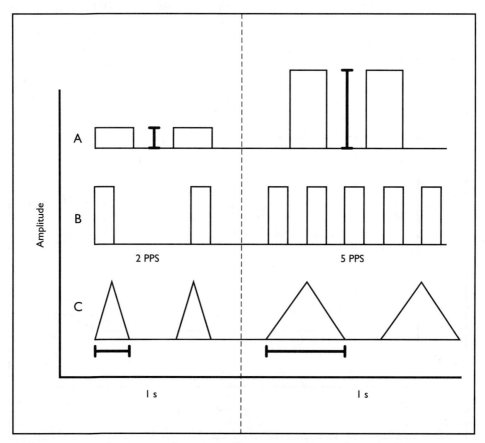

Figure 10–21. Total current can be increased by increasing (*A*) peak amplitude, (*B*) pulse frequency, and/or (*C*) phase duration.

phase duration affect the strength of the pulse charge. Changes in phase duration and pulse frequency affect the length of the interpulse interval.

A safe range of total current to the patient is considered to be 1 to 4 mA/cm² electrode area.[38] The lowest level of stimulation producing the desired response is the current level used. Small electrodes must not be used with machines capable of delivering high total current. The Russian stimulator is an example of a commercial machine capable of delivering high total current. The use of small electrodes, e.g., 1 x 1 inch, would be inappropriate and dangerous with this unit.

MODULATION

Modulation is varying one or more of the electrical parameters of the pulse or current as a whole over time while delivering the stimulus. Amplitude and duration can be modulated in the pulse. Modulations of the whole current or pulse train include frequency modulation, ramping, mode of current delivery, on-off time, and bursting.

Amplitude, phase or pulse duration, and frequency can be modulated individually or in combination, changed intermittently, or varied sequentially. Figure 10–22 illustrates the intermittent modulations of these parameters.

Sweep is a term used by manufacturers to denote sequential modulation of

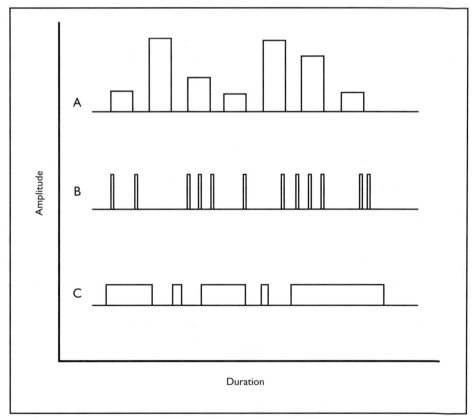

Figure 10–22. Intermittent modulation of (*A*) peak amplitude, (*B*) pulse frequency, and (*C*) phase duration.

pulse frequency. This feature gives the option of a constant sequential modulation (sweep) of the entire available frequency range or portions of it.

Amplitude and frequency may also be modulated in AC. *Surged AC* is an old term applied to the sequential modulation of amplitude of AC.

Ramping is the sequential modulation of phase charge by changing the phase duration or amplitude. *Ramp time* has been discussed and is amplitude modulation (see Fig. 10–20).

Current is delivered continuously or with interruption. The ability of the machine to do both is an important feature for versatility of treatment. On *continuous* mode, the current is delivered without interruption for the length of the treatment. The current ceases for a specific period of time of at least one second to allow relaxation when *interrupted*. Interruption may be fixed in intervals by the manufacture or variable within a range using on-off time controls. Many manufacturers unfortunately label the interruption control SURGE, using the same term describing continuous amplitude modulation of AC. *Surge mode* and *reciprocate mode* are commercial labels describing the delivery of interrupted current to all leads or alternating between leads, respectively.

DELIVERY OF ELECTRICAL STIMULATION

The power source for the delivery of electrical stimulation can be either DC from a battery or conventional AC from a 115-V 60-Hz wall outlet. The current or voltage, depending on stimulator output, is converted from the power source current into the appropriate therapeutic current waveforms. Oscillator circuits within the machine allow independent control of the different treatment variables such as frequency, phase duration, and duty cycle.

Electrical stimulation is delivered to the body through electrodes. A lead wire connects the generator to the electrode. Electrodes have two functions. They can apply a stimulating current to the body tissue to excite or they can record and detect the presence of an electrical signal in the body. The principles of electrode use and placement are discussed in more detail in Chapter 16.

The electrical current can be introduced through *transcutaneous* electrodes in contact with the skin or through *subcutaneous* electrodes. The subcutaneous electrode is invasive and can be inserted through the skin via a wire or needle electrode *percutaneously* or surgically implanted on excitable tissue.[39] The percutaneous method is often used to assess the patient's response and reactions to the electrical stimulation prior to implantation.

OVERVIEW: USAGE OF ELECTRICAL STIMULATION

This section discusses the general indications and treatment restrictions of electrical stimulation.

INDICATIONS

The indications for electrical stimulation encompass most systems of the body including the musculoskeletal, gynecologic, urologic, and neurologic systems. Electricity can be applied to the body to treat (commercial stimulators) or to diagnose (nerve conduction tests). Electricity from the body can be recorded to treat (biofeedback) or to diagnose (electromyography). Many indications have already been addressed in the section on therapeutic goals.

Electrotherapy has been long associated with pain management, muscle strengthening, and stimulation of denervated muscle. It also has a place in wound care, fracture healing, promotion of circulation, and edema management. It has been used to increase joint range of motion, deliver medications through the skin (iontophoresis), replace orthotics, reduce spasm, and reduce scoliosis.

CONTRAINDICATIONS

The contraindications of electrical stimulation are relatively few. Pregnancy should be considered a contraindication even when applied to an area distant from the abdomen. Pain management with electrical current during labor is occasionally used.

Electrical current can interfere with the functioning of a pacemaker. A demand pacemaker senses the heart activity and responds accordingly. A pulse from an external stimulator could deceive a demand pacemaker into suppressing needed rhythms or creating abnormal rhythms.[23] Fixed pacemakers could be affected by signals through the leads.

Electrical stimulation should not be used in the presence of other electrical implanted stimulators, in patients with cardiac arrhythmic instability, or in cases with cardiac conduction disturbances. A stable cardiac patient with a history of angina or myocardial infarction may receive electrical stimulation, but electrodes must be placed cautiously avoiding current flow across midline in the chest area. The patient should be monitored with an ECG initially and then closely monitored during treatment. Some therapists do not apply electrical stimulation to a patient with cardiac disease, stable or not.

Cancer is treated as a contraindication because of the risk of metastasis. This contraindication is sometimes waived in favor of the pain relief when patients are in advanced stages.

Stimulation should not be performed adjacent to or distal to an area of thrombophlebitis or phlebothrombosis because of risk of emboli. Many therapists treat these conditions as totally contraindicated for an electrical stimulation treatment.

Electrical stimulation should not be used in the presence of active tuberculosis. It should not be done over the carotid sinus or in areas of active hemorrhage.

PRECAUTIONS

Electrical stimulation should be used cautiously in the presence of obesity. Fat is an electrical insulator and stimulation is generally not well tolerated. Greater-than-normal current levels are often required to achieve the desired physiologic effect.[23]

Caution should be exercised in areas of absent or diminished sensation. Areas of abnormal impedance should be avoided. Electrical currents can exacerbate eczema, psoriasis, acne, dermatitis, and can spread infections.[20] Patients including those with diabetes with thin fragile skin could be at risk for breakdown.

Peripheral neuropathies may prevent generation of muscle contractions at stimulation levels that are comfortable and safe.[23] Areas of denervation will not respond to any form of current other than DC.

In the presence of metal, either internal or external fixation devices, electrodes should be positioned with the metal well outside the pathway of current.

The patient should be cleared for active exercise in protocols requiring motor levels of stimulation. Care should be taken that the force of contraction is within a tolerated and permitted range of motion.[23]

Judgment is necessary to determine if electrical stimulation should be applied to any patient who is unable to follow instructions or provide feedback to the therapist. The treatment must be closely supervised if the decision is made to deliver the electrical stimulation.

Stimulation to patients with spinal cord injury may enhance an episode of dysreflexia.[23]

CLINICAL TREATMENT DECISIONS

SAFETY OF THE TREATMENT ENVIRONMENT

Equipment and User

Electrical shock is the response of the body to any electrical exposure that places the person within the circuit. This statement has just described treatment with electrical stimulation. The clinician must be aware of the potential dangers of applying electrical current and the measures assuring safe treatment.

The magnitude of electrical shock depends on the amount of *current* (amperes) forced into the body. Currents between 100 and 200 mA are lethal.[40] Physiologic reactions to current intensities follow a progression of sensation, muscle contraction, fibrillation, defibrillation, burns.[41] Electrical shock is first perceived as a faint tingling by sensory nerves around 1 mA. Current levels as low as several microamperes have been perceived by the finger tips.[35] Motor response usually occurs at levels above 5 mA. *Let-go current* is the maximum current level allowing the voluntary release of the current source and emphasizes the danger of AC over DC. The motor response to DC is a twitch, whereas AC causes a holding or tetanizing contraction. The ability to *let go* may be lost at current levels around 20 mA.[42] This value increases with pulsatile currents. The intrapulse and interpulse intervals provide current interruptions. Breathing can become labored at 20 mA and cease before 75 mA.[40] Uncoordinated twitching of the heart's ventricles (ventricular fibrillation) occurs at levels greater than 80 mA.[39] The heart will maintain a sustained contraction (ventricular defibrillation) at 6 A (6000 mA) and return to normal rhythm if exposure to current at that level is of short duration.[43] Burns occur at current levels above 12 A.

Electrical shock is either *macroshock* or *microshock*. Macroshock is a perceptible current at levels of greater or equal to 1 mA.[39] It occurs when current is introduced to the body through the skin and enters the body cavity. Microshock is below perceptible range and result from exposure to currents below 1 mA applied directly to the myocardium.[39] The current bypasses skin and enters the heart directly through cardiac catheter tips or myocardial electrodes. Pacemakers can be very susceptible to microshock through the pacemaker wires. The upper safety limit margin of current passing directly to the heart is 10 μA.[42]

Body tissues offer resistance to the passage of current. Skin resistance protects internal organs from shock and determines how much current enters. This resistance varies between people and varies within the individual depending on point of contact and skin hydration. Dry skin offers around 500,000 Ω of resistance, whereas moist skin offers approximately 1000 Ω.[40] This protective resistance is bypassed when an invasive electrode is used, but the use of this type of electrode is not common practice clinically.

Electric power is delivered to the machine through the ends of two wires having an electrical potential of 115 V between them. The *live* (hot) wire has the high potential. The *neutral* wire has 0 potential and connects to the ground. The term *ground* refers to anything with an electrical connection to the earth. Earth is an inexhaustible source of electrons and is capable of accepting or donating large quantities of charge.[16] Generally, current flows from the live wire through the electrical unit back to the neutral wire and earth.[14] An exchange occurs between charged bodies and earth. A positively charged body will take electrons and a negatively charged body will give electrons to earth. Current flows. *Grounded* means there is no difference in potential between the conductor and earth, so current will not flow.

One potential clinical hazard is direct contact with the live wire circuit through a frayed power cord or an outlet problem.[42] Another possible hazard, *earth shock*, results from an indirect connection made between the live wire and the ground.[14] The live wire, possibly because of faulty or old insulation, makes contact inside of the machine with its casing. A person touching the casing and standing on the ground draws this current and completes a circuit between the live wire and the ground. Newer machines are now usually cased in plastic or other insulating material. Earth shock can also result from a phenomenon called *leakage* or *stray* current. It is an inherent flow of a small amount of current from the live circuit along an insulating surface such as the casing or accessories. Electric shocks can also result from contact with grounded objects such as water pipes, damp floor, and radiators during electrical treatments.

Earth shock can be avoided by a grounding wire that provides the path of least resistance from the machine casing to earth. The grounding wire, normally not conducting current, triggers a fuse on the live wire when electrical problems cause current to flow through it. This stops current flow and alert the operator to a problem. A polarized outlet and three-pronged plug provide this grounding circuit. The outlet receptacle has three slots, a small rectangular one for the live wire connection, a larger rectangular one for the neutral wire connection, and a round opening for the ground wire connection. This protective round pin is longer than the rectangular prongs, assuring that the ground wire is the first wire connected to the circuit and the last unplugged.[20]

Failure of the grounding wire to be connected in the building to a ground source or breaking of the ground wire in the receptacle can go undetected, creating a potential hazard. The electrical system is believed to be safe when in actuality the grounding circuit is nonfunctional. A ground fault interrupter (GFI) is a sensor shutting down the electrical circuit when it senses changes in electrical potentials, impedance, or an increase in normal leakage current levels.

Preventive maintenance is necessary to assure electrical safety in the treatment area. New equipment purchased should have the Underwriters' Laboratory (UL) approval seal, assuring the maximum degree of safety.[16] Table 10–5 outlines other safety guidelines that should be observed in the clinic. Electrical safety comes with awareness and knowledge. The clinician should always read the manufacturer's manual and be sure that he or she understands the limitations of the unit as well as its safety features.

Table 10–5 **Electrical Safety in the Clinic**

Replacement of standard outlets with ground fault interrupters (GFI).

Replacement of plugs with hospital-grade UL (Underwriters' Laboratory) plugs with green dot.

Yearly maintenance checks of all electrical equipment by biomedical engineer.

Dated inspection sticker affixed to all electrical units.

Unplug equipment not in use.

Disconnect machines from outlet receptacles by plug not cord.

Frequently check the integrity of plugs, cords, and electrical stimulation leads for fraying or disruptions.

Report loose-gripping connections between plug and outlet receptacles.

Never use extension cords.

Never use cheater adapters allowing three-pronged plugs to be used in two-pronged receptacles.

Do not use electrical equipment near objects or environments that draw current.

Post sign notifying usage of equipment that may interfere with pacemakers.

Patient Factors

Patient Education   The public is familiar with electricity and the potential for shock and electrocution. Many patients may be initially fearful of treatment. A patient may be anxious or reluctant to place their foot in a tub of water containing two electrical pads.

The key to successful treatment is patient education and cooperation. The questions concerning patient education that must be posed are *what* and *how much*. It has been proven that information can sometimes increase and develop stressful feelings that might not have been present ordinarily.[44] Two types of coping styles are identified. There are those people who seek information to get through an aversive event and there are those people who would rather not know anything. Patients treated according to their coping style exhibited increased tolerance levels to electrical stimulation.[44]

Certain safety instructions are necessary. Information that must be given includes the sensation of treatment and instructions concerning touching of controls, changing body position, and calling the therapist when there is a problem or change in sensation. Informational material includes the goal and expected outcome of treatment, number of expected treatment sessions, and the treatment time. Patients using the unit at home require more detailed instructions on how the unit works, application of electrodes, purpose and consequence of dial adjustments, how to protect the skin and inspect area before and after treatment, and under what circumstances to discontinue treatment. Written instructions should be given, especially diagrams of electrode placement.[45]

Equipment Positioning   Electrical stimulation delivered by a line-powered unit (versus battery unit) should be administered in a predetermined area within the clinical setting where appropriate outlets (GFIs) have been installed. Electrical equipment generates heat and should be well ventilated. Equipment should not be placed next to water pipes, radiators, or other sources that may draw current, creating a shock hazard. The machine should be situated close to the wall outlet to avoid tension on the cord and possible tripping over cords. Positioning of the electrical stimulation unit must allow easy access to the therapist for adjustment of controls as well as avoiding excessive tension on lead wires or a situation where the patient is able to adjust parameters without supervision. The patient should be informed as to which dial controls the amplitude and how to turn it down. The current interruption switch should be easily accessed.

Skin Inspection The intensity of stimulation is guided by the patient's response and tolerance level. A sensory assessment of the treatment area is essential to establish patient reliability. The skin must be carefully inspected before electrodes are applied. Skin tone and color should be assessed for indications of circulatory impairment and fragility that could result in breakdown or tissue damage. The skin should be examined for conditions affecting skin impedance such as edema, ischemia, scars, skin lesions, and abrasions. Areas of abnormally high impedance require increased current levels for penetration. Areas of abnormally low impedance draw current and increase total current in a small area. Tissue damage could result from either situation. Abrasions and open areas that cannot be insulated with petroleum jelly should not be treated unless treatment objective is wound healing.

Patient Positioning

The basic tenets of positioning are patient comfort and accessibility to the treatment area. There are several considerations specific to electrical stimulation. Positioning should permit enough slack in lead wires from machine to electrodes so that connections will not disengage during treatment. Firm contact and securing of electrodes will influence choice of position. Some placement sites may require the patient's body weight on the electrodes. The patient must be in a position to use a call button or disengage the machine if a problem arises.

The Treatment

A training period may be necessary with electrical stimulation, and required stimulation levels may not be achieved during the first session. Patient anxiety can sometimes be relieved by allowing the patient control of increasing the amplitude dial.

Muscle contraction time can be limited to 5- to 7-second peaks with low-level repetitions of 10 to 15 contractions the first treatment to prevent initial soreness.[34] On and off times have a high ratio initially but are reduced in subsequent treatments with conditioning.

The patient should be asked if he or she feels tingling in all areas of the electrode. The electrode could be secured improperly or losing its conductivity if the answer is no. If the patient is not feeling any sensation at all as amplitude is increased past a point where sensory fibers should fire, stop immediately and *drop the amplitude control back down to zero before making any adjustments.* Most contemporary machines have reset controls to protect against high levels of current surging into the patient when machines are energized with current levels up. These types of controls require that amplitude dials be clicked off prior to increasing the amplitude. Never increase amplitude during the off phase of the current cycle.

Clinical judgment must be exercised as to when a treatment should be discontinued because of physical or mental intolerance, preventing the safe achievement of intended goals.

The electrical stimulation treatment can be divided into pretreatment, delivery, posttreatment, and recording steps. Patient comfort, tolerance, and safety are priorities. The manufacturer's instruction manual must be carefully read, understood, and followed. The following general guidelines will only assist with sequencing the treatment.

Pretreatment

- Machine wires and electrode check (inspection dates should be periodically checked).
- Patient education.
- Machine is plugged into the wall.
- Turn the machine power switch on.
- Patient is positioned.
- Skin in treatment area is inspected; gross assessment of sensation.
- Electrical stimulation machine is positioned.
- Electrode placement sites are determined.
- Treatment area is washed; electrodes are prepared and secured.
- Preset parameters on machine area adjusted such as frequency, pulse and phase duration, delivery mode (interrupted or continuous), on-off time, ramp, choice of polarity, treatment timer.
- Make sure amplitude dials are on zero.

Delivery

- Increase amplitude to stimulation level but always within patient's tolerance.
- Ask patient *what do they feel* and *where do they feel it.*
- Adjust any parameters requiring modification.
- Stay with patient for several minutes to monitor reaction, tolerance, and appropriate amplitude level.
- Continue to monitor patient reaction and tolerance periodically through treatment.

Posttreatment

- Turn amplitude to zero.
- Remove electrodes.
- Turn machine power off.
- Inspect treatment area.
- Note all variables set for treatment and document.
- Unplug unit from wall receptacle.

Documentation   Documentation must be thorough and inclusive. Notes must stand up under close scrutiny in this age of liability and reimbursement. The written note assures consistent replication of treatment; is a written record describing the patient's physical state, reactions, and progress; validates treatment success or failure to determine effectiveness; and justifies treatment for appropriate reimbursement.

The general elements of the electrotherapy note include the problem, goal, treatment given, skin status, electrode technique, electrode size, number and placement of electrodes, commercial stimulation unit used, electrical parameters of treatment, treatment time, and response to treatment.

An electrical parameter that can be set on the machine or determined from a readout must be documented. Give specific settings for all parameters adjusted. Documented parameters may include, but are not limited to, current type (AC, DC, pulsed), waveform (*monophasic*, *biphasic*, polyphasic), peak amplitude (amperes or volts), frequency, phase duration, delivery mode (continuous, interrupted), on-off times, phase charge, polarity, specific modulations used (bursts, ramps), and clinical stimulation level (subsensory, sensory, motor, or noxious).

SUMMARY

Each electrical parameter dictates a specific response in the body and intimately relates to many other parameters. The pulse and current variables form a delicate web of cause and effect.

An electrical stimulation unit must be assessed in terms of its electrical features as "yes, effective to accomplish goal" or "no, lacking the necessary features for this use."

The electrotherapeutic field is growing and changing. New current waveforms, stimulator units, treatment features, and applications will be a part of this growth. The clinician who understands the basic concepts of electricity, terminology, relationships between electrical parameters, and effect on body tissue will be able to execute treatment confidently.

DISCUSSION QUESTIONS

1. What electrical parameters affect the sensation of current?

2. An electrical stimulation treatment requires a small charge accumulation in the tissues. Discuss the reasons for choosing or not choosing the different waveforms.

3. Discuss the different relationships interplaying between phase duration, frequency, interpulse interval, peak amplitude, total current, and phase charge. Which of these terms describe the single pulse and which a series of pulses?

4. Distinguish the difference between the following terms: (a) ramp time and rise time; (b) intrapulse interval, interpulse interval, and off times; (c) pulse and burst.

5. How does Ohm's law apply to constant-current and constant-voltage output stimulators?

REFERENCES

1.   Watkins, AL: A Manual of Electrotherapy. Lea & Febiger, Philadelphia, 1962.

2.   Electrotherapy Standards Committee of the Section on Clinical Electrophysiology of the American Physical Therapy Association: Electrotherapeutic Terminology in Physical Therapy. Section on Clinical Electrophysiology and the American Physical Therapy Association, Alexandria, 1990.

3.   McNeal, DR: 2000 years of electrical stimulation. In Hambrect, T and Reswick, JB (eds): Functional Electrical Stimulation: Application in Neural Prosthesis, vol 3. Marcel Dekker, New York, 1977.

4.   Geddes, LA: A short history of the electrical stimulation of excitable tissue. Physiologist (Suppl) 27:S-1, 1984.

5.   Licht, S: History of electrotherapy. In Stillwell, GK (ed): Therapeutic Electricity and Ultraviolet Radiation, ed 3. Williams & Wilkins, Baltimore/London, 1983.

6.   Licht, S: History of electrodiagnosis. In Licht, S (ed): Electrodiagnosis and Electromyography, ed 3. Elizabeth Licht, New Haven, 1971.

7.   Marcello, P: The Ambiguous Frog: The Galvani-Volta Controversy on Animal Electricity. Translated by Mandelbaum, J. Princeton University Press, Princeton, 1992.

8.   Bleese, PK, et al: Implanted cardiac pacemakers: Clinical experience and evaluation. Med Prog Technol 1:69, 1972.

9.   Ko, WH: Instrumentation for neuromuscular stimulation. In Hambrect, T and Reswick, JB (eds): Functional Electrical Stimulation: Application in Neural Prosthesis. Marcel Dekker, New York, 1977.

10.   Nashold, BS, Somjen, G, and Friedman, H: The effects of stimulating the dorsal columns of man. Med Prog Technol 1:89, 1972.

11.   Shealy, CN: Electrical control of the nervous system. Med Progr Technol 2:71, 1974.

12.   Mills, PM, Deakin, M, and Kiff, ES: Percutaneous electrical stimulation for ano-rectal incontinence. Physiother 76:433, 1990.

13.   Shelley, T: Implanted stimulators for the control of urinary incontinence: The physicians and patients standpoint. Med Prog Technol 1:82, 1972.

14.   Forster, A and Palastanga, N: Clayton's Electrotherapy: Theory and Practice, ed 8. Bailliere Tindall Books, London, 1981.

15.   Kukulka, CG: Principles of neuromuscular excitation. In Gersh, MR (ed): Electrotherapy in Rehabilitation. FA Davis, Philadelphia, 1992.

16.   Buban, P and Schmitt, M: Technical Electricity and Electronics, ed 2. McGraw-Hill, New York, 1977.

17.   Patterson, RP: Instrumentation for electrotherapy. In Stillwell, GK (ed): Therapeutic Electricity and Ultraviolet Radiation, ed 3. Williams & Wilkins, Baltimore, 1983.

18.   Binder, SA: Applications of low- and high-voltage electrotherapeutic currents. In Wolf, SL: Electrotherapy. Churchill Livingston, Edinburgh, 1981.

19.   Killian, CB: Basic electricity overview: Seminar on high voltage galvanic stimulation theory and practice. 1984.

20.   Wadsworth, J and Chanmugam, A: Electrophysical Agents in Physiotherapy: Therapeutic and Diagnostic Use, 2d ed. Science Press, Marrickville, 1983.

21.   Alon, G and De Domenico, G: High Voltage Stimulation: An Integrated Approach to Clinical Electrotherapy. Chattanooga Corporation, Chattanooga, 1987.

22. Kahn, AR and Maveus, TC: Technical aspects of electrical stimulation devices. Med Prog Technol 1:58, 1972.

23. Benton, LA, et al.: Functional Electrical Stimulation: A Practical Clinical Guide, ed 2. Ranchos Los Amigos Rehabilitation Engineering Center, Downey, CA, 1981.

24. Ross, CR and Segal, D: High voltage galvanic stimulation: An aid to post-operative healing. Curr Podiatr, reprint May 1981.

25. Gracanin, F and Trnkoxzy, A: Optimal stimulation parameters for minimum pain in the chronic stimulation of innervated muscle. Arch Phys Med Rehabil 56:243, 1975.

26. Baker, LL, et al.: Effect of carrier frequency on comfort with medium frequency electrical stimulation (abstract). Phys Ther 69:373, 1979.

27. Bowman, BR and Baker, LL: Effects of waveform parameters on comfort during transcutaneous neuromuscular electrical stimulation. Ann Biomed Eng 13:59, 1985.

28. Delitto, A and Rose, SJ: Comparative comfort of three waveforms used in electrically eliciting quadriceps femoris muscle contractions. Phys Ther 66:1704, 1986.

29. Baker, LL, et al: Waveform and comfort of electrical stimulation in the upper extremity (abstract). Phys Ther 69:372, 1989.

30. Alon, G: High voltage stimulation: Effects of electrode size on basic excitatory responses. Phys Ther 65:890, 1985.

31. Honert, C and Mortimer, JT: The response to the myelinated nerve fiber to short duration biphasic stimulating currents. Ann Biomed Eng 7:117, 1979.

32. Li, CL and Bak, A: Excitability characteristics of the A- and C-fibers in a peripheral nerve. Exp Neurol 50:67, 1976.

33. Howson, DC: Peripheral neural excitability: Implications for transcutaneous electrical nerve stimulation. Phys Ther 58:1467, 1978.

34. Alon, G: Northeast Seminars: Electrosynthesis (A Lab Course). Course Publication, 1993.

35. Reilly, JP: Electrical Stimulation and Electropathology. Cambridge University Press, USA/Victoria, 1992.

36. Charman, RA: Cellular reception and emission of electromagnetic signals. Physiotherapy 76:509, 1990.

37. Crago, PE, et al: The choice of pulse duration for chronic electrical stimulation via surface, nerve and intramuscular electrodes. Ann Biomed Eng 2:252, 1974.

38. Ray, CD and Maurer, DD: A review of neural stimulator system components useful in pain alleviation. Med Prog Technol 2:121, 1974.

39. Myklebust, BM and Kloth, L: Electrodiagnostic and electrotherapeutic instrumentation: Characteristics of recording and stimulation systems and principles of safety. In Gersh, MR (ed): Electrotherapy in Rehabilitation. FA Davis, Philadelphia, 1992.

40. Clinic Notes: The fatal current. Phys Ther 46:968, 1966.

41. Sances, A, et al: Electrical injuries. Surg Gynecol Obstet 149:97, 1979.

42. Berger, WH: Electrical shock hazards in the physical therapy department. Clin Manag 5:24, 1994.

43. Bruner, JM and Leonard, PF: Electricity, Safety and the Patient. Yearbook, Chicago, 1989.

44. Delitto, A, et al: A study of discomfort with electrical stimulation. Phys Ther 72:11, 1992.

45. Lampe, GN: Introduction to the use of transcutaneous electrical nerve stimulation devices. Phys Ther 58:1450, 1978.

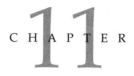

Physiologic Basis of Electrical Stimulation

Cecilia Mullin, PTA
Elizabeth R. Gardner, MS, PT, NCS

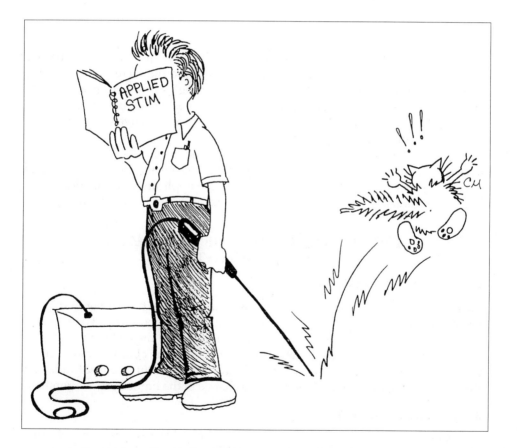

CHAPTER OBJECTIVES

- Review the physiologic basis of nerve and muscle excitation.
- Outline and describe the influencing factors of stimulatory currents.
- Describe the principles of safe and efficacious use of electrical stimulation.

The purpose of this chapter is twofold: first, to review the physiologic basis of nerve and muscle excitation, and second, to describe the factors that influence whether a stimulating current being delivered through surface electrodes is sufficient to cause excitation. An understanding of the mechanism by which electrical stimulation affects tissues in its current path is critical to delivering appropriate, effective, comfortable, and safe treatment.

Prior knowledge of the muscular system and neurophysiology is expected as a basis for reading this chapter. It is the intention of the authors to highlight important aspects of physiology as they relate to the application of electrical stimulation. Additional readings have been suggested at the end of the chapter.

PHYSIOLOGIC BASIS OF NERVE AND MUSCLE EXCITATION

CHARACTERISTICS OF EXCITABLE CELLS

There are unique properties that distinguish excitable cells from other living cells. Nerve and muscle cells are examples of excitable cells, as opposed to fat or bone cells, which are not excitable. These unique properties include the ability to maintain a large electrical potential across the cell membrane and the ability to have this potential altered. This alteration occurs rapidly and transiently in response to adequate thermal, mechanical, chemical, or electrical change in the immediate environment.

Resting Membrane Potential

Although all living cells possess membranes capable of separating electrical charges, the charge across an excitable membrane is greater in magnitude. It is on the order of -60 to -90 millivolts (mV) for nerve and muscle cell membranes, with the inside negative in relationship to the outside. This resting membrane potential is the result of the unequal distribution of ions across the cell membrane. Each ion will try to equalize its concentration across the membrane. There are several factors that prevent this from happening, thereby contributing to an unequal distribution of ions across the cell membrane as depicted in Figure 11–1.

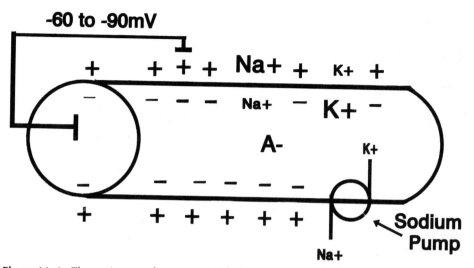

Figure 11–1. The resting membrane potential of a nerve axon, which results from the unequal ionic distribution across the membrane because of membrane permeability and an active sodium pump.

The cell membrane has an inherent permeability that causes it to act as a barrier to sodium (Na^+) while allowing potassium (K^+) to cross more freely. Since the membrane is about 20 times more permeable to K^+ than to Na^+, the resting membrane potential is close to the equilibrium potential for K^+, which is -90 mV. Also, large ions that are negatively charged are trapped within the cell, adding to the negative internal charge. The presence of an active sodium pump causes Na^+ to pump out the cell's interior against its electrochemical and concentration gradients. In this way, excitable cells actually expend metabolic energy to maintain the resting membrane potential. It is this resting membrane potential with a large electrochemical gradient for Na^+ that provides a ready source of potential energy for excitation.

Action Potential

As mentioned earlier, two properties unique to excitable membrane are the resting membrane potential and the ability to rapidly and transiently alter the potential across the membrane. Given a stimulus, the cell membrane will increase its permeability to Na^+. This is called a local excitatory response. As the number of Na^+ ions entering the cell increases, a reduction in negative charge called *depolarization* occurs. If this alteration in charge reaches a certain critical level, then the permeability to Na^+ will increase explosively; this critical level of depolarization is called the *threshold*. The rapid reversal of electrical potential that ensues following stimulation at threshold level or greater is called an *action potential* (AP); this is depicted in Figure 11–2.

The action potential is a brief event lasting only 1 to 2 milliseconds. During this event, the membrane potential rapidly changes from -70 to $+35$ mV as Na^+ rushes into the cell. When the permeability increases for Na^+, it also increases for K^+, but this change takes place more slowly and reaches its peak after the permeability to Na^+ has shut down. This causes the membrane to become hyperpolarized for a brief period as K^+ approaches its equilibrium potential of -90 mV. The potential across the membrane during this time is more negative than during the resting state. These changes in membrane permeability just described are transient. Following the action potential, the cell reverts to its previous permeability and the

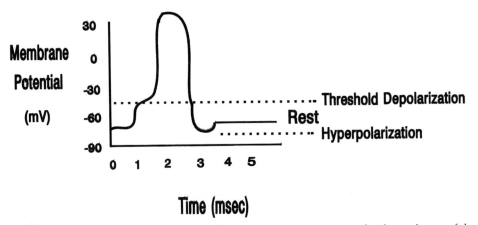

Figure 11–2. Changes in the membrane potential and the time course for these changes following application of a threshold stimulus to an excitable membrane.

sodium pump, through active transport, quickly restores the cell to its original resting membrane potential.

The depolarization phase of the action potential is called the *absolute refractory period*. Even in the presence of a threshold stimulus, another action potential cannot occur during this time. During the hyperpolarization phase, called the *relative refractory period*, the cell is capable of generating an action potential, but the stimulus has to be greater (suprathreshold) to compensate for the hyperpolarization. It is important to point out that the action potential is an "all-or-none" phenomenon, the amplitude of the action potential is always the same regardless of the strength of the stimulus. Once a threshold level of stimulation is reached, an action potential will occur. Additional increase of the stimulus amplitude will not change the size of the action potential.

PERIPHERAL NERVE STRUCTURE AND FUNCTION

Description of Structure

The neuron is the structural and functional unit of the nervous system. It is highly specialized to generate and transmit electrical signals. A peripheral nerve is one that lies outside of the brain or spinal cord. It comprises many nerve fibers (cells), called *neurons*, which can be sensory (afferent) or motor (efferent) in nature. As shown in Figure 11-3, the three main components of a neuron are its cell body, dendrites, and axon.

A neuron is confined by the cell membrane that provides its shape. The cell membrane controls the entry, transportation, and exit of material and helps to regulate the resting potential and the action potentials mentioned earlier. The entire cell is controlled by the central portion, called the *nucleus*. Information enters the cell through the dendrites, while the action of the axon is to send information from the cell body. Together the dendrites and the axon are known as *nerve fibers* or *nerve processes*.

All peripheral nerve axons are covered by a tube or sheath that is formed by Schwann cells. This sheath is called the *neurolemma* and provides structural support and protection for the axon. Some axons are myelinated, which means that they have a fatty (lipoprotein) layer in between the Schwann cell and the axon membrane. This fatty layer acts as an insulator. As shown in Figure 11–3, the myelin sheath is discontinuous, in other words, there are gaps at regular intervals. These gaps are known as *nodes of Ranvier*. Action potentials occur at nodes. The im-

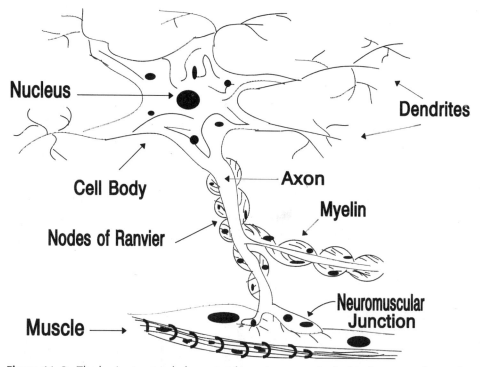

Figure 11–3. The basic structural elements of a motor nerve, including its connection to the muscle and the neuromuscular junction.

pulse moves along from node to node as if jumping; this phenomenon is termed *saltatory conduction.* An unmyelinated nerve fiber, on the other hand, does not have fat insulation and so does not have gaps (nodes), so movement of the impulse along these axons is continuous but slow.

For messages to travel from neuron to neuron, there is a junction called a *synapse,* and the impulse must cross this gap for it to continue along the nerve pathway. This occurs via release of a chemical neurotransmitter. When the nerve fiber meets the muscle fiber, another junction is formed, called the *neuromuscular junction* or the *motor endplate.* At this junction, the nerve fiber forms nerve terminals that lie within the muscle just above the muscle fiber membrane. As with the nerve-to-nerve junction, the message is transmitted across the nerve-to-muscle junction via a neurotransmitter. A muscle contraction occurs when there is adequate depolarization of the muscle membrane by the motor nerve at the neuromuscular junction.

Classification

A peripheral nerve was described earlier as carrying sensory information, motor information, or both. The major differences among peripheral nerve axons relate to physical size and membrane properties. Nerve fibers are generally classed into three categories known as A, B, and C. The A fibers are the largest, are myelinated, and are motor and sensory in function. B fibers, also myelinated, are smaller and carry motor and sensory visceral information. C fibers are the smallest and are unmyelinated. A good example of information carried by a C fiber is poorly localized pain that you feel when you scratch your skin (cutaneous), or pain from within the body cavity (visceral) (Table 11–1).

Table 11-1 Mammalian Nerve Fiber Types and Characteristics

Fiber Type	Fiber Diameter (μm)	Conduction Velocity (m/sec)	Spike Duration (ms)	Absolute Refactory Period (ms)	Peripheral Organ	Receptor Organ	Function
A fibers (motor)							
alpha	12–20	70–120	0.4–0.5	0.4–1	Muscle		Somatic motor
gamma	3–6	15–30					Motor to muscle spindle
A fibers (sensory)							
Group Ia						Annulospiral spindle endings	
Group Ib	12–20	70–120	0.4–0.5	0.4–1	Muscle	Tendon organs of Golgi	Proprioception

Group II						
beta	5–12	30–70	0.4–0.5	0.4–1	1. Extensor muscles	Flower spray of spindle
					2. Flexor muscles	Flower spray of spindle
					3. Skin	Touch pressure receptors
Group III					1. Muscle	Unknown pain receptors(?)
delta	5–12	12–30	0.4–0.5	0.4–1	2. Skin	Pain
B fibers	1–3	3–15	1.2	1.2		
C fibers						
Group IV	0.5–1	0.5–2	2	2	Muscle and skin	Pain

Touch, pressure, vibratory receptors

Pain—(fast?), temperature (cold, heat)

Preganglionic sympathetic

Pain—(slow), temperature, mechanoreceptors

Source: From Baker, L., et al,[2] p 8, with permission.

These differences in nerve fibers have a functional impact. In general, the greater the fiber diameter, the faster the conduction velocity, the lower the threshold, the larger the action potential, and the shorter the duration of the action potential and refractory period. Since these different nerve fibers often travel together, application of an electrical stimulus may cause the desired motor response, but it may also cause excitation of autonomic fibers (which can cause goosebumps or sweating), or pain fibers (which can hurt) if the stimulus is sufficiently strong. So, when you apply an electrical stimulus to a peripheral nerve, you tend to recruit nearby large sensory fibers first (proprioceptive), followed by large motor nerve fibers that supply many muscle fibers. As you continue to increase the stimulus intensity, you will meet or exceed threshold for more and more nerve fibers, including small pain fibers and possibly autonomic fibers. This is why electrical stimulation can be perceived as painful; however, careful choice of stimulus parameters can minimize this discomfort. This is discussed in more detail in Chapters 10 and 12.

Propagation

Propagation is a movement or a cause of movement through a medium. In this case, it is the electrical impulse (action potential) that is moving along the nerve membrane. Propagation allows the nerve impulse to travel to another nerve or to a muscle to create a contraction. At rest, a cell membrane is positive on the outside and negative on the inside. Reversal of this polarity (charge) accompanying an action potential leads to local current flow in both directions away from the initial point of depolarization. This triggers an action potential along the length of the cell membrane. The local current flow initiated by the original action potential is called an *eddy current*. This is depicted in Figure 11–4A. These currents cause threshold depolarization of the neighboring membrane, initiating an adjacent action potential. In this way, the entire surface of the cell membrane will gradually become excited and the impulse can be propagated along the entire cell.

The distance that the current will spread depends on the membrane resistance, the internal longitudinal resistance of the nerve fiber (axoplasmic resistance), and the radius of the nerve fiber. It follows according to this formula:

$$\text{Propagation distance} = \text{fiber radius} \times \text{membrane resistance} / \text{axoplasmic resistance.}$$

Large nerve fibers have a greater radius and less axoplasmic resistance and, therefore, they have greater longitudinal conduction. In addition, myelin acts to increase the membrane resistance, thereby increasing the distance the current will flow.

The speed of propagation varies with nerve characteristics, including size and myelination. Myelination acts to increase speed of propagation because eddy currents do not have to cross the membrane except at the nodes of Ranvier, where the myelin is thin (Fig. 11–4B). The time it takes for a voltage change to occur across the membrane is determined by the product of its resistance and capacitance (charge storing capability) called the *time constant*. Since a large nerve axon has a lower longitudinal resistance compared to a smaller axons, the membrane can become depolarized more quickly and therefore the current can spread faster. In addition, myelination acts to decrease the capacitance of large nerves, which also increases conduction velocity.

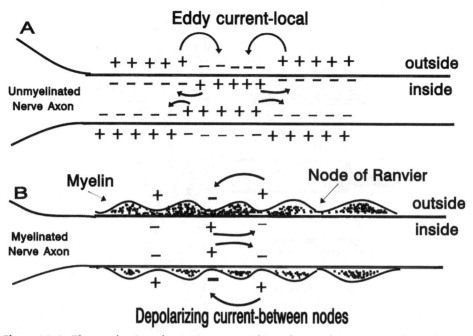

Figure 11–4. The conduction of an action potential impulse *(A)* along an unmyelinated nerve via local eddy current and *(B)* along a myelinated nerve via saltatory conduction.

SKELETAL MUSCLE STRUCTURE AND PHYSIOLOGY OF CONTRACTION

Skeletal Muscle Structure and Organization

Our skeletal muscles enable us to move. These muscles are attached to bones via tendons and in combination produce movement that our nervous system controls. Muscles contract in order to allow us to remain upright against the force of gravity (postural control) and they act to move us from place to place. In order to better understand how a muscle produces movement, it is necessary to understand its intricate structural organization (Fig. 11–5).

A skeletal muscle is made up of thousands of small muscle fibers. Each muscle fiber is covered by a cell membrane called the *sarcolemma,* and within the interior of the muscle fiber, there are bundles of protein called *myofibrils.* Up to several thousand myofibrils can be contained in a muscle fiber. They are described as having a banded appearance or striated appearance, which can be seen throughout the entire length of the myofibril. The striation is cause by the interchange of light and dark bands called *myofilaments* that contain the contractile proteins actin (thin) and myosin (thick). Each myofibril contains two types of myofilaments that are thin or thick in size and is divided along its length into many sections called *sarcomeres.* The beginning and end of each sarcomere is marked by dark Z disk. The thin myofilaments are attached to the Z disk and they extend less than half of the length of the sarcomere. The thick myofilaments are in the middle of the sarcomere and are interdigitated with the thin filaments.

Motor Unit

The basic functional unit of a muscle is the motor unit. A motor unit comprises a motoneuron and all the muscle fibers supplied by that neuron. In the absence of

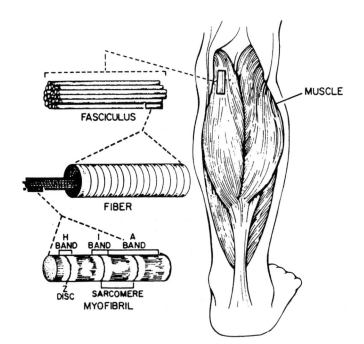

Figure 11–5. Successive levels of the structural organization of muscle. (*From Baker, L, et al,*[2] *p 14, with permission.*)

pathology, the activation of one motor unit is the minimum level of contraction obtainable. Motor units vary in size according to their specific function. Small motor units are found in muscles where fine control of movement is necessary, such as those of the face. In a small motor unit, a single neuron may supply only a few muscle fibers; therefore, the movement generated can be very precisely controlled. There may be up to several thousand muscle fibers in a large motor unit. Large motor units are typically found in muscles where force production is more important than fine control such as in the leg muscles.

Excitation and Contraction of the Muscle

The structural organization of the muscle fiber forms the basis for function, that is, how the muscle contracts. Muscle shortening results from the thin myofilaments sliding between the thick myofilaments. In order to accomplish this, the thick filaments have tiny bridges that link them with the thin filaments. These bridges, like oars in a rowboat, break contact with the thin filaments and reconnect at a site closer to the center to pull them closer together; this is known as the sliding filament theory. Thus, the length of each sarcomere shortens, causing the length of the entire muscle to decrease. At rest, the muscle is at its optimum length to develop tension. It is assumed that the resting length of the muscle provides optimal overlap of the thick and thin filaments. If the muscle is stretched beyond its resting length, the tension it can develop will decrease because there will be less overlap between the filaments. Conversely, if the muscle is shorter than the resting length (on slack), it will again develop less tension, which is an important consideration when designing a neuromuscular stimulation program.

Adequate stimulation from a motor nerve initiates a muscle action potential that results in a muscle contraction. This excitation occurs at a specialized site called the *neuromuscular junction* (Fig. 11–6). The nerve action potential causes acetylcholine, a neurotransmitter, to be released. Acetylcholine crosses the synapse and causes depolarization of the muscle cell membrane. It is excitation of the muscle cell membrane that causes the chain of events that allows actin and myosin to bind so that the muscle contracts.

When a nerve action potential initiates a muscle action potential, the excitation is propagated by the sarcolemma, which surrounds each muscle fiber through an elaborate membrane system called the T system (tubule system). This system is responsible for conducting current to the interior of the muscle fiber. Within the muscle fiber, each myofibril is wrapped in a sleeve called the *sarcoplasmic reticulum*. At regular intervals, there are sacs along the sleeve that contain calcium and the action potential is carried along the T-system to the sacs of the sarcoplasmic reticulum causing them to release this calcium. It is this release that allows the formation of cross bridges leading to shortening of the muscle (Fig. 11-7).

A twitch is a contraction of the muscle fiber. This happens when adequate membrane depolarization of the muscle occurs as a result of a nerve action potential. This twitch response of a muscle fiber to a single threshold stimulus is from its motor nerve and cannot be graded by varying the intensity of the stimulus; however, the magnitude of a single fiber response can be altered by the timing of the excitatory stimulus. This is because the contraction time of a muscle is much slower than its action potential. The action potential of a muscle lasts a few milliseconds, whereas, depending on the muscle fiber type, the twitch may last 25 to 75 milliseconds. As shown in Figure 11–8, if one action potential is immediately followed by another, the second twitch can occur before the first one has time to relax. If the tension developed during one twitch overlaps (fuses) with the next

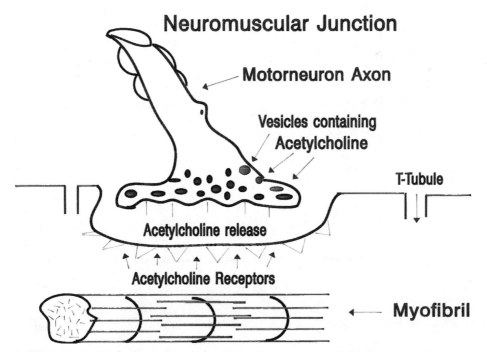

Figure 11–6. The basic structural elements of the neuromuscular junction are shown.

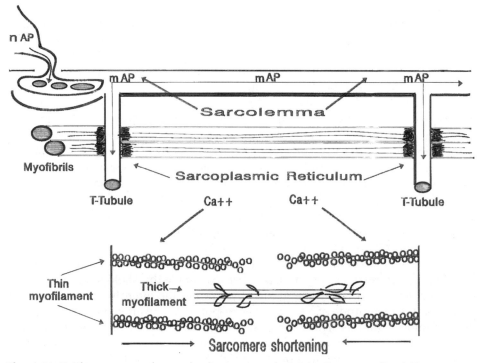

Figure 11–7. The sequence of events leading to a muscle contraction are outlined. First, a nerve action potential (nAP) generates a muscle action potential (mAP), which is propagated along the T system. This causes the sarcoplasmic reticulum to release calcium, which allows the actin (thin myofilament) and myosin (thick myofilament) to bind and the muscle to shorten.

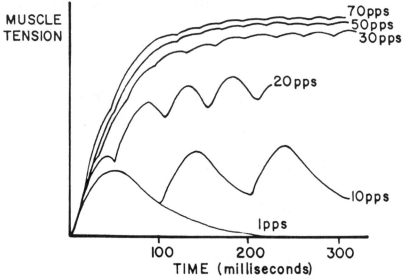

Figure 11–8. A single muscle twitch is shown in the lower left-hand corner. This is followed by successive muscle twitches at various frequencies. As the interval between the stimuli is shortened, the muscle does not have time to relax between stimuli. When the stimuli become sufficiently frequent, the twitches fuse and cannot be individually distinguished. *(From Baker, L, et al,[2] p 16, with permission.)*

successive twitch, the tension will be cumulative. If successive twitches are completely fused, the contraction is said to be tetanic.

The frequency of stimuli necessary for a tetanic contraction is said to be the critical fusion frequency and depends on the duration of the muscle twitch. This is different for muscle fibers that primarily use oxygen for metabolism (type I) compared to those that use glycogen (type II). Type I (slow-twitch) fibers have a twitch time of about 75 milliseconds, so fusion occurs at about 13 hertz (Hz). Type II (fast-twitch) fibers have a twitch time of 25 milliseconds, so fusion occurs at about 40 Hz. Therefore, increasing the frequency of stimulation beyond 50 to 60 Hz will not produce much of an increase in muscle force (tension), because the twitches are already maximally overlapped.

Motor Unit Recruitment

The strength of a contraction is graded by the number of motor units that are recruited. For instance, when the amplitude of electrical stimulation is increased, more motor units are recruited because the stimulus reaches threshold for more and more motor units. As this occurs, the strength of the contraction becomes greater because more muscle fibers are contracting.

When we voluntarily contract a muscle, we recruit small motor units first, so that smooth and gradual tension will be developed. Also, small motor units are usually made up of type I muscle fibers and tend to be fatigue resistant, so that the first motor units to be recruited may sustain the longest contraction. Large motor units are recruited as contraction strength increases. However, the order of motor unit recruitment is reversed with electrical stimulation. Large, superficial motor units are recruited first; these tend to be made up of fast-twitch muscle fibers (type II). Development of tension is therefore not as gradual as it is with voluntary contraction, and these motor units tend to fatigue rapidly.

There is another difference between contractions evoked by electrical stimulation compared to those produced voluntarily. During a voluntary contraction, motor units are activated asynchronously. While a voluntarily contraction is maintained, motor units are constantly turning on and off in an alternate fashion. This is highly energy efficient and delays fatigue. Asynchronous firing of motor units also helps to maintain smooth steady tension. On the other hand, as long as an electrically stimulated contraction is maintained, active motor units are constantly responding to the stimulus. This is called synchronous recruitment, and unlike asynchronous contraction, is very fatiguing to the muscle. The combination of reversed recruitment order and synchronous recruitment makes electrically stimulated contractions very inefficient. Therefore to avoid unnecessary fatigue, careful choice of stimulus parameters is an important consideration when designing neuromuscular stimulation programs.

ADEQUATE STIMULUS LIMITS ON MEMBRANE EXCITABILITY

In order to generate an action potential, the electrical stimulus must be of sufficient intensity and duration to equal or exceed the threshold of excitation for the tissue being stimulated. The permeability of the membrane must be altered in such a way as to allow a certain critical number of Na^+ ions to move into the cell in excess of those being pumped out by active transport. The stimulus must last long enough (duration) and be strong enough (intensity) for the local excitatory process to reach threshold.

Excitable cells have certain inherent membrane properties that set limits on their ability to respond to an electrical stimulus; two of these properties are membrane resistance and capacitance. The membrane's resistance is its ability to oppose current flow. Excitable cell membranes are also capable of storing an electrical charge; this is called *capacitance.* If the membrane resistance is multiplied by its capacitance, it yields a value known as the time constant. The time constant sets the rate at which a charge across the membrane is altered by an electrical stimulus. The time constant of a membrane represents the minimum time that a stimulus must be applied before depolarization will occur.

Because of membrane properties such as resistance and capacitance, there is a certain minimum intensity and duration of stimulation required for nerve and muscle to reach threshold. If the stimulation is applied at an intensity or duration below these minimum values, no action potential will occur. These values are different for nerves of different diameter and for muscle. If an infinitely long stimulus duration is applied, which is defined as 300 milliseconds, the minimum current amplitude that will produce excitation is called *rheobase.* If the rheobase intensity is doubled, the amount of time (pulse duration) that current must flow to achieve excitation is called *chronaxie.* If one gradually decreases the stimulus duration below 300 milliseconds and records the minimum intensity of stimulation required to generate a threshold response, a curve can be plotted representing the tissue's excitability, which is called the strength–duration (S–D) curve.

S–D curves for various nerve fibers and for denervated muscle are depicted in Figure 11–9. (Concepts of S-D were presented in Chapter 10.) A denervated muscle is a muscle without its nerve supply. As indicated in the figure, large motor and sensory nerves (type A) are capable of responding to shorter stimulus pulse durations with a lower intensity of current compared to other nerves or compared to muscle. It is this difference that forms the basis for selection of stimulus parameters to achieve a particular therapeutic goal. For instance, the use of sensory level stimulation for pain management (also called TENS) typically employs stimulus pulses that are very short in order to selectively activate large proprioceptive sensory fibers (type A) while avoiding stimulation of small pain sensory fibers (type C). Differences in excitability between nerve and denervated muscle also form the basis for using the S-D test, which is a diagnostic tool for determining the innervation status of a muscle.

Accommodation

There are conditions under which a nerve cell will not generate an action potential even in the presence of what would normally be considered a threshold stimulus. These conditions include subthreshold depolarization of the nerve prior to delivery of a threshold stimulus or presenting the nerve with a stimulus that has a slowly rising intensity. These situations allow the critical firing level (threshold) of the nerve cell to rise so that it takes a suprathreshold (greater than threshold) stimulus to elicit an action potential (Fig. 11–10A). This property (Fig. 11–10B and C) is called *accommodation* and it is unique to nerve cells. The ability of muscle cells to accommodate is minimal. In addition to meeting certain minimal excitation requirements of the nerve, the current must reach its maximum intensity rapidly in order to avoid the effects of accommodation; otherwise, the stimulus will be ineffective in generating an action potential.

AMPLITUDE

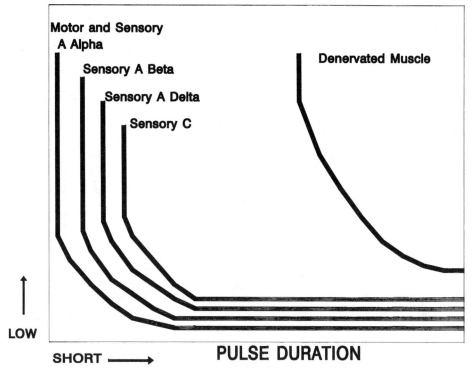

Figure 11–9. Strength–duration curves for various nerve fibers and muscle. Note that large sensory and motor nerves are most excitable in contrast to denervated muscle, which requires a much longer pulse duration and increased amplitude of stimulation to respond.

PRINCIPLES OF ELECTRICAL STIMULATION

ION FLOW IN RESPONSE TO ELECTRICAL CURRENT

By convention, current is defined as flowing from the point of high electrical potential, or the positive pole, to the point of low potential, which is the negative pole. You may wish to review this in Chapter 10. The positive pole is referred to as the anode and the negative pole is the cathode. Remember that at rest, the neuron is negatively charged on the inside and positively charged on the outside. Creating a positive charge on the outside of the nerve would cause hyperpolarization, making it less excitable, while creating a negative charge would cause depolarization. Similar charges repel each other and dissimilar charges are attracted. Figure 11–11 depicts the flow of current from surface electrodes through skin, fat, and other tissues to our target of stimulation, the underlying motor nerve. As electrical current is delivered through electrodes on the surface of the skin, positively charged ions in the body are repelled from the positive pole and attracted to the negative pole, and therefore, the nerve becomes hyperpolarized (less excitable) at the anode. Depolarization of the nerve takes place primarily at the cathode, since positive ions are being pulled away from the nerve toward the negative electrode, rendering the outside less positive. Although both the anode and cathode are necessary to form a complete circuit, the cathode is often referred to as the active elec-

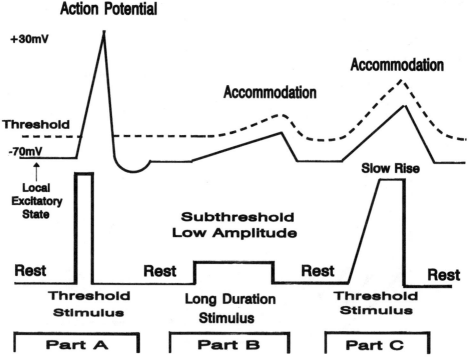

Figure 11–10. The response of a nerve to various stimuli is depicted. *(A)* A rectangular threshold current pulse results in a nerve action potential. *(B)* A rectangular subthreshold pulse results in a rise in the nerve threshold (accommodation) but no action potential is generated. *(C)* A slowly rising threshold pulse results in accommodation and no action potential is generated.

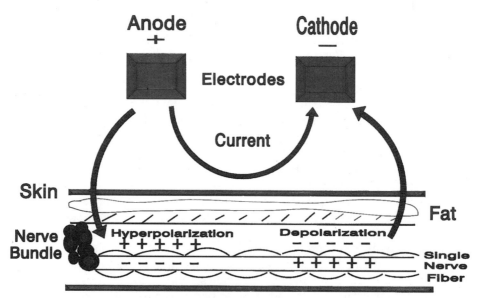

Figure 11–11. The flow of current from surface electrodes to an underlying motor nerve is shown. Hyperpolarization takes place under the anode because positive ions are driven away from this electrode into surrounding tissues. Depolarization, which can lead to an action potential, takes place under the cathode.

trode because nerve activation (excitation) takes place under this electrode. Conversely, the anode is often referred to as the inactive dispersive electrode.

Consider the example in Figure 11–11. If the electrode leads were reversed, then nerve excitation would now take place under the electrode to the left, which was previously the anode. This reverses the polarity of the circuit. By reversing the leads, the site of nerve activation has been reversed. Various stimulus waveforms have been discussed in the previous chapter. Polarity is a critical issue when applying asymmetrical pulsed waveforms because one electrode, the cathode, is the site of greatest nerve excitation. However, it should be noted that when a symmetrical biphasic pulsed waveform is applied, polarity is constantly reversing in equal amounts with each pulse of current. Therefore, nearly equal depolarization will occur under both electrodes and the concept of an anode and cathode loses relevance.

RESISTANCE AND IMPEDANCE

When electrical stimulation is delivered through the skin, many factors can interfere with flow of the current to the desired site. Tissue impedance causing opposition to current flow is undesirable, since it limits the amount of current reaching the tissue to be stimulated. Excitable tissues and nonexcitable tissues possess an inherent resistance. Skin and fat, for instance, are good insulators; this means that they offer considerable resistance to the flow of electrical current. This resistance can dramatically influence the ability to generate an adequate sensory and/or motor response in response to the underlying muscle. For instance, it would require a greater intensity of current to obtain a motor response in an area covered by adipose tissue (such as the gluteus maximus muscle) compared to an area with little fat (such as the anterior tibialis muscle). Increasing the current intensity to a level sufficient to drive current through the adipose to the nerve may make the sensation of the stimulation unbearable for the patient. This may rule out stimulation as a treatment option, or limit its effectiveness, depending on the goals of treatment. Minimizing impedance is important for all applications of stimulation because this allows current intensity to be reduced, which may increase patient comfort.

With adequate patient and equipment preparation, impedance can be minimized, increasing the effectiveness for treatment. Cleaning the skin surface with alcohol prior to electrode application will remove dirt and body oils and will decrease impedance; removing excess body hair beneath electrodes will also reduce impedance, as will warming the region to be stimulated or warming the electrode gel. Use of low-impedance electrodes, such as silicon rubber electrodes, with adequate conductive gel also minimizes impedance. Self-adhering electrodes are currently a popular choice for delivery of surface stimulation because of their ease of application and removal. Electrode manufacturers can provide information about electrode impedance. This is important, since a good skin–electrode interface is one of the best ways in which to reduce impedance when applying surface stimulation. Firmly and evenly adhered electrodes ensure even current distribution with less impedance. Finally, electrode size affects impedance, as will be discussed in the next section.

ELECTRODE SIZE AND ORIENTATION

Current Density

Current density is a measure of the quantity of charged ions that has moved through a cross-sectional area of a tissue. It is expressed as the number of milliamperes per square centimeter.

Current density is usually highest at the skin–electrode interface and decreases with the distance from the electrodes. Remember that skin is highly innervated with sensory nerves. Since current density is highest at the skin–electrode interface and sensory nerves are close to the skin surface, electrical stimulation is felt at amplitudes much lower than those needed to generate a muscle contraction.

There is an inverse relationship between electrode size and current density; the current density at an electrode increases as the size of the electrode decreases. If you were to drive the same amount of electrical current through different-sized electrodes, the greatest current density would occur under the smallest electrode. The relationship between electrode size and current density is an important consideration when planning treatment. If current density is low, it may be insufficient to cause excitation of the tissue. If it is too high, it may cause the sensation of the stimulation to be intolerable.

Specificity of Response

Electrode size is one factor that dictates the specificity of the obtained stimulated response. By decreasing the size of an electrode, one can obtain an isolated contraction from very small muscles, such as those of the thenar eminence of the thumb. However, small electrodes offer more resistance than larger ones and the current density will be greater under the small electrodes. Benefits such as specificity must be weighed against costs such as increased impedance and current density, which can increase discomfort. It is important to determine the size of the area to be stimulated and to choose the electrode size accordingly. For example, the quadriceps muscle is relatively large, and to get an adequate contraction from this muscle one should choose large electrodes. Choice of small electrodes for this application could lead to inadequate recruitment with decreased comfort for the patient. Conversely, choice of electrodes that are too large may distribute the flow of current over too great an area and compromise the desired response or recruit additional undesired muscle groups.

Depth of Current Penetration

As a rule, closely spaced electrodes will result in more superficial stimulation, while electrodes spaced far apart will allow deeper current penetration. If electrodes are spaced at too great a distance over a thin area (such as the forearm), it is possible to mistakenly stimulate muscles on the opposite side of the extremity. For example, finger flexors can be inappropriately stimulated if electrodes placed on the extensor surface are placed at too great a distance from each another. In contrast, closely spaced electrodes over a large muscle may not allow adequate depth of current penetration to reach the target muscle. An additional word of caution regarding closely spaced electrodes is that discomfort will greatly increase when the edges of the electrodes are close to each other. This will cause an increase in current density between the electrodes.

SUMMARY

In this chapter the structure and function of nerve and muscle as it is related to the use of electrical stimulation have been reviewed in this chapter. This should serve as a basis for understanding the effect of electrical current on excitable tissues and for establishing appropriate stimulation programs based on sound rationale. Resources used for preparing this chapter are provided and are recommended readings.

DISCUSSION QUESTIONS

1. Action potentials occur in both nerve and muscle fibers. Explain how these are related to one another and describe the end result of the action potential.

2. Describe differences between the three major types of nerve fibers. Discuss how recruitment via electrical stimulation is affected by differences such as size.

3. What factors influence propagation of an action potential?

4. What factors should be considered when choosing an electrode to be used for neuromuscular stimulation?

5. What are some ways to minimize impedance when initiating an electrical stimulation program? Why is it important to minimize impedance?

REFERENCES

1. APTA, Section on Electrophysiology: Electrotherapeutic Terminology in PT. APTA, Alexandria, VA, 1990.

2. Baker, L, et al: Neuromuscular Electrical Stimulation: A Practical Guide, ed 3. Los Amigos Research and Education Institute, Downey, CA, 1993, pp 7–44.

3. Bishop, B: Basic Neurophysiology. Medical Examination Publishing Company, New York, 1982, pp 34–86.

4. Noback, C, et al: The Human Nervous System, ed 4. Lea & Febiger, Philadelphia, 1991, pp 15–56.

5. Pansky, B and Allen, DJ: Review of Neuroscience. Unit 3: Sections 61–67. Macmillan, New York, 1980.

6. Snyder-Mackler, L and Robinson, AJ: Clinical Electrophysiology. Williams & Wilkins, Baltimore, 1989, pp 61–94.

7. Wolf, SL: Electrotherapy. Churchill Livingston, New York, 1981, pp 1–24.

ACKNOWLEDGMENTS

The authors would like to thank Jean Scofield from Rancho Los Amigos for her assistance with figure permission; Kathy Goodstein from Shriners Hospital for slide reproduction; the members of the Research Department at Shriners Hospital, Philadelphia Unit, in particular, Carolyn Barbieri, Esther Halden, Mike Ignatowski, Megan Moynahan, MJ Mulcahey, and Bonnie Perilstien for their computer knowledge, editorial assistance, support, and guidance. Also, Betsy Butterworth, PTA, Vicki Vanartsdalen, PTA, and Joy Cohn for their editorial recommendations. We are dedicating this chapter to the memory of Thomas Steffa.

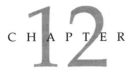

12

Neuromuscular Applications for Electrical Stimulation

Joy C. Cohn, PT
Cecilia Mullin, PTA

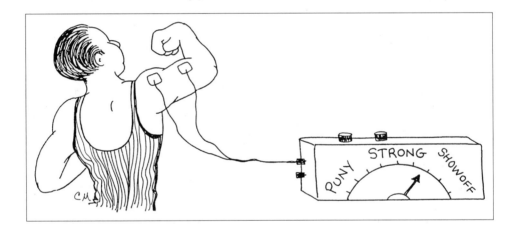

CHAPTER OBJECTIVES

- Discuss the specific clinical applications for NMES for strengthening and endurance, range of motion, facilitation of muscle function, management of muscle spasms and spasticity, edema reduction, and orthotic substitution.
- Outline treatment techniques for patient problems.
- Discuss the factors that determine whether or not NMES would be appropriate for a patient.
- Discuss the clinical decision making process for determining the effectiveness of the use of NMES and whether or not modifications should be made.

CHAPTER OUTLINE

Identifying Appropriate Patients

Therapeutic Current Characteristics
Waveforms
Amplitude
Pulse Duration
Pulse Rate
Timing Modulation Duty Cycle
    On-Off Ratio
Ramp Modulation

**General Guidelines for Clinical
    Applications**
Patient Positioning
    Electrodes
Duration and Frequency of Treatment

Specific Clinical Applications
Strengthening and Endurance
Range of Motion
Facilitation or Retraining of Muscle

Management of Muscle Spasms and
    Spasticity
Edema Reduction
Orthotic Substitution
Partial Denervation

Safety Considerations
Equipment
Patient Factors
    Medical History
    Skin Condition and Sensation
    Cognitive Issues

Patient Education
Expected Outcomes

Clinical Decision Making
Evaluating Treatment Effectiveness and
    Modifying Treatment
Documenting Treatment

The purpose of this chapter is to demonstrate the clinical use of surface electrical stimulation (ES) to accomplish a variety of therapeutic goals and to explore the guidelines for clinical decision making and treatment.

Technological development of ES devices and the treatment of human ills have progressed hand in hand to the present day, but not without confusion. To utilize ES devices effectively, it is important to focus on the treatment outcome expected. Although the technology for ES may change over time, the goal of treatment will probably remain the same.

This chapter considers the use of neuromuscular electrical stimulation (NMES) in treatment programs. NMES is defined as "the use of electrical stimulation for activation of muscle through stimulation of the intact peripheral nerve."[1] Functional electrical stimulation (FES) and functional neuromuscular stimulation (FNS) are forms of NMES. They are used as a substitute for an orthosis to activate muscle contractions in paretic or paralyzed muscles to assist in functional activities, such as standing or grasping an object. Other potential uses of electrical stimulation, such as wound healing, are covered in other chapters of this text.

IDENTIFYING APPROPRIATE PATIENTS

NMES requires an intact, or at least partially intact, peripheral nerve to respond to the stimulation. A stimulated muscle contraction will always be generated via the innervating peripheral nerve, if intact. In the case of partial denervation because of a peripheral neuropathy of metabolic or neurologic origin (e.g., diabetes or Guillan-Barré), it may not be possible to stimulate a contraction of any more strength than the patient is able to produce voluntarily as a result of diffuse denervation commonly associated with these diseases. Electrical muscle stimulation

(EMS) is pulsed monophasic current that is used to activate denervated muscle directly. EMS is considered to be of questionable value[2] and will not be covered in this chapter. Innervation status, if in doubt, is determined via history, physical examination, and a strength–duration test (S–D test) or an electroneuromyographic (EMG) evaluation. There is a questionable role for NMES in the presence of primary muscle disease such as muscular dystrophy. Further study is required.

There are a few contraindications to NMES.[3] The presence of a cardiac demand pacemaker is an absolute contraindication because of the possibility that the electrical current will interfere with the electronics of the pacemaker. Use of NMES with any other pacemaker should be undertaken with great caution, and the supervising physician should be contacted prior to use if ES is seen to be an essential part of the treatment plan. Precautions for NMES include:[4,5]

1. Elderly patients should be monitored closely for heart rate and blood pressure responses during initiation of a stimulation program to rule out unknown cardiac problems in response to exercise.

2. The effect of NMES during pregnancy on the fetus is unknown. It may induce labor in a woman in her third trimester, and therefore should be avoided.

3. Superficial metal (i.e., staples, pins, external fixation devices) will be a site of concentration for the current delivered to the skin in the vicinity and can cause discomfort. Orthopedic metal implants (i.e., total hip replacement) are generally located too deep beneath the skin surface to be cause for concern.

4. Absent or impaired skin sensation is *not* a contraindication, but requires close monitoring of the skin response, careful choice of and application of electrodes, and in general, usage of biphasic and short-duration waveforms to avoid the potential tissue damage associated with direct current. Safety issues in the use of electronic equipment will be considered later in the chapter and have been thoroughly discussed in Chapter 10.

THERAPEUTIC CURRENT CHARACTERISTICS

Individuals may respond negatively when first introduced to a stimulation program because of an innate fear of electricity or discomfort with stimulation. However, careful explanation of the goals of treatment, gradual introduction of the stimulation amplitude, and readiness to consider a change in stimulation waveform or parameters can lead to success in most cases. This chapter contains a brief review of therapeutic treatments. The reader is urged to refer to Chapters 10 and 11 for a more detailed description of terminology.

The two main concerns in planning a program of NMES are: (1) the quality of the stimulated muscle contraction and (2) patient comfort leading to cooperation with the treatment plan. Both are greatly affected by the stimulation parameters. The success of the treatment program is not based on the stimulator chosen; many different stimulators have been used effectively. It is a knowledge of the "features" (i.e., parameters) of a particular stimulator that should most affect treatment planning.

WAVEFORMS

Patient comfort has been investigated in many studies. Three studies of note investigated comparative comfort with differing waveforms. Delitto and Rose[6] found that there was no clear choice among three symmetrical biphasic waveforms, and that different preferences existed for different patients. In a comparison of symmetrical and asymmetrical biphasic waveforms, Bowman and Baker[7] found that normal female subjects preferred the symmetrical waveform when a large muscle group (quadriceps) was stimulated. But in another similar study,[8] it was found that when the target muscle groups were small (wrist flexors and extensors) normal subjects preferred an asymmetrical biphasic waveform. In a study comparing current frequencies with a symmetrical biphasic waveform,[9] the authors demonstrated a preference for higher frequencies when 30, 50, and 100 pulses per second (pps) were tested in stimulation of a tetanic contraction of the quadriceps muscle.

AMPLITUDE

Current amplitude (intensity) must be gradually increased when first introducing a stimulation program to a patient. A patient will become comfortable with the sensation of stimulation within the first 15 minutes of a gradually introduced stimulus amplitude, thereby becoming able to tolerate an increase in amplitude to achieve the desired muscle response. The desired muscle response can usually be accomplished within one or two sessions.

The quality of a stimulated muscle contraction is determined by a combination of many parameters, including stimulus amplitude, pulse duration, stimulus frequency, and duty cycle. Increasing the stimulus amplitude causes recruitment of additional nerve fibers (smaller fibers and fibers further from the electrode), leading to increased force of muscle contraction. There is a limit to the force increase observed once most of the muscle fibers have been recruited. Since most portable electrical stimulation devices use an arbitrary 0 to 10 scale for the amplitude control, it is difficult to quantify the amount of current delivered to the patient, and the therapist must rely on the muscular response seen and the patient's sensory tolerance. The amplitude of current needed to achieve the desired response will also vary from patient to patient because of differences in resistance (impedance). In obese patients it may not be possible to achieve the desired muscle response because the motor nerve may be too "insulated" by the intervening layer of fatty tissue to allow sufficient stimulation without painful stimulation of the sensory nerves in the skin.

PULSE DURATION

The pulse duration has a corresponding relationship with stimulus amplitude. This relationship can be seen by examination of a strength–duration curve. A short pulse duration (below 40 μs) requires a much higher stimulus amplitude. A high stimulus amplitude is necessary to elicit a muscular response until a pulse duration over 40 μs is chosen. When the pulse duration is set between 40 and 500 μs, an increase in amplitude between 15 and 40 mA (a relatively small range) will give you the full range of muscular responses. Increasing the pulse duration above 500 μs will not improve muscular responses (Fig. 12–1).

One of the primary differences between stimulators lies in the pulse duration available for use. High-voltage pulsed-current stimulators have short and usually fixed pulse durations (generally not above 200 μs). Most other units appropriate for NMES have pulse durations generally between 20 and 500 μs. Whether the pulse duration is adjustable varies from unit to unit. A unit that has a pulse dura-

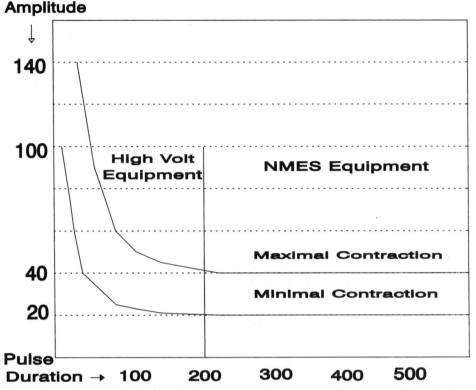

Figure 12–1. This annotated strength–duration curve demonstrates the inverse relationship between the amplitude of current and the pulse duration. The range of pulse duration available is one of the primary determinants of different classes of clinically available stimulation units.

tion between 200 and 400 μs will be more than adequate for NMES applications. Further similarities and differences among devices are discussed in Chapter 15.

PULSE RATE

On many NMES units, the primary controls regulate amplitude and pulse rate (frequency). As pulse rate increases, the rate of motor nerve firing rises and the overlapping twitch response leads to a stronger contraction. However, one must recognize the difference between voluntary and an electrically induced contraction (see Chap. 11). An electrically induced contraction results in reverse motor unit recruitment (large superficial motor units are usually recruited first) with synchronous activity of nerve and muscle fibers. This relationship causes action potentials of nerve and muscle to be dependent on frequency; higher frequency leads to more rapid fatigue. To minimize fatigue, lower the pulse rate. Fused tetany can occur at frequencies as low as 12 pps, depending on the muscle.

TIMING MODULATION DUTY CYCLE ON-OFF RATIO

Another stimulus parameter that affects fatigue is the duty cycle or on-off ratio. Duty cycle is defined as "the ratio of on time to the total time of the trains of pulses or bursts."[10] Duty cycle is expressed as a percentage and calculated by dividing the on time by the total cycle time (on time + off time) and multiplying by 100. The on-off ratio is expressed in seconds and is calculated by dividing the on time by the off time. An example of a 1:3 ratio is where the on time is 4 seconds, and the off time is 12 seconds. (4/12 = 1:3).

The off time of the stimulation program represents the time during which a muscle is able to recover from the previous contraction and rest. Insufficient rest leads to rapid fatigue and limited success in achieving various treatment goals. The majority of clinical treatment paradigms utilize a 1:3 or 1:5 on-off ratio with the typical on time being 2 to 10 seconds. Total contractions for a typical 30-minute treatment session when a 1:5 on-off ratio is chosen are reduced by one half. Knowledge of this fact should influence the length of the treatment session.[11] The on time chosen can often affect patient comfort as well. Since there is a range of on times from 2 to 10 seconds, documentation should include both the ratio and the actual on time. Patients generally find a contraction of 8 to 12 seconds in length to be very uncomfortable, sometimes likening it to a "charley horse" or cramp.

RAMP MODULATION

A ramp is another possible modulation of the therapeutic current chosen. The current is gradually increasing or decreasing with a "plateau" of stimulation.[12] The ramping of the current can be achieved by (1) a gradual increase of the amplitude, or (2) increase of pulse duration from zero to the maximum setting over a set time interval. The perceived difference between a ramp of amplitude or pulse duration is "virtually indistinguishable"[12] and therefore is determined by the manufacturer in most devices and not often clearly identified for the user. The user must be aware that many devices include ramp time within the chosen on time. Therefore, to assure that the stimulus reaches peak amplitude, the ramp time must be less than the on time. The usefulness of a ramp lies in the ability to "grade" the muscular response as it begins and ends with stimulation. Rarely do muscular movements occur abruptly. They are more commonly graded in intensity as the muscle fibers are recruited. This type of stimulated contraction is usually much more comfortable for a patient. A "ramp down" of the stimulation allows a more controlled return of the limb to its resting position than would a sudden drop that occurs if the stimulation ends abruptly. When determining the on-off ratio of a stimulation program, the on time is considered to be only the time of the "plateau" of maximum stimulation and the off time should be set accordingly. In most clinical paradigms, a ramp of 2 or less seconds is sufficient. Ramps of greater than 2 seconds are generally chosen when there is a very high level of stimulation required or with a spastic muscle that is sensitive to a rapid stretch.

GENERAL GUIDELINES FOR CLINICAL APPLICATIONS

PATIENT POSITIONING

The patient should be positioned for comfort. A comfortable patient is best able to attend to the treatment program and can participate in reaching the therapeutic goals established. It is always worth the few extra minutes taken to achieve a comfortable starting position. Whenever possible, position a patient to allow him or her to see the results of a stimulated contraction. Visual feedback for the patient enhances sensory information and learning. Varying the patient's position during the course of treatment will also enhance learning. For example, if the goal of treatment is to achieve independent ankle dorsiflexion, the muscles for dorsiflexion might be stimulated first in a supported long sitting position; progress to sitting with feet on the floor; then progress to standing. Finally the contraction could be timed to coincide with the correct phase of the gait cycle.

When stimulating weakened muscles, careful attention to limb position can take advantage of the length–tension relationship (see Chap. 11) to enhance muscular performance. For example, a quadriceps contraction would be enhanced with stimulation if the patient was positioned semireclined with a bolster under the knee. In this position the quadriceps is mildly stretched and more likely to achieve a visible limb movement.

The treatment program must take into account range-of-motion (ROM) limitations either imposed by a joint instability or dictated by a surgeon following a reconstruction. For example, in the early phase of rehabilitation following an anterior cruciate ligament reconstruction of the knee, patients may not actively or passively extend the knee beyond a position of 45° of flexion to avoid stressing the newly repaired ligament. Patients can safely perform stimulation augmented quadriceps and hamstring exercises by utilizing isokinetic equipment, which allows for range limitations and/or "locking" the limb into fixed positions for isometric exercise (Fig. 12–2).

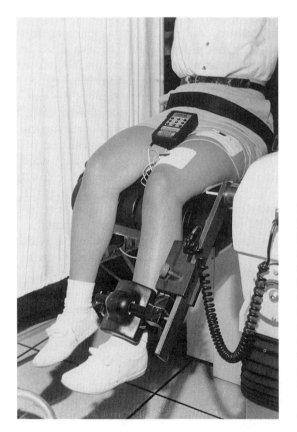

Figure 12–2. This patient setup illustrates how to exercise the quadriceps isometrically without endangering a recent ACL repair. This setup can be used for isometric quadriceps contractions or cocontractions of the hamstrings and quadriceps. Note the carbon rubber electrodes secured by self-adhesive foam patches over the quadriceps muscle. Hamstring electrodes are not visible. (Ultra Stim model 650-01, Neuromedics, Inc., Clute, TX.) *(Photo courtesy of Kathy Goodstein, Shriners Hospital, Philadelphia Unit.)*

Electrodes

Three decisions must be made with regard to electrodes: type, size, and placement. These issues are discussed in Chapter 15.

A stimulated contraction will be most effective in meeting your goals if it closely approximates a "normal" contraction. In addition to the current modulations already discussed, it is important to attempt to achieve a "balanced" movement at the joint most affected by the muscle contraction. For example, in stimulating the wrist extensors, the goal is extension of the wrist without excessive ulnar or radial deviation. A balanced contraction most closely approximates a functional movement in most cases and provides the patient with the best opportunity to re-experience normal movement. Careful electrode placement with a small negative electrode over the (small) target muscle and an asymmetric biphasic waveform will offer the best chance of success.

DURATION AND FREQUENCY OF TREATMENT

Clinical decision making becomes most difficult when considering the duration and frequency of treatment. It is very dependent on the short-term goals, expected outcome, and the patient response to treatment. Frequent reassessments will guide the decision to continue treatment. The duration of treatment will vary from as much as 6 weeks if the goal is muscle endurance, to as little as one treatment for muscle facilitation. A patient with an orthopedic injury and a "normal" nervous system will generally respond more quickly than the patient with a neurologic disease or injury.

SPECIFIC CLINICAL APPLICATIONS

STRENGTHENING AND ENDURANCE

The interest in using NMES to increase muscle strength only really began after Russian athletes were observed being treated with ES during the 1976 Olympics. In 1977, a USSR physician, Dr. Kots, gave a series of lectures in Canada making claims that ES with a "Russian current" stimulation protocol could lead to a 10% to 30% increase in muscular strength above what an athlete could achieve by conventional exercise regimens. The Russian current he described has been investigated with mixed results. However, Kots's claims led to renewed interest in using other more familiar NMES devices and protocols to achieve strength gains in normal as well as patient populations.

Conventional exercise programs to increase strength are based on the overload principle of eliciting a small number of high-intensity contractions (at least 70% of a maximal contraction × 10 repetitions or less) in a treatment session performed three to five times per week for 2 to 3 weeks. The same parameters of exercise apply when utilizing NMES to augment strength in healthy and healthy-but-injured patient populations. Research has yielded little compelling evidence that NMES adds to the strength gains that normal individuals can achieve through conventional training programs alone.[13,14] However, in the treatment of limited traumatic or orthopedic injuries, NMES has been shown to lead to greater strength gains than those achieved with conventional exercise.[15,16]

Candidates for NMES can be any patient with multiple areas of weakness and deconditioning. These patients frequently benefit from a program that emphasizes endurance of the muscle or muscles of interest. This emphasis on endurance spotlights the other major function of a muscle, the ability to produce a force repetitively. Conventional endurance exercise programs consist of a decreased force of contraction and high repetitions (a Fair to Fair Plus contraction and a total of "30 to 60 minutes of stimulated contraction per day"[17]) in treatment sessions five to seven times per week for 2 to 10 weeks. Several shorter sessions during the course of the day make the exercise programs more manageable, but total time of cycled stimulation must take into account the total on time (in this instance, including the ramp time).

A typical orthopedic patient would be a woman with a reconstruction of her anterior cruciate ligament (ACL) because of a skiing injury. This patient would not be allowed to fully extend her knee beyond 45° of flexion in the early weeks of rehabilitation. One example of a treatment plan:

1. Conventional exercise program to maintain right hip and ankle strength and overall aerobic capacity.
2. NMES to increase isometric strength of the right quadriceps and hamstring muscles.
3. Ice to the right knee to control edema after exercise.

Results of studies using NMES have shown that superior isometric strengthening can be achieved in comparison to conventional isometric exercises.[17,18] The NMES program can be carried out in two ways: Simultaneous stimulation of the quadriceps and hamstrings to achieve cocontraction with no net extention force or NMES to the quadriceps with the knee held in 45° or more of flexion. In both instances, the use of an isokinetic machine to limit ROM and monitor the force produced by the stimulation program allows for safe exercise and quantitative information regarding improvement in force production (see Fig. 12–2).

If the hamstrings and quadriceps are both stimulated, the two channels of stimulation must by synchronized and balanced for comfort and force production. Stimulation of the quadriceps alone requires only one channel of stimulation. Amplitude is adjusted to achieve a maximally tolerated isometric contraction.

A typical neurologic patient is a woman with a left middle cerebral artery infarct who had a flaccid right hemiplegia initially but progressed to walking with a straight cane and molded ankle-foot orthosis (MAFO) on the right leg. She is able to ambulate without the MAFO, but her ankle dorsiflexors on the right fatigue within 20 feet. A typical treatment plan:

1. General conditioning exercises to improve overall fitness level
2. Traditional strengthening exercises for all right leg muscle groups
3. Closed-chain exercises, including use of a biomechanical ankle platform
4. NMES endurance program for the right ankle dorsiflexors

It is important to achieve a "balanced" response in the foot (Fig. 12–3) and an ankle with a neutral position relative to inversion and eversion without clawing or hyperextension of the toes (Fig. 12–4). A portable NMES unit would be ideal to allow this patient to continue stimulation at home on a daily basis because endurance training requires an extended treatment protocol.

The following represents a suggested patient handout for using NMES at home:

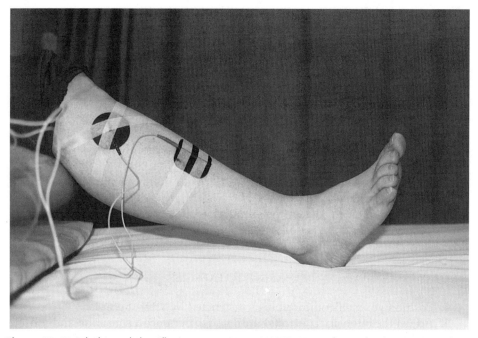

Figure 12–3. A balanced dorsiflexion response to NMES. Note electrode placement and extremity positioning.

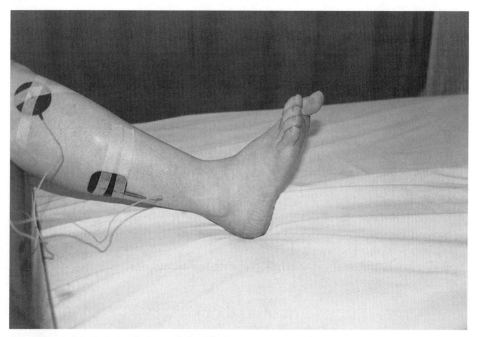

Figure 12–4. An unbalanced dorsiflexion response with excessive toe extension.

INSTRUCTIONS FOR HOME USE OF STIMULATOR

Your treatment time is ____ minutes ____ times per day.

Your response to the treatment is dependent on your effort to adhere to the suggested program.

PREPARING TO USE THE STIMULATOR

1. Clean the skin with mild soap and water in the area where you will place your electrodes.
2. Prepare your electrodes as instructed by your therapist and apply securely to the designed areas.
3. Connect the electrodes to the stimulator—be sure to insert all plugs completely so that there is no exposed metal.

PREPARING TO EXERCISE

4. Position yourself comfortably as instructed by your therapist.
5. Adjust the intensity control(s) until you experience a sensation and muscle response similar to your supervised exercise with your therapist.
6. Exercise for the length of time designated above.

ENDING YOUR EXERCISE SESSION

7. Turn the intensity control(s) to OFF.
8. Disconnect all of the wires by pulling on the plugs (*Do not pull on the wires!*).
9. Remove the electrodes and clean/store as instructed by your therapist.

PRECAUTIONS FOR STIMULATOR USAGE

1. The stimulator is preprogrammed for your personal use *only* and should not be used on another part of your body or any other person.
2. Carefully inspect your skin in the electrode area before and after you apply the electrodes. Do not apply the electrodes to broken or irritated skin. Slight reddening of the skin under the electrodes is normal after stimulation. If you experience persistent skin irritation, stop using the stimulator until you see your therapist.
3. Do not bathe or shower while wearing the stimulator.

TROUBLESHOOTING

1. No stimulation felt—
   a. recheck all connections
   b. recheck electrode contact with skin
   c. recheck or replace batteries

2. Stimulation uncomfortable—
   a. recheck electrode contact with skin
   b. readjust intensity controls
   c. check skin under electrode for irritation
3. Stimulation intermittent—
   a. check wires for a break
   b. check connections
   c. check electrode contact to skin

It is recommended that the patient also be given a diagram of electrode placement or preferably a photograph.

RANGE OF MOTION

Methods to maintain ROM for some neurologically impaired and orthopedic patients are often taught to patients and their families. Passive ROM for neurologically impaired patients with mild spastic tone often has a good outcome. However, patients with moderate to severe spasticity tend to have difficulty making gains with passive ROM that may limit their daily functions. Orthopedic patients differ in that they have limited ROM as a result of immobilization of a muscle and or a joint or pain.

The typical orthopedic patient would be a male who has just had a cast removed because of a tibial fracture and is unable to fully extend his knee. An example of a treatment plan:
1. NMES of quadriceps muscle to achieve increased knee extension
2. Home exercise program

It is important to avoid excessive knee joint compression when initiating this program to prevent increased joint irritation.

The typical neurologic patient would be a young woman with a closed head injury. The patient exhibits bilateral biceps spasticity with elbow flexion contractures. An example of a treatment plan: Serial casting along with NMES to the triceps muscle to restore elbow extension. In order to not limit her daily functions, such as self-feeding, the nondominant arm is treated first. The patient is casted in the available extension range, blocking flexion but not limiting extension while using NMES (Fig. 12–5). The time of ramp-up must be extended in this instance because of the spasticity present in the opposing muscle group. A ramp-up time of 6 to 8 seconds may be necessary to achieve a slow, effective stretch without increasing spasticity in the biceps by a quick stretch. Each week the serial cast should be removed and ROM measurements taken to document improvement. The serial cast is again applied in the available extension range, blocking flexion but not limiting extension to continue NMES sessions. In some instances a fabricated splint is preferred.

FACILITATION OR RETRAINING OF MUSCLE

Following a neurologic injury or surgery (especially orthopedic surgery) a patient may have difficulty in initiating movement in a muscle group. This is especially the case if the patient has been unable to use the muscle for any length of time, leading to disuse atrophy, weakness, or pain. The central nervous system (CNS) relies heavily on the many forms of sensory feedback received to modulate per-

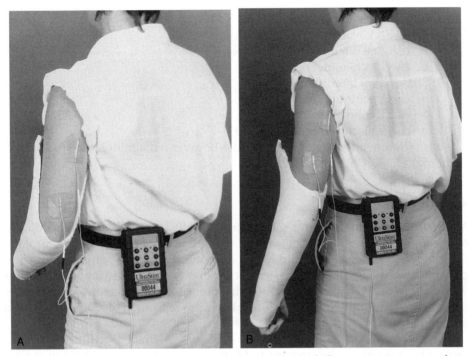

Figure 12–5. The "drop-out" cast required to achieve improved elbow extension range of motion. On the left side of the figure, elbow flexion is blocked by the front of the cast. On the right side of the figure, elbow extension is stimulated with the electrode placements illustrated to gain additional extension range. (Ultra Stim model 650-01, Neuromedics, Inc., Clute, TX; Pals Reusable Neurostimulation Electrodes, Axelgaard Mfg. Co., Ltd, Fallbrook, CA.) *(Photo courtesy of Kathy Goodstein, Shriners Hospital, Philadelphia Unit.)*

formance. In the case of a neurologic injury, that feedback can be greatly affected by sensory loss or distortion and/or change in available movement strategies and tone. In the case of surgery, the motoneuron pool can be directly inhibited by the pain efferents, and it has been suggested that cutting of a joint capsule during surgery can affect the normal proprioceptor activity.[18]

The desired response is a voluntary contraction that is enhanced by the NMES to increase CNS feedback and motor learning. Timing and coordination are crucial to the relearning of motor skills. Therefore, it is important that the NMES occurs at the correct time in the anticipated motor response. The timing of the stimulus must be controlled by the therapist or patient by use of an external trigger that is generally a foot or hand switch.

Sometimes the contraction must be initiated by NMES, but in other situations the stimulation is used to augment a weak voluntary response or to allow stabilization via stimulation of a related muscle group. This type of NMES program is not generally used by patients independently, but it represents a powerful adjunct for the therapist during a treatment session. Facilitation, to be most effective, requires patient cooperation and timing of stimulation within functional tasks.

A typical orthopedic patient would be a female who is status post a left total knee replacement (TKR). In attempting to teach the woman quadriceps isometric exercises, you realize that she, despite a strong effort, is unable to activate her quadriceps effectively. One example of a treatment plan:

1. NMES to facilitate quadriceps activity
2. Conventional exercises to maintain ipsilateral hip and ankle strength and prevent circulatory stasis
3. Protected weightbearing and gait training with appropriate assistive device when indicated
4. Ice to the left knee to control edema after exercise

The location of the distal electrode over the quadriceps may have to be modified if staples are still present at the incision site because electrical current can concentrate around superficial metal and cause pain. The distal electrode should be moved more proximally (leaving a gap of at least 1 inch between the electrode and staples) so that the staples are not within the main current path. An alternative is to use an asymmetric biphasic waveform and place the anode posteriorly on the hamstrings. This should ensure a comfortable stimulus for the patient. If not, NMES should be reconsidered, if needed, once the staples are removed. Close observations of the incision site is called for with treatment to ensure that there is not excessive pull on a healing incision. If there is, a decreased amplitude may still be effective in giving a sensory cue for a quadriceps contraction. It is expected that this type of facilitation will be needed for only a short period of time because this patient has a normal CNS requiring possibly only one or two sessions of 15 to 20 minutes each before the patient is able to continue strengthening exercises on her own.

A typical neurologic patient would be a woman who had a left middle cerebral artery thrombosis 3 months prior to her initial evaluation. She has returned for additional therapy because she states that she has begun to move the fingers of her right hand. As part of a complete evaluation, it is found that she can actively flex and extend her fingers (though not through a complete range), but she cannot actively extend and stabilize the wrist, limiting her ability to produce a functional grasp. One example of a treatment plan:

1. Conventional rehabilitation to maximize motor learning for functional independence
2. NMES to facilitate voluntary movement in right wrist extensors
3. Functional training in conjunction with NMES as appropriate.

It is important to cue this patient visually so that she can receive visual, kinesthetic, and cutaneous feedback and coordinate stimulation with volitional prehension activities.

The wrist and finger muscles are very close in the forearm and careful placement can include or eliminate activity in the fingers as desired. "Balanced" wrist extension without excessive ulnar or radial deviation is optimal. This patient has an abnormal CNS and may have increased difficulty in recruiting some muscle groups. Therefore, she may require more experience with NMES to be capable of activating her wrist extensors independently and appropriately. The treatment time could be as limited as 15 to 20 minutes per session, but the duration of treatment might be as long as a week or two, especially if an effort is made to vary the motor learning experience by attempting functional activities such as grasp and release or different upper extremity positioning during wrist extension activation. If a patient is not successful with a trial of NMES because of her evolving neurologic status, it may be appropriate to try again at another time in the treatment course.

MANAGEMENT OF MUSCLE SPASMS AND SPASTICITY

NMES is widely utilized to address pain by reducing the tension in a muscle in spasm because of injury. However, if the mechanism of improvement is not clear, high-frequency stimulation can lead to rapid muscle fatigue in a constantly active muscle. It is possible to break the so-called pain-spasm-pain cycle with relief of pain for up to several hours post treatment. This allows one to improve ROM and treat the particular areas of injury effectively.

In a neurologically impaired patient, stimulating a spastic muscle causes relaxation similar to that of a muscle in spasm; however, the relaxation period is brief because of the continued underlying abnormality in the CNS. During this brief relaxation period, the extremity can be repositioned to allow casting or bracing to be applied effectively.

A typical orthopedic patient would be a secretary with muscle spasms of the right upper trapezius and rhomboids and limited rotation and forward flexion of the cervical spine with pain upon movement. When evaluated, the patient demonstrates acute muscle spasms with limited rotation and forward flexion because of pain with movement. One example of a treatment plan:

1. Pulsed current (see Fig. 12–6 for an example of this device) to trapezius muscles
2. Heat or ice is frequently used in conjunction with stimulation
3. Home exercise program
4. Patient education on sitting posture

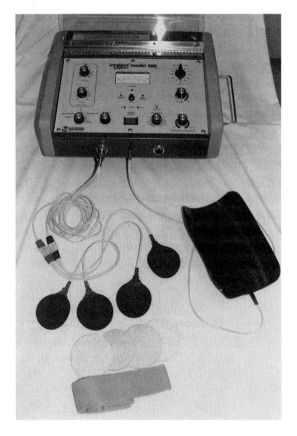

Figure 12–6. This unit illustrates the available adjustable parameters and electrode selection with one version of a clinical High Volt Pulsed Current Stimulation Unit (Intelect model 500, Chattanooga Corp, Chattanooga, TN)

This patient could benefit from either a bipolar or monopolar electrode placement (see Chap. 16). Documentation of the time frame of pain relief after treatment will assist in determining the necessity to continue the electrical stimulation treatment.

EDEMA REDUCTION

Acute edema develops because of trauma to the blood vessels with leakage of blood cells and plasma proteins into the interstitial space. These blood components are negatively charged and when exposed to a negative polarity they are repelled from the area.[19] As a result, the excess fluid, because of its attachment to the negatively charged proteins, is also shifted from the area.[20] Chronic edema requires venous and lymphatic drainage that is enhanced by cyclic muscle contractions. Treatment of edema (both chronic and acute) typically includes ice application or cool water immersion, elevation, and compression. NMES can be an effective adjunct to these standard treatments.

A typical patient would be a construction worker who sustained a crush injury to the left hand 3 days ago. There were no fractures, but the patient has severe edema with limited ROM. An example of a treatment plan:

1. Ice bath
2. NMES while in water
3. Elevation for exercising and rest
4. AROM exercises as tolerated

The treatment setup is somewhat unusual in this instance. The patient is positioned with the arm up to the mid-forearm in a nonmetallic bath of cool water (10° to 20°C). One pair of electrodes are placed in the bath bracketing but not touching the hand or a negative electrode in the water with a positive electrode affixed to the dorsal forearm outside the water. The reduction of edema will be most effective if the muscles within the hand (the intrinsics) contract, so the active electrode should be moved to maximize the intrinsic activity. The current should be adjusted to elicit a brief but effective contraction of the local muscles (frequency of 20 to 50 pps). Continuation of treatment is based on edema reduction.

ORTHOTIC SUBSTITUTION

The ability to activate innervated but inactive, paretic, or paralyzed muscle has proven to be an effective replacement for orthotics in the management of deformity, or to assist purposeful movement. Beginning in the 1960s, a great deal of research took place with what has come to be called functional electrical stimulation, or FES. This continuing research explores many areas, including the restoration of standing and ambulation in paraplegic patients (Fig. 12–7), a dorsiflexion assist for hemiplegic patients, and surface stimulation to substitute for bracing in idiopathic scoliosis.[21-23] Many of the functional activities in which FES offers promise are complex activities (such as walking) requiring multiple channels of stimulation and feedback to allow the stimulation to be modulated to meet varying conditions. These crude systems are experimental presently.

Electrical stimulation to activate the ankle dorsiflexors in the swing phase of the gait cycle is widely used in the clinic because of the repetitive, rarely varying nature of the movement (Fig.12–8). The system requires a portable electrical stimulator with an external switch under the heel and one channel of stimulation (Fig. 12–9). The

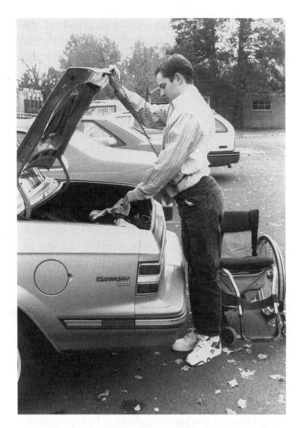

Figure 12–7. This research participant is a T4 level paraplegic who is pictured using an experimental, multichannel neuromuscular stimulator (worn at his waist) to achieve standing without bracing. *(Photo courtesy of Kathy Goodstein, Shriners Hospitals, Philadelphia Unit)*

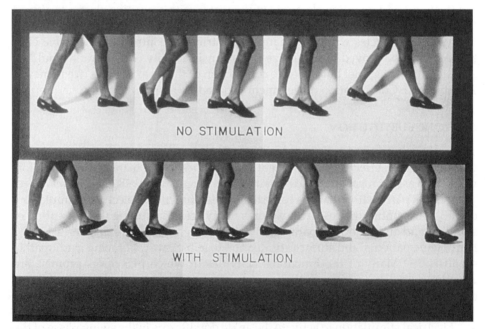

Figure 12–8. This is a comparison of the swing phase of the right lower extremity with and without the aide of timed NMES. The patient seen here had experimental implanted electrodes instead of the clinically used surface electrodes. *(From Los Amigos Research and Education Institute, Downey, CA, with permission)*

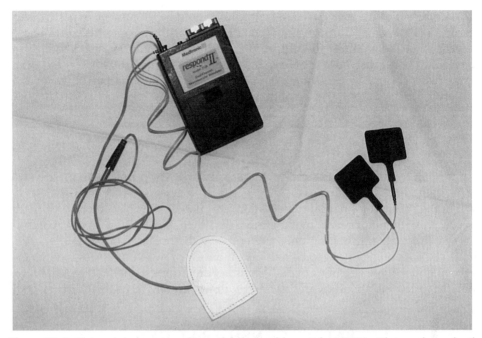

Figure 12–9. This unit is a commonly available portable unit for NMES with two channels of stimulation and an optional external heel switch to time the stimulated contraction with the gait cycle (Respond II FES Unit, Model 90003108, Medtronic Corp, San Diego, CA).

stimulation is activated by the heel rising off the floor at the end of stance leading to stimulation of the ankle dorsiflexors to allow toe clearance during swing.

Because of the repetitive nature of the muscular activity necessary to achieve long-term substitution for orthotics, any clinical application of NMES as an orthotic substitute first requires the development of muscular endurance described earlier in this chapter. Baker and associates[23] have clearly described an FES program to address shoulder subluxation, which can accompany the flaccid paralysis of a cerebral vascular accident.

PARTIAL DENERVATION

NMES can be effective in retraining a muscle that is recovering its innervation following a peripheral nerve injury. The reinnervation process following a nerve injury is slow, unpredictable, and seldom complete. The degree of expected function is difficult to predict and depends on many factors including: (1) the degree of atrophy, (2) the mechanism and extent of the nerve injury, and (3) the time since the injury. With the paresis or paralysis associated with a peripheral nerve injury comes a "disconnection" of the CNS to the particular muscle(s). With reinnervation, many patients find that they are no longer able to activate the muscle without the sensory cues associated with NMES: cutaneous, kinesthetic, and visual. The otherwise normal CNS readily accommodates allowing the patient to begin to "reconnect" and initiate movement. In addition the muscle strength can increase, usually within only a few sessions. It is difficult, however, to predict the muscular response achievable, given limited knowledge of the innervation status.

A typical patient with partial denervation would be a man who experienced a peroneal nerve injury during a right total knee replacement 9 months ago. The patient has needed an ankle-foot arthrosis (AFO) on the right because a foot drop since surgery because he is unable to actively dorsiflex the right ankle. According to the results of an EMG, the tibialis anterior muscle is reinnervating; however, the patient is unable to perform a volitional contraction. An example of a treatment plan:

1. NMES to re-educate reinnervating muscle
2. Conventional strengthening exercises if patient learns to contract voluntarily
3. Gait training with externally triggered NMES if appropriate to progress to ambulation without AFO.

In the presence of partial denervation, the motor point placement is difficult to predict with motor points moving more distally in most instances.[25,26] A stimulus with a longer pulse duration is preferable in the presence of partial denervation. The patient may have to be followed monthly or quarterly to assess reinnervation status until a Fair– or Fair contraction can be generated volitionally. Reinnervation is difficult to predict and requires frequent re-evaluation.

SAFETY CONSIDERATIONS

EQUIPMENT

It is the clinician's responsibility to assure the safety and proper operation of all equipment. Inspection of equipment before use is an important safety measure that should be implemented as routine. A professional inspection of equipment should be scheduled yearly with a sticker clearly showing the date of the last inspection.

Every piece of equipment comes with an operating manual. Take the time to read the manual, which should be readily available. Equipment should never be operated if the user is not thoroughly familiar with its operation. Although the clinician's safety is an important factor when using electrical equipment, the patient's safety is obviously paramount. Refer to Chapter 10 for details on safety conditions.

PATIENT FACTORS

Medical History

It is recommended that before treatment the patient should be questioned relative to the indications and contraindications of the modality being utilized. At the time of the evaluation, the patient may have forgotten to mention a possible problem, or may have developed a problem that may make the application of the modality questionable. Thus it is good practice to interview the patient prior to all treatments. If the patient does disclose additional relevant information, you must report that information to the evaluating therapist before treatment.

Skin Condition and Sensation

A visual inspection of the area to be treated will identify both normal and abnormal skin conditions. Normal findings may include birthmarks or other skin discolorations that will remain after a treatment is given. Observations should be clearly documented in the patient's medical chart to inform other therapists who may provide treatment and to enable the treating therapist to identify any change in skin conditions that may result from a treatment.

After treatment, the stimulated skin area may be pink in color as a result of an increase in the superficial blood flow that results from a treatment. These changes should resolve within 30 to 60 minutes following the treatment. If the treated area remains quite red and/or color changes do not resolve, one should consult the therapist immediately. An electrical burn will cause black or brown skin spots. If an electrical burn has occurred, the patient must be treated immediately with the appropriate first aid. Maintenance of a good interface between the electrode and the patient by using an adequate amount of gel, complete contact of the electrode with the skin, and adequate fixation will prevent tissue damage.

Your communication with and observation of the patient and the area being treated is critical. Careful selection of waveform, pulse duration, and electrodes will prevent tissue damage from stimulation electrodes.

Cognitive Issues

Cognition, psychologic abilities, and neuromuscular performance are interdependent. Impairment of cognition may be identified during the evaluation and relayed to you or you may identify cognitive impairment through your careful observations and good communication. Cognitive impairments include a decreased ability to learn or understand instructions or an inability to translate instructions into expected outcomes. Clear and concise communication is essential. The use of visual and tactile cues will be beneficial. Demonstration and feeling a normal muscular contraction on an unaffected body part may be one way to explain the goal of muscle re-education clearly. Remember, most patients do not have medical backgrounds. Using laypersons' terms to describe procedures is important.

Cognitive dysfunction can be incorrectly translated to poor motivation. Clinicians must continuously encourage and reinforce positive results throughout treatment. Patient understanding can be determined by asking the patient to repeat the instructions, the process, and the expected outcomes. Most important, help the patient understand why the treatment is needed and how it will relate to his or her everyday activities.

Lack of cognition does not prohibit the use of electrical stimulation. Electrical stimulation has been found to be very effective in decreasing spasticity and improving ROM in comatose patients.[27] Careful observation is mandatory for safety in this application.

PATIENT EDUCATION

EXPECTED OUTCOMES

Expected outcomes are directly related to the patient's education and understanding before, during, and after treatment. Patients must understand the reason for the treatment, the process of the treatment, and the outcomes and benefits of the treatment. Explaining the rationale for treatment will allow the patient the opportunity to communicate his or her needs, which then can be incorporated into the treatment plan. The reason for treatment is usually identified or most understood in functional terms. Electrical stimulation for muscle re-education to the quadriceps may benefit the patient in transfers or ambulation potential. It is important to communicate with the evaluating therapist to be sure that you understand the expected outcome and not provide false hope to the patient.

Explaining procedures utilized during the treatment process and the expected sensations will reduce the patient's fears and anxieties. Education and understanding of these procedures and sensations will allow the patient to better communicate and give the therapist feedback with which to maximize the treatment.

Proper education of the expected outcomes and benefits is crucial. Clinicians must understand these outcomes prior to the initiation of treatment and appropriately utilize them with each patient. Electrical stimulation has many uses in physical therapy as was previously discussed. Electrical stimulation may be used for muscle relaxation as in the case of spasticity. Achievement of this relaxation may assist antagonist muscles to function, or improve mobility through increased ROM. Muscle re-education is commonly seen with the use of electrical stimulation. Increased strength and utilization of extremities is often seen as volitional control is redeveloped. Reduction of swelling and edema through the utilization of electrical stimulation can also enhance range of motion and use of extremities in all facets of activities of daily living.

CLINICAL DECISION MAKING

EVALUATING TREATMENT EFFECTIVENESS AND MODIFYING TREATMENT

Treatment goals should be realistically and reliably achieved. A thorough understanding of the application of electrotherapy is very important to its use, especially since it is not a modality that is readily understood by many physicians or insurance companies, much less the patients who will experience it. It is equally important to be able to assess the outcome of treatment once initiated. It is impossible to do so without timely, appropriate, and reliable measurements of the patient's physical status before, during, and after treatment. Clear and timely communication between the evaluating therapist and assistant will ensure effective and appropriate treatments. On a daily basis, it is important to assess skin integrity, patient's response to the last treatment, and any complaints of discomfort or change in symptoms.

DOCUMENTING TREATMENT

At evaluation and subsequent regular reassessments, other measurements of status are made. Although the issue of reliability of clinical measurements is beyond the scope of this chapter, certain types of measurement have been accepted as generally reliable. Isokinetic assessments of strength are frequently used and in many cases have been shown to be very reliable for the assessment of strength and endurance.[28,29] Active and passive ROM measurements are very useful in documenting progress in contracture management and motor control. It is frequently important to measure both active and passive ROM. In the assessment of edema and hypertrophy, girth measurements have been frequently used. Volumetric measurements of the amount of water displaced by a limb are preferable when realistic to perform. Accurate descriptions of gait or movement patterns and measurement of the temporal aspects of gait with a stopwatch are all useful, and when available, videotaping of the patient's performance is especially helpful.

The use of NMES to address the wide variety of patient scenarios presented in this chapter requires a familiarity with the equipment available in your facility and the characteristics of the available waveforms and stimulation parameters available with that equipment. Portable equipment in general will be less powerful, have fewer adjustable parameters, and can be more prone to damage. Clinical models will be potentially more versatile (for applications such as iontophoresis and wound healing, which are beyond the scope of this chapter), but less portable and more powerful, with a greater likelihood of causing tissue damage.

As stated previously, patient comfort is of primary importance because a treatment that cannot be tolerated is an ineffective treatment. It is very important for the assistant to monitor the patient closely during the initial treatment sessions to assess comfort and communicate immediately with the evaluating therapist if a change in parameters should be considered.

SUMMARY

In this chapter the application of neuromuscular electrical stimulation (NMES) as a clinical modality has been briefly reviewed. Understanding the rationale for using NMES when making clinical decisions for your patients will ultimately be reflected in their progress. This broad topic merits additional study through further reading.

DISCUSSION QUESTIONS

1. What are the sensory and motor effects of altering current, amplitude, and pulse duration?

2. When stimulating a patient, what is the importance of the current path?

3. If a patient has external metal on his or her skin such as staples, can electrical stimulation be used and why should your placement of the electrodes be carefully considered?

4. When stimulating the ankle, should you be concerned with deviations such as inversion and eversion? What can you do to address these deviations produced by the electrical stimulation?

5. What size surface electrode would you choose when stimulating the gluteus maximus, and why is the size of the surface electrode important?

REFERENCES

1. Electrotherapeutic Terminology in Physical Therapy. Section on Clinical Electrophysiology: American Physical Therapy Association, Alexandria, VA, 1990, p 29.

2. Nelson, RM and Currier, DP: Clinical Electrotherapy. Appleton and Lange, Norwalk, CT, 1987, p 110.

3. Baker, LL, et al: Neuromuscular Electrical Stimulation: A Practical Clinical Guide, ed 3. Los Amigos Research and Education Institute, Downey, CA, 1993, p 73.

4. Baker, LL, et al: Neuromuscular Electrical Stimulation: A Practical Clinical Guide, ed 3. Los Amigos Research and Education Institute, Downey, CA, 1993, p 75.

5. Snyder-Mackler, L and Robinson, AJ: Clinical Electrophysiology—Electrotherapy and Electrophysiologic Testing. Williams & Wilkins, Baltimore, 1989, p 131.

6. Delitto, A and Rose, SJ: Comparative comfort of three waveforms used in electrically eliciting quadriceps femoris muscle contractions. Phys Ther 66:1704, 1986.

7. Bowman, BR and Baker, LL: Effects of waveform parameters on comfort during transcutaneous neuromuscular electrical stimulation. Ann Biomed Eng 13:59, 1974.

8. Baker, LL, Bowan, BR, and McNeal, DR: Effects of waveform on comfort during neuromuscular electrical stimulation. Clin Orthop Related Res 233:75, 1988.

9. McNeal, DR, et al: Subject preference for pulse frequency with cutaneous stimulation of the quadriceps. Proc Rehabil Eng Soc North Am 9:273, 1986.

10. Electrotherapeutic Terminology in Physical Therapy. Section on Clinical Electrophysiology: American Physical Therapy Association, Alexandria, VA, 1990, p 25.

11. Baker, LL, et al: Neuromuscular Electrical Stimulation: A Practical Clinical Guide, ed 3. Los Amigos Research and Education Institute, Downey, CA, 1993, p 87.

12. Electrotherapeutic Terminology in Physical Therapy. Section on Clinical Electrophysiology: American Physical Therapy Association, Alexandria, VA, 1990, p 21.

13. Currier, DP, and Mann, R: Muscular strength development by electrical stimulation in healthy individuals. Phys Ther 63:915, 1983.

14. Robinson, AJ and Snyder-Mackler, L (eds): Clinical Electrophysiology—Electrotherapy and Electrophysiologic Testing, ed 2. Williams & Wilkins, Baltimore, 1995, pp 129–130.

15. Delitto, A, et al: Electrically elicited co-contraction of thigh musculature after anterior cruciate ligament surgery. Phys Ther 68:45, 1988.

16. Selkowitz, DM: Improvement in isometric strength of the quadriceps femoris muscle after training with electrical stimulation. Phys Ther 6:186, 1985.

17. Baker, LL, et al: Neuromuscular Electrical Stimulation: A Practical Clinical Guide, ed 3. Los Amigos Research and Education Institute, Downey, CA, 1993, p 51.

18. Draper, V and Ballard, L: Electrical stimulation versus electromyographic biofeedback in the recovery of quadriceps femoris muscle function following anterior cruciate ligament surgery. Phys Ther 71:455, 1991.

19. Sawyer, P (ed): Biophysical Mechanisms in Homeostasis and Intravascular Thrombosis. Appleton-Century-Crofts, New York, 1965.

20. Nelson, RM and Currier, DP: Clinical Electrotherapy. Appleton and Lange, Norwalk, CT, 1987, p 176.

21. Phillips, CA: Functional electrical stimulation and lower extremity bracing for ambulation exercise of the spinal cord injured individual: A medically prescribed system. Phys Ther 69:842, 1989.

22. Baker, LL: Neuromuscular electrical stimulation in the restoration of purposeful limb movements. In Wolf, SL (ed): Clinics in Physical Therapy—Electrotherapy. Churchill Livingston, New York, 1981, p 25.

23. Eckerson, LF and Axelgaard, J: Lateral electrical surface stimulation as an alternative to bracing in the treatment of idiopathic scoliosis. Phys Ther 64:483, 1984.

24. Baker, LL and Parker, K: Neuromuscular electrical stimulation of the muscles surrounding the shoulder. Phys Ther 66:1930, 1986.

25. Richardson, AT and Wynn-Parry, CB: The theory and practice of electrodiagnosis. Ann Phys Med 4:3, 1957.

26. Wynn-Parry, CB: Strength duration curves. In Licht, S (ed): Electrodiagnosis and Electromyography, ed 2. Elizabeth Licht, 1961, p 241.

27. Baker, LL, Parker, K, and Sanderson, D: Neuromuscular electrical stimulation for the head injured patient. Phys Ther 63:1967, 1983.

28. Farrell, M, and Richards, JG: Analysis of the reliability and validity of the kinetic communicator exercise device. Med Sci Sports Exer 18:44, 1986.

ACKNOWLEDGMENTS

The authors would like to thank Jean Scofield from Rancho Los Amigos for her assistance with photo permission; Kathy Goodstein from Shriners Hospitals, Philadelphia Unit, for photography; Shriners Hospitals, Philadelphia Unit, Research Department for their support; and Elizabeth R. Gardner, MS PT NCS, Linda Baird-Jansen, MS PT, Betsy Butterworth, PTA, Vicki Vanartsdalen, PTA, and Sophia Mullin Selgrath for their editorial recommendations. Most importantly, thanks to Andy, Alex, and Ellen for their understanding, love, and support.

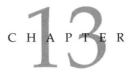

Tissue Healing with Electrical Stimulation: Wound Care and Iontophoresis

Mary Ann Dalzell, PT

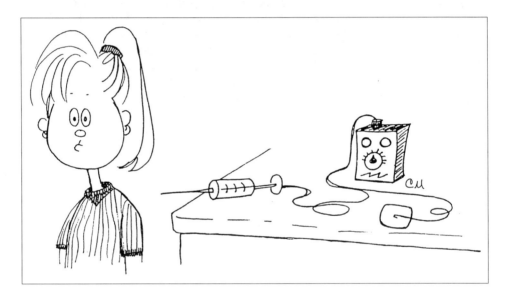

CHAPTER OBJECTIVES

- Describe the use of electrical stimulation for medication delivery.
- Describe the ionic properties of direct current.
- Outline the procedures for phoretic delivery of medications.
- Differentiate between iontophoretic drug delivery and injection.
- Outline the medications utilized and their polarity.
- Discuss the classifications of wounds.
- Discuss the electrical potentials of normal and injured tissues.
- Outline the application of electrical stimulation to promote tissue repair.
- Discuss documentation of or electrical stimulation for wound care.

Electrical stimulation for tissue repair (ESTR) encompasses management of open wounds, transcutaneous drug delivery, that is, iontophoresis, and reduction of edema. This chapter will focus on the uses of electrical stimulation for wound healing and for drug delivery. Edema control has been covered elsewhere in this text.

ELECTRICAL STIMULATION FOR WOUND HEALING

GENERAL HISTORICAL PERSPECTIVE

Injured tissue produces an electrically measurable signal that varies according to the nature of the injury and the type of tissue injured.[1,2] This "current of injury" became the basis for the development of diagnostic tools as well as electrical currents for the healing of tissues.[3] It is only within the past 20 to 30 years that clinicians have produced controlled studies on animals and humans examining the ability of electrical currents to heal tissue. Three areas of research have dominated the literature on tissue healing with electrical stimulation: bone healing, wound healing, and the mechanisms underlying the effect of an externally applied electrical field on the process of healing. In addition, muscle, tendon, and ligament healing have more recently been investigated by several authors who hoped to reproduce the same results with different soft tissues.[4,5] However, the stimulation parameters for facilitation of healing appear to vary between tissues with different cellular compositions, and thus more research is needed to identify the specific electrical properties of these tissues before consistent and reproducible results can be obtained.

Healing of nonunion fractures and osteonecrosis in both pediatric and adult populations has been shown to be improved by electrical stimulation.[6] Initially, variable results reported by different authors made the orthopedic community skeptical about using this modality of treatment, but, more recently, a statistically significant healing of type I and type II nonunion fractures of the tibia has been demonstrated.[7] In addition, core decompression of osteonecrotic femoral heads has been studied to determine the potential benefits of electrical stimulation. Electrical stimulation produced greater vascularization of necrotic bone.[8] As stimulation parameters continue to be defined, other authors have had success in increasing the mineralization of osteogenic tissue, increasing the calcification of connective tissue, and inhibiting necrosis and collagen degradation.[10,11] However, these results have been obtained in bone that did not follow the normal course of healing, and it remains uncertain as to whether fractures healing normally without complication would be enhanced by electrical stimulation.

Studies on wound healing focus on chronic ulcerations complicated by vascular deficiencies, neurologic impairment, or endocrine pathologies.[12] These wounds have been conclusively shown to heal faster when electrically stimulated.[13] However, studies on acute, uncomplicated wounds appear to indicate that the normal process of healing cannot be accelerated.[14–16]

This section will briefly review the literature pertinent to the therapeutic application of electrical currents to chronic wounds. In addition, it will elaborate on the principles of treatment, the rationale for selection, and procedural protocols for application.

WOUNDS: BRIEF HISTORICAL PERSPECTIVE

As far back as 1688, it was noted that smallpox lesions treated with applications of charged gold leaf healed without scarring.[17] More recently, evidence suggests that the microcurrents generated by the electrostatic charge from gold leaf may enhance wound healing. These microcurrents mimic the bioelectrical currents associated with injury and thereby trigger the healing process.[18]

In 1940, Burr and associates [19] measured the electrical potentials of abdominal incisions post surgery and found that they varied from positive to negative until healing was complete. This "current of injury" was further studied by Becker[20] in the 1960s and found to trigger biological repair. Furthermore, he found that artificially augmenting the negative polarity of regenerating salamander limbs accelerated the healing process. Within the same decade, Smith[21] succeeded in partially regenerating frog limbs and Becker and Spodero[22] extended Becker's experiment to other mammals.

In 1969, Wolcott and colleagues[23] accelerated the healing of skin ulcers by stimulating the wounds with 100 to 1000 μA. A program of direct current 7 days a week was used. Seventy-five percent of the wounds healed completely in an average of 9.6 weeks.

Further investigations on the precise nature and source of healing wounds have continued over the past few decades alongside further clinical studies on the effectiveness of different stimulation parameters for promotion of healing of chronic open wounds.[24]

MECHANISMS OF EFFECTIVENESS

Animal and human studies have been conducted measuring specific voltage gradients across the epidermis.[25] Incisions were shown to generate lateral intraepidermal currents that peaked in close proximity to the wound and declined with distance from the wound. This so-called skin battery is thought to be the source of currents for healing wounds.

Another theory suggests that the body possesses currents within the vascular interstitial tissues.[26] In 1983, Nordenstrom[26] proposed that the walls of blood vessels, insulating tissue matrix, transcapillary junctions, interstitial fluid, and intravascular plasma are all capable of conducting bioelectricity. The combined direct current (DC) potentials of the skin, subcutaneous tissue, and vascular system may contribute to a total current of injury. This current stimulates the cellular activity necessary to debride damaged tissues, stimulate tissue regeneration, and remodels these tissues in response to functional needs.[27] Depending upon the characteristics of the electrical current, artificial stimulation may be capable of nonspecifically stimulating the process or specifically guiding cellular activity.

Cellular Responses to Healing

Many experiments on the effects of electrical field exposure have demonstrated that individual cells migrate toward electrodes (galvanotaxis) and that the speed and direction of migration is determined by the strength of the field and the polarity of the electrodes.[13] Migration to the cathode resulted from electric field exposure in fibroblast, epidermal, myoblast, and neurite cell cultures. Specific frequencies of pulsed currents caused alterations in cellular biosynthesis and differentiation.[28]

Human fibroblasts were exposed to current densities of 40 V/cm for 20 minutes at a frequency of 100 Hz and a significant increase in protein and DNA synthesis was precipitated by the stimulation. The effect was maximized within specific frequency ranges and minimized when greater current densities were applied. There is also evidence showing that electrical currents can inhibit bacterial growth. Experiments revealed that the growth of *Pseudomonas aeruginosa*[29] and *Staphylococcus aureus*[31] are inhibited by the application of cathodal stimulation. A human study showed that bacterial contamination of burns was inhibited by low-voltage stimulation.[31] In addition, it has been found that anodal stimulation can reduce the growth of hypertrophic scars[32] and thrombose the veins of dogs, whereas cathodal stimulation increases blood flow[33] and facilitates the debridement of necrotic wound tissue.[34]

In summary, the current research supports the belief that different parameters of electrical stimulation have specific effects upon the cellular responses to healing.[24] Negative polarity has been shown to increase vascularity and stimulate fibroblastic growth and collagen production, induce epidermal cell migration, and inhibit bacterial infiltration. Positive currents attract macrophages, promote epithelial growth, and act as vasoconstrictors.[2] In addition, current density and frequency are capable of facilitating or inhibiting cellular activity, depending upon their intensity.[24]

Human Studies

Electrical stimulation is likely to be beneficial in skin healing.[2] The rates of healing vary between studies, and in a few experimental projects very little benefit was reported.[35,36] Failure to carefully duplicate and control the parameters of stimulation has contributed to the present ambiguity.[24] The parameters of treatment constitute the dosage, which must be standardized to permit cross-evaluation of the literature. Therefore, the literature on human studies must be interpreted with great caution in order to avoid generalization. In 1969, Wolcott and colleagues[23] reported a mean healing rate of 13.4% per week for 75 chronic ulcers that were treated with a constant DC current in the range of 200 to 800 μA. These investigators used a negative polarity until asepsis was obtained and then switched to positive polarity.

Using the same parameters of stimulation, two other groups of investigators attempted to duplicate the results of Wolcott. One hundred patients with ischemic ulcers were treated and reported a healing rate of 29% in the treatment group versus 14% in the control group.[37] Studies using a larger number of controls and fewer hours of treatment per week reported an 18% versus 9% healing rates in treatment versus control groups.[38] Of particular interest is the series of patients with bilateral ulcers which was reported in each of these studies. Given a controlled comparison, stimulated ulcers in these subgroups of patients showed differences in healing rates ranging from 15% to 22% greater.

More recently, high-voltage monophasic pulsed currents have been used in a series of studies on decubitus ulcers.[39,40] However, it is difficult to compare the results of these initial studies given the small patient population and lack of control groups. A well-controlled study was conducted in 1988 on 16 subjects with stage II ulcers where a reported 46% healing rate for stimulated ulcers occurred versus 11.6% for the controls.[41] In fact, the control ulcers increased in size despite regular wound care, and when a small group of these control ulcers were stimulated following the study, they healed an average of 38% per week. Once again, it was found that changing the polarity during treatment optimized the results.

The effects of high-voltage pulsed currents in a randomized placebo-controlled group of 17 patients who had been unresponsive to traditional wound care were studied. There was a statistically significant difference in healing rates.[42] A new pulsed galvanic electrical stimulation device (Dermapulse, Staodyne Corp., Longmont, CO) was tested in two studies on patients with nonhealing stage III and IV ulcers. These well-controlled studies once again demonstrated that healing rates were greater than twice that of the sham (electrodes applied, but no current delivered) treated groups.[43] Moreover, when the sham group was crossed over to active stimulation at the end of the trial, healing rates greater than 3.5 times that of the previous 4 weeks were reported.

In summary, the human studies provide support for the benefits of electrical stimulation for chronic wound healing despite some of the variations in protocols and parameters used for stimulation. No adverse effects have been noted,[13] less debridement is necessary, and in fact, highly contaminated wounds became less contaminated.[3,29] Although ideal dosages remain to be defined, it is nonetheless apparent that patients who are debilitated by various medical problems (vascular deficiencies, diabetes, neurologic deficits) respond dramatically to the stimulus of an electric current that triggers healing.[40]

Animal Studies

Interestingly, there are greater variations in the outcome of many of the animal studies that traditionally provide better controlled environments for verification of the effectiveness of treatment. This phenomenon likely arises from the fact that stimulation parameters varied more greatly in the animal studies, and more importantly, it is difficult for these investigators to duplicate the debilitated medical state of human patients who were involved in the studies on electrical stimulation.[44]

When anodal (+) stimulation was used, treated wounds had fibrous connec-

tive tissue with the collagen fibers aligned perpendicular to the surface. Cathodal
(−) stimulation produced larger denser scars with the collagen fibers aligned parallel to the surface. More recent studies[47–49] have emphasized the importance of
polarity in determining the quality of healing. The effects of changing polarity
over the course of treatment have been evaluated in a series of studies using high-
voltage stimulation, with no differences between control and treated groups.
However, alternating the polarity from negative to positive after 3 days of stimulation produced 87% healing rates and higher rates of epithelialization in the
treated animals.[31,51,52]

A recent study specifically evaluated the effects of polarity on epithelialization
of wounds. The best results were obtained by initiating treatment with negative
stimulation followed by positive. Alternating polarity daily produced the poorest
results.[53] The acute incisional wounds studied may differ in polarity over the progressive healing stages from those of chronic wounds.

In summary, the tensile strength and structure of fibrous tissue appears to be
normalized and enhanced by electrical stimulation provided that the appropriate
dosage parameters are used. Twenty-four hours of stimulation per day may *not*
improve healing,[48,54] whereas one hour of stimulation per day has repeatedly been
shown to be beneficial.[32,36] Varying polarity is thus more effective in speeding
wound healing than maintaining the same polarity. Current densities that take
into consideration the effective duty cycle as well as the duration of treatment will
have to be specifically controlled in future studies to permit greater consistency in
study design and the capacity to cross-evaluate results.[24]

PRINCIPLES AND METHODS OF TREATMENT

Chronic wounds are difficult to manage and represent a major cost to the medical
community. The principle cause of these wounds is a lack of adequate blood supply (ischemia) combined with damage to the nervous system (insensitivity), complicated by a lack of mobility and poor general metabolism. Thus, the groups of
patients most vulnerable to the development of chronic wounds are spinal-cord-
injured patients, patients with peripheral vascular disease, and geriatric patients.
The rationale underlying treatment is to facilitate the healing process by optimizing the conditions that prevail during normal wound closure.

Some of the key factors that contribute to a homeostatic wound environment
have been reviewed in detail by McCulloch and associates[44] in a text devoted to
the management of chronic wounds. They emphasized the importance of wound
moisture, sufficient blood perfusion, the availability of oxygen, the prevention of
wound contamination by bacteria, and the maintenance of voltage gradients between the wound and the adjacent skin.

A moist wound environment has been shown to stimulate epidermal cell migration[55] and can maintain the lateral voltage gradients that are thought to control
the direction of epidermal cell migration. Dehydrated and scabbed wounds increase the resistance to wound closure by obstruction with dead tissue which must
be debrided before normal granulation tissue can develop. Debridement or the removal of necrotic and devitalized tissue from wounds must be done manually by
saline irrigation or whirlpool jets directed at the wound unless large amounts of
necrotic tissue prevent the use of these simple methods.

The oxygen and nutrient supply to wounds is as critical as fuel is to automobiles. When blood flow to a given tissue is impaired, the tissue suffers irreversible cell damage. Furthermore, tissues that are inflamed or in the process of healing need an even greater supply of oxygen and nutrients because of the increase in metabolism associated with these processes. It is not surprising that patients with either circulatory supply problems (i.e., arterial insufficiency) or circulatory return problems (i.e., venous insufficiency) need to have the circulation local to the skin wound primed and re-established before healing can take place.

One of the most common causes of skin breakdown is mechanical pressure or friction that inhibits blood flow. These pressure sores or decubitus ulcers usually occur over bony prominences and in areas that are difficult to decompress. Treatment of these pressure-induced skin ulcerations must include pressure-relieving devices such as cushions, mattresses, or water-flotation pads as well as careful nursing to ensure that patients unable to move themselves are repositioned frequently.

Open wounds are also very susceptible to contamination with bacteria from air exposure, contact with bedding, and continuous handling of occlusive dressings. Therefore controlling the wound environment must include the application of antimicrobial solutions such as hydrogen peroxide, acetic acid solution, sodium hypochlorite solution, or topical bactericidal agents such as neosporin ointment, silvadene, furacin, and zinc oxide. The choice of solutions or ointments is dependent upon the specific bacterial invasion present or anticipated. Treatment principles for chronic wounds are outlined in Table 13–1.

Indications for Use

The global objective underlying the use of electrical stimulation is to catalyze and accelerate the rate of chronic wound healing. Specifically, based upon the review of the literature presented in the first section of this chapter, electrical stimulation can be used to debride necrotic material, attract neutrophils and macrophages, increase blood flow, stimulate growth of fibroblasts, inhibit bacteria, and induce epidermal cell migration.

In combination with other conservative methods of treatment that include manual or mechanical debridement, pressure-relieving devices, and antibacterial serums or ointments, electrical stimulation can form a very strong ally to the forces necessary to repair chronic wounds. The indications for use include decreasing pressure ulcers in patients with vascular insufficiencies, diabetic ulcerations, ulcers due to neurologic deficiencies, and burns that are relatively localized.

Table 13–1 **Principles of Treating Chronic Wounds**

1. Maintain wound moisture.
2. Prevent scab formation.
3. Debride necrotic material.
4. Increase blood flow.
5. Prevent contamination by bacteria.
6. Promote the development of granulation tissue.
7. Promote re-epithelialization.

Contraindications for Use

In addition to the general precautions and contraindications for the use of electrical stimulation discussed in Chapter 10, there are some other considerations to the use of electrical stimulation for wound healing. The knowledge that electrical currents act as electrical catalysts to stimulate tissues in a relatively nondifferential manner gives rise to several contraindications for use. Particular attention must be paid to the past and present medical history of the patient before applying an electrical current. Any present or past history of cancer or a localized malignancy is an absolute contraindication to use of these devices. In addition, any past or suspicious present history of a potential osteomyelitis (particularly when an ulceration has exposed or infiltrated a bony prominence) is a contraindication to use until lab tests can rule out this possibility. Finally, any indication of thrombosis underlying an ulceration of circulatory origin is a contraindication for use, given the increase in local blood flow and at a distance from the electrical stimulators that may potentially embolize the thrombus.

Clinical interactions with either oral or locally applied medications is a cause for significant concern when dealing with patients who are likely to be in a debilitated state of health. Medications that systemically influence ionic balance and regulation, such as diuretics, may cause patients to be more sensitive to electrical currents. In particular, it has been noted that iodine-based products being used to cleanse or medicate chronic wounds interact with electrical currents and produce an irritation or burns depending on the concentration of the solution and the strength of the current. Clinicians must ensure that wounds are well cleansed before applying these devices, and, ideally, alternative bactericidal solutions should be used during this period of treatment.

Precautions

To avoid potential skin irritations, several precautions should be taken when using electrical stimulation. Liberal irrigation of wounds with saline before beginning treatment will ensure that topically applied ointments or solutions will not interact with the current to be applied.

The generally friable, poorly nurtured skin of patients with chronic wounds must be taken into consideration when dosage parameters are being selected. Tissue damage can occur if the wound dressings are too small because of a concentration of current over a localized area. Tissue damage can occur if the electrical current is too intense or applied for too long a period of time. It is important to increase dosage parameters gradually in order to assess the skin tolerance before full protocol currents are applied. It is of equal importance to follow protocols over time and not manipulate dosage parameters at liberty. The final precaution is to avoid application during pregnancy given the fact that safety has not been established during fetal development.

Wound Safety Considerations

To prevent bacterial contamination, dressings are to be disposed of following one use and electrode dispensers should be dedicated to use by one patient only. Finally, the cables of each stimulator should be wiped clean with alcohol following use to avoid transmission of bacteria from one patient to another.

Treatment Techniques

Therapy strategies should be based upon the depth and extent of soft tissue necrosis present in the wound to be treated. Wounds may vary in grade from one part to another and it is essential to treat the most severe condition present in the wound at any given time. Adjustments of the parameters of treatment are made as the most severe condition is resolved. Therefore, before elaborating upon protocols for treatment, a brief description of the wound stages will enable the practitioner to recognize when the ulcer status is improving or deteriorating and provide a basis for selection of dosage parameters. Table 13–2 outlines ulcer categories and descriptions.

For more indepth guidelines on identifying wound stages that must be documented throughout treatment, it is recommended that the clinician consult a comprehensive text on standards and protocols for ulcer care.[60]

Ulcer Preparation and Concomitant Therapy

An appropriate healing environment must set the stage for wound care, otherwise treatment efforts become an exercise in futility. Nutritional assessments and vitamin therapy will improve the general health status of the patient. Laboratory studies for serum albumin and glucose will determine whether underlying metabolic

Table 13–2 Ulcer Categories and Character Descriptions

Four distinct wound categories have been defined, ranging from minor preulcerative skin states to defects that include skin, soft tissue, and bone.[59] These categories are described as follows:

Category I: Wounds retain an intact epidermis but show signs of redness and chronic irritation. Skin discoloration persists despite transient pressure alterations and is highly susceptible to breakdown.

Category II: Defects are relatively superficial and involve the epidermis and/or the dermis. This partial-thickness skin loss is characterized by a clear serous drainage, a cream-colored ground substance, and fragile granulation tissue around the wound edges.

Category III: Defects extend into subcutaneous tissue and involve damage or necrosis that may extend to the underlying fascia. If contaminated, a purulent yellow or green/brown exudate of foul odor fills the defect. These full-thickness skin losses heal by becoming pink initially, followed by a "beefy red" serosanguinous stage that is the precursor of healthy granulation tissue.

Category IV: Defects extend not only into subcutaneous superficial tissue but also into muscle, bone, or joint. These full-thickness skin losses induce significant damage to supporting structures and great caution must be exercised before conservative treatment is implemented. Surgical debridement is indicated when the margin of the eschar is fused with the rim. When bones are visibly exposed, biopsies or x-rays must rule out osteomyelitis. When sinus tracts or tunnels into wounds are present, the clinician must proceed with caution and ideally consult with the referring physician.

Electrical stimulation is indicated when a partial eschar with purulent or nonpurulent drainage is present. Healing progressions are once again identified by alterations in the quantity and quality of drainage from brown-green to yellow, to "beefy red," and from thick to a watery serosanguinous oozing that precedes the development of granulation tissue.

problems exist. Air mattresses, sheep skin, and special beds relieve continuous pressure, which impairs the circulation and retards healing. In addition, x-rays or biopsies must be taken when there is suspicion of bone exposure. Wound cultures will determine whether defects are contaminated and identify the bacterial organism. All of these steps must be taken before and during treatment to ensure that wound healing is enhanced (Tables 13–3 and 13–4).

The following protocol is suggested based upon a recent series of studies on chronic wound healing.[24,41,43] Low-intensity pulsed current of negative polarity should be used in the initial stimulation phase for approximately 1 hour per day until healing is complete. The pulsed rather than continuous currents allow higher current densities without irritation or burning and improve vascular support, particularly when delivered with negative polarity. The most effective absolute charge density is thought to be in the range of 1 to 2 mA/cm^2, which takes into consideration the electrode size, area through which current is being conducted, and the strength of the current. Kloth[41] suggests that once the wound has been debrided of necrotic and purulent material, switching to a high-voltage pulsed current of positive polarity alternating with negative polarity when a healing plateau is evident may maximize wound closure.

Documentation

Pretreatment measurements of wound location, size, depth, and shape must be recorded before each stimulation session. Clinical tools available to facilitate measurement are transparent tracings on film or gridded acetates, photographs and tape measurements. A sterile-tipped applicator can be inserted into the wound, removed, and measured for an indication of sinus, tunnel, or wound depth.

The degree of inflammation or infection is also important to document. Pain, swelling, redness, and increased temperature provide information on the degree of generalized inflammation and infection and precise descriptions of the odor, color, amount and consistency of any wound drainage will more specifically provide a record of the degree of contamination.

Treatment parameters must be recorded to ensure consistency between treatments and the progression of parameters utilized. The size of electrodes, space between electrodes, polarity of the active electrode, and position of application must

---

Table 13–3 **Wound Care Procedures for Electrical Stimulation**

> Wound care procedures that must continually accompany the electrical stimulation sessions include:
>
> 1. Specific or nonspecific debridement (enzymatic and surgical versus whirlpool jet agitation and wound irrigation)
>
> 2. Topical antibiotic therapy
>
> 3. Saline- and gauze-soaked dressings for defects including tunnels and sinuses
>
> 4. Occlusive dressings when the "beefy red" pregranulation stage develops
>
> Throughout treatment, it is imperative to avoid adhesive dressings, never remove skin buds, minimize pressure dressings, and above all, ensure that a moist environment is maintained.[55]

Table 13–4   Treatment Steps with Electrical Stimulation for Wound Healing

Step 1. Before treating a patient with electrical stimulation, the wound must be irrigated with copious amounts of normal saline, particularly if ointments, creams, or lotions have been used to medicate the ulceration. Interactions between topical medications and the electrical stimulation can cause severe irritation or burns.

Step 2. Place a saline-saturated gauze dressing into the ulcer bed to keep it moist and ensure that the current will be conducted to all parts of the wound. Blot the surrounding skin dry.

Note: It is possible to provide stimulation through hydrocolloid (hydrated) dressings.[61] The dressings must be throughly hydrated. Furthermore, any dressing with resistance greater than $5 \times 10 \ \Omega/cm^2$ will prevent passage of the minimum amount of current required to stimulate healing. Therefore polyurethane film or foam dressings must be removed during treatment.

Step 3. The active electrode is placed onto the ulcer bed and the dispersive electrode is placed between 15 and 25 cm (6 to 8 inches) away from the ulcer over intact skin or a large muscle mass. Ideally, the cathode is placed caudal (inferior) to the anode to amplify the "current of injury."

When necrotic or purulent material fills the ulcer defect, cathodal stimulation is used until the infection clears. As mentioned previously, the cathode has been shown to have the capacity to solubilize necrotic tissue; destroy bacterial cell membranes; increase vascularity; and cause migration of macrophages, neutrophils, and leucocytes to the wound site.

When the exudate becomes clear and more sanguinous, anodal stimulation can commence. It is unclear as to whether chronic wounds are favored by maintaining anodal stimulation until healing is complete or continuously alternating polarity whenever a plateau in healing is observed. Further research is needed to clarify this important detail.

Step 4. Set the stimulation parameters.

Step 5. Remove the electrodes and use a sterile technique to reapply medications and dressings.

be documented. In addition, the type of current (continuous DC, low-voltage pulsed, or high-voltage pulsed currents), current amplitude, and time of stimulation must be recorded.

In summary, the status of the wound over time and the progressions of treatment must be documented to ensure that the electrical stimulation is of continuous benefit to the patient. This information will be used by the treating practitioner and other clinicians responsible for the continuous care of the patient. A consistent body of knowledge emerges from the large numbers of wounds treated via electrical stimulation to ensure that further developments on ideal treatment parameters be made to optimize results.

IONTOPHORESIS

BRIEF HISTORY

Iontophoresis is the introduction of ionic substances into the body for therapeutic purposes by means of a direct current. Transdermal ion migration deposits ions subcutaneously via an electromotive force. The dosage of drug delivered is dependent upon the polarity of application, the force of the current, the mobility of the ion, and the resistance of soft tissues to which the drug is being applied. Therapeutic results are dependent upon the choice of drug in relation to the pathology as well as the capacity to deliver sufficient quantities of medication to the affected tissues.

Iontophoresis was employed clinically in the early twentieth century.[62,63] Subsequently, it became less favored and was utilized principally as a research tool.[64] More recently, a renewed surge of interest has been sparked by the search for methods of drug delivery that are associated with less general metabolic complications, less pain, and less trauma. Iontophoresis is often capable of localizing medication to the tissues of interest, but precise dosage delivery through adjustments of electrical stimulation parameters remain to be clarified.

CURRENT RESEARCH WITH IONTOPHORESIS

Development of stimulation units and electrode accessories designed specifically for iontophoretic drug delivery have greatly facilitated the process of application.[65] At present, iontophoresis is being used in a wide variety of domains, which include dermatology, ophthalmology, dentistry, and physical medicine.[66] Research efforts have varied between the basic science efforts to maximize iontophoretic delivery of given solutes,[6] and the clinicians' efforts at developing painless local anaesthetic procedures, relieving chronic pain, and reducing the inflammation associated with common musculoskeletal conditions.[68]

Basic Science Research

The process of skin permeation is complicated by the skin's resistance to both ionized and nonionized species in solution. During iontophoresis, the greatest concentration of ions moves toward skin pores, hair follicles, or regions of skin damage.[69] The size and molecular weight of the ions will determine the degree of penetration via this path.

More recently,[66] it has been noted that the mechanisms underlying the absorption of ions in solution are not exclusively pore-dependent. Transport also occurs through paracellular current pathways.[70] When ions of large molecular size and weight are inhibited from pore or hair follicle penetration, other mechanisms may compensate for this inhibition.

The polarity question once again dominates the literature on iontophoresis as it did with electrical stimulation for wound healing.[67,69,70] Transdermal ion migration is possible because like charges repel one another. Solutions that contain primarily positive ions must be driven through the skin with a negative current and vice versa. Ions of the same charge (coions) and ions of the opposite charge (counterions) will compete for skin penetration when present within the iontophoretic solution.[67]

The various layers of skin, namely the stratum corneum and the remaining layers of epidermis have been determined to be primarily of negative charge or positive charge, respectively.[70] These factors will play a role in determining the absolute concentration of medication delivered by this method.

In summary, the principal factors that determine the fluctuations in penetration capacity of solutes and between individuals treated with the same dosage parameters appear to be related to physiochemical factors that include the charge of the solute, the ionic strength, the pH of the solution, and the size and chemical structure of the solute; physiologic factors that include age, sex, region and skin hydration; and electrical factors.[5]

Clinical Research

Despite a relatively large volume of early literature on the clinical use of iontophoresis, very few well-controlled studies have been carried out in this field.[71] Many case reports and anecdotal publications have made the assumption that medications delivered by iontophoresis will have the same effect as those delivered by injection or oral administration despite the potential interactions between ionic solutions, skin barriers, buffering agents, and the direct current itself. Comparative studies between oral medications, injections, and iontophoresis as well as between traditional physical therapy procedures and iontophoresis must be carried out before clinicians can be certain that this procedure is cost-effective.

Anti-Inflammatory Medication   The effect of dexamethasone iontophoresis on delayed muscle soreness and function following strenuous bouts of exercise was studied in 18 untrained subjects. Subjects were subdivided into three groups of 6 and received either iontophoresis, sham treatment, or no treatment.[68] Following one treatment, the subjects in the experimental group had significantly less discomfort and had no adverse reactions to treatment. It remains to be proven if multiple applications enhance the duration and degree of effectiveness.

In a study on a variety of knee inflammatory conditions,[72] including osteoarthritis, synovitis, and patellofemoral joint problems, dexamethasone (Decadron) iontophoresis was capable of relieving pain and inflammation in 72% to 75% of the subjects. Functional improvements coincided with these results and the authors concluded that the procedure was much less traumatic than injection of corticosteroids. However, the effect of electrically driven corticosteroids on the health of soft tissues must be studied in comparison with injection or electrical stimulation alone.

More recently, a prospective nonrandomized study of iontophoresis, wrist splinting, and anti-inflammatory medications in the treatment of work-induced carpal tunnel syndrome suggested that iontophoresis and injections resulted in improvement of 57% of patients as compared to 17% of subjects responding to splinting alone.[74] These results compare with those obtained by others who studied tendinitis[74] of the upper limb and a variety of musculoskeletal problems.[75]

Three methods of treatment for myofascial syndrome were compared including analgesic and muscle relaxant medications (oral), heat and ultrasound, and iontophoresis with dexamethasone combined with lidocaine. Iontophoresis was reported to be the most effective treatment, but no statistical analysis of the data were presented.[76]

Local Anesthetics   The principal research on local anesthesia provided by iontophoresis is found in the domains of dental; ear, nose and throat (ENT); and ophthalmologic literature. A comparative study that evaluated the effect of lidocaine infiltration, iontophoresis, and topical application concluded that injection and iontophoresis provided the same degree of anesthesia.[77] Lidocaine iontophoresis has also been used for producing external ear canal anesthesia[78,79] and prior to tooth extraction,[80] and found to be equivalent in effectiveness to local injection.

Dermatologic Conditions One of the most successful and popular applications of iontophoresis is for the treatment of hyperhydrosis (excessive sweating).[81,82] Anticholinergics or simple tapwater can obstruct the sweat ducts when applied via an electrical current.[83] Sweat production has been objectively measured by perspirant paper tracings and quantified by image analysis to prove that this treatment is effective. Interestingly, several daily treatment sessions over a span of 2 weeks are necessary before results are obvious, and this fact has led to great speculation on the mechanisms underlying the effectiveness of this treatment. Palmar, plantar, and axillary hyperhydrosis have been successfully treated by this technique.[66]

Zinc oxide iontophoresis has been used to facilitate the closure of small ischemic ulcers less than 1 cm in diameter.[84] Thirty minutes of stimulation per day over a span of 20 days is the average treatment time reported.

Miscellaneous Applications A great number of metallic and nonmetallic ions have been delivered by iontophoresis. Copper, zinc, magnesium, calcium, iodine, and silver have been used to treat conditions ranging from fungal infections of the hand[85] to osteomyelitis.[86] Unfortunately, no controlled studies have been published and treatment effectiveness remains to be proven.

More intensive research has been sparked by the possibility of delivering insulin via iontophoresis using pulsed current.[87] Even though this application falls out of the realm of physical rehabilitation, it is an interesting prospect for the future. The potential benefits of this treatment could significantly enhance the injection-dependent lives of people with diabetes.

PRINCIPLES OF THERAPEUTIC APPLICATION

The process of ionization occurs when ionizable substances in solution dissociate into their component ions. These electrolytic solutions are capable of conducting an electrical current because of the migration of dissociated ions. Iontophoresis is therefore the process of specific ion transfer from an electrolytic solution by means of an externally applied current.[66]

The number of ions transferred out of solution to the skin interface is dependent upon the current density of the active electrode, the duration of current flow, and the concentration of ions in solution. A continuous direct current assures maximum ion transfer with the exception of large macromolecular substances (insulin) in solution, which appear to respond better to a pulsed direct current.[65]

Dissociation of positive and negative ions occurs in response to the polarity of the active electrode. Like ions will be driven away from the active electrode and oppositely charged ions will be attracted to the electrode. Therefore, matching of the therapeutically effective ions to the polarity of the active electrode is a major principle of application.[69]

The number of ions transferred through the superficial layers of the skin to underlying tissues is dependent upon the number of ions transferred out of solution, the chemical combinations, and the dispersion of ions via the local circulation. The conductivity of soft tissues is directly equivalent to their water content.[67]

Several factors determine the duration of time needed to depose adequate concentrations of ions to target tissues. The lag time for diffusion of materials across the skin is dependent upon solvent drag and the skin resistance to permeation. Solvent drag is the result of the fact that an electrical current drives not only a flow of ions but also a flow of water (electro-osmosis) out of solution, and skin resistance to these combined forces may be greater.

Indications for Use

Iontophoresis has a wide variety of indications for use, dependent upon the ions selected. In general, this procedure is applied with minimal discomfort or adverse metabolic reactions as compared with infiltration or medications. Dosage requirements to produce therapeutic benefits are minimal in comparison with other treatment methods and can be highly localized to produce results[71] (Table 13–5).

Contraindications for Use

The use of iontophoresis as a treatment modality is the use of electrical stimulation. For this reason, precautions and contraindications to the use of electrical stimulation must be observed (review Chapter 10). In addition, a lack of skin sensation, new skin tissue, allergies to medication, and the concomitant use of oral medications that may negatively interact with the ions introduced locally must be avoided.

Precautions

Chemical burns from the excessive formation of sodium hydroxide at the cathode[71] and heat burns secondary to anatomic regions of high resistance must be prevented by taking additional precautions when applying this modality. Skin should be washed prior to application and electrodes applied with constant uniform pressure. Increased resistance and potential burns can occur when electrodes are not sufficiently moist or if wrinkles create a concentrated focus of current.

Current intensities should be gradually increased over the treatment time to allow accommodation to the ionization process. Moreover, the application of two chemicals under the same electrode or the administration of ions of opposite polarity will reduce the effectiveness of treatment or result in the synthesis of antagonistic ions.[70]

Electrodes should never be moved or rearranged when the current is on. Failure to take this precaution may result in an uncomfortable sensation or "shock" being imparted to the patient or the hands of the therapist.

Sequencing with Other Modalities

The interventions of other biophysical modalities either before or after iontophoresis render it difficult to predict skin and soft tissue penetration of ions. Increased skin permeability may enhance the transport of ions to the target tissue.

Table 13–5 **Indications for the Use of Iontophoresis**

1. Local anaesthesia for tissues highly sensitive to infiltration (conjuctiva, external auditory canal, tympanic membrane).[77–79]
2. Reduction of inflammation of peripheral articulations and soft tissues.[72–75]
3. Treatment of hyperhydrosis, fungus infections, and small open ulcers.[81–85]
4. Reduction of the size of calcium deposits or breakdown scar tissue that inhibits normal function.[76]

However, increased circulation and vasodilation may dilute ionic concentrations and render the treatment ineffective.

Pending further research into the effect of concomitant use of other modalities, iontophoresis should be the sole intervention with the exception of mild exercise or passive soft tissue mobilizations.

Topically Applied Medications

A list of commonly applied ions and their source, polarity, and indications for use is included in Table 13–6. Selection of the appropriate ion for the pathology is essential to the success of treatment. In addition, consideration of the electrochemical and electrophysiologic properties of the ion as well as the specific parameters of treatment that will enhance delivery of the ion must be taken before treatment commences.[66]

Equipment

There are a variety of devices that can be used for iontophoresis ranging from some of the original DC generators used for stimulation of denervated muscle to small portable units designed specifically for the safe and convenient application of iontophoresis[73] (Fig. 13–1).

Table 13–6

Solution/Medication	Polarity	Indications for Use
1 mL 0.4% Decadron Dexamethasone sodium phosphate	–	Musculoskeletal conditions: Anti-inflammatory, i.e., osteoarthritis, frozen shoulder
1 mL 0.4 Decadron 2 mL 4% Hydrocyhloride	–	Musculoskeletal conditions: Analgesic and anti-inflammatory, i.e., epicondylitis, bursitis
2% Acetic acid solution	–	Musculoskeletal conditions: Calcium deposits, i.e., calcific tendonitis, myositis, ossificans
2% Sodium chloride	–	Sclerotic: Scars, adhesions
Wydase (hyaluronidase)	+	Swelling: Sprains, strains
Mecholyl ointment	+	Neurologic conditions: Vasodilator, analgesic, i.e., neuritis, neurovascular deficits
2% Copper sulfate	+	Dermatology: Anti-bacterial, i.e., fungus infections, athletes' foot
2 mL Lidocaine hydrochloride	+	Ophthalmology, ENT, dentistry: Analgesic, i.e., minor surgeries

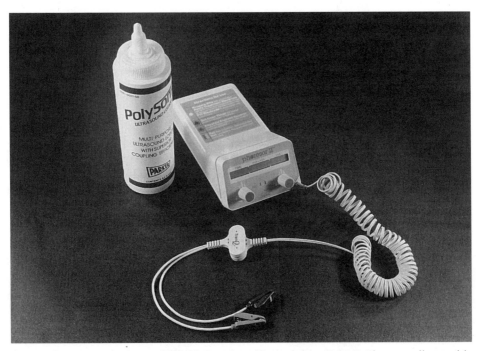

Figure 13–1. Demonstration of the relative size of an iotophoresis unit. These small, portable units are battery operated. The coiled lead wire is bifurcated into two clamps that attach to single-use electrodes. The ultrasound couplant bottle is shown for its size relative to the iontophoresis unit.

Units generally consist of a power source (electrical, battery) that can generate either a continuous or pulsed DC output. The intensity of output must range between 1 and 5 mA of current and iontophoresis devices should be constantcurrent devices capable of delivering these low-amplitude doses of DC without fluctuation.

Electrodes that deliver a uniform current density are essential to safe application of iontophoresis. Skin burns are principally caused by uneven distributions of current in the tissues beneath the electrodes.[71] Sophisticated disposable electrodes have been developed that are capable of being filled with the electrolytic solution and even contain an ion-exchange membrane that prevents the flow of unwanted products into the skin (Sanderson, SR, de Rail: Method for iontophoretic drug delivery, U.S. patent pending, 1986).

Future units will be capable of measuring the degree of skin contact between the device and the skin and delivering specific doses despite variations in skin resistance. Combined with improving the portability of devices, iontophoresis units will be capable of providing medication in a precisely controlled and safe manner.

Treatment Procedure

Treatments with iontophoresis should be carefully administered, observing all contraindications and precautions. This form of treatment differs from other forms of electrical stimulation since a chemical substance is being delivered to the tissues via the flow of electrical current. Because of the use of DC, which causes polar effects underneath the electrodes, additional care should be taken when administering iontophoresis.[88] Table 13–7 outlines the steps involved for treatment with iontophoresis.

Table 13–7 **Steps for Treating with Iontophoresis**

Step 1: Patient preparation

Skin condition must be evaluated before application. Irritated or broken skin is a contraindication to use.

Skin sensation must be tested. Desensitized skin is a contraindication to use.

The skin local to the site of application must be cleansed with alcohol prior to applying electrodes. Excess hair may be trimmed with scissors or electric clippers with care to ensure that the skin is not irritated or broken in the process. Shaving is discouraged, since it may cause skin irritation.

Patients should be positioned to avoid pressure on the electrodes and ensure that they are comfortable for the duration of treatment.

Patients should be counseled to minimize movement of the part being treated and take care not to lean on electrodes or touch them with their hands.

Patients should be educated with respect to the sensations associated with treatment and the abnormal sensations associated with chemical or heat burns.

Step 2: Electrode preparation

Thoroughly rinse sponges or other electrode interface materials (towels, gauze) before soaking in the ionic solution. If an ionic ointment is being used, massage the ointment into the skin overlying the pathology and place the thoroughly rinsed sponges, towel pads, or gauze pads over the area.

Place the active electrode over the pathology and the indifferent proximal or distal to the active.

Note: The negative electrode should be twice as large as the positive regardless of which electrode is active.

Secure electrodes in place with an even distribution of pressure.

Ensure all dials are set at zero. Connect the electrodes to the current generator.

Step 3: Set the stimulation parameters

Selector switch must be set to continuous direct current on multipurpose stimulators.

Set the polarity switch to the same polarity of the ion being introduced.

Set the output to a continuous or pulsed mode.

Gradually increase the current intensity to 2 to 3 mA. Allow the skin to accommodate to this current for approximately 10 minutes. Increase the intensity to a maximum of 5 mA for the remainder of the treatment time (20 minutes).

Note: Check for skin irritation periodically to ensure that a burn is not developing, particularly when regular electrodes combined with multipurpose stimulators are being used. Current intensities may vary more greatly at the low end of the output scale.

Step 4: Treatment termination

Turn the generator off slowly.

Remove the electrodes and thoroughly inspect the skin underlying both electrodes.

Apply a soothing lotion or an astringent solution to the areas.

The treatment should be repeated every 48 to 72 hours (2 to 3 days) to a maximum of 6 to 10 sessions. Results are frequently obtained within the first 3 to 5 sessions. Patients should be evaluated for decreased pain, tenderness, and increased function prior to each treatment session. Failure to have any improvement within the first 3 sessions may indicate that the treatment intensity may need adjustment (5 mA for 20 minutes) provided that skin irritation has not developed. Alternatively, the medication being applied should be re-evaluated.

Documentation

Pretreatment measurements of pain on movement, with resistance or on palpation must be recorded for musculoskeletal conditions. Clinical tools available to facilitate objective recording include goniometers, tensiometers, and dolorimeters that measure either range of movement or pain associated with a measurable degree of resistance or pressure. Precise treatment parameters must be recorded to ensure consistency between treatment and progressions of parameters, electrode size, placement, polarity, and type (disposable versus carbon-carbon versus metal) should be documented. Current intensity and time of application as well as the concentration of the drug solution constitute the dosage and must be recorded after each treatment.

Skin reactions should be recorded and can range from a slight erythema to skin breakdown. In the event that skin breakdown occurred during treatment, an incident report must be completed and the patient evaluated by a medical practitioner to prevent future litigation.

SUMMARY

Electrical stimulation has been discussed in this chapter as a treatment modality to promote wound healing and deliver medications through the skin. These applications are similar to other applications of electrical stimulation in that the same precautions and contraindications to the use of electrical stimulation must be observed. The applications differ in that due to the fragility and sensitivity of the tissues being treated, additional precautions for skin care must be considered.

DISCUSSION QUESTIONS

1. Why would there be additional considerations to the use of either iontophoresis or low-intensity electrical stimulation for wound healing in addition to the general precautions and contraindications?
2. Explain how electrical stimulation for wound healing would be incorporated into a treatment plan for a patient.
3. In terms that a patient would understand, explain why electrical stimulation may promote wound healing.
4. In terms that a patient would understand, explain how iontophoresis delivers a medication transdermally.

REFERENCES

1. Adams, G: An essay on electricity. Edited by W Jones. Dillon and Co, London, 1799, pp 482–575.

2. Gentzkow, GD and Miller, KH: Electrical stimulation for dermal wound healing. Clin Pod Med Surg 8:827,1991.

3. Cunliffe-Barnes, T: Healing rate of human skin determined by measurement of electric potential of experimental abrasions. Am J Surg 69:82, 1945.

4. Owoeye, I, Sielholz, NT, and Nelson, AJ: Low intensity pulsed galvanic current and the healing of tenotomized rat Achilles tendons: Preliminary report using load-to-breaking measurements. Arch Phys Med Rehabil 68:296, 1987.

5. Akai, M, et al: Electrical stimulation of wound healing: An experimental study of the patellar ligament of rabbits. Clin Orthop 235:296, 1988.

6. Brighton, CT: Bioelectric effects on bone and cartilage. Clin Orthop 12:204, 1977.

7. Bassett, CAL and Schink-Ascani, M: Long-term pulsed electromagnetic field results in congenital pseudarthrosis. Calcif Tissue Int 49:216, 1991.

8. Aaron, PK, Lennox, D, and Bunce,GE: The conservative treatment of osteonecrosis of the femoral head: A comparison of core decompression and pulsing electromagnetic fields. Clin Orthop 249:209, 1989.

9. Bassett, CAL, Schink-Ascani, M, and Lewis, SM: Effects of pulsed electromagnetic fields on Steinberg rating of femoral head osteonecrosis. Clin Orthop 246:172, 1989.

10. Sharand, WJW: A double-blind trial of pulsing electromagnetic fields for delayed fracture union. Orthop Trans 12:555, 1988.

11. Trock, DH, et al: A double-blind trial of the clinical effects of pulsed electromagnetic fields in orteoarthritis. J Rheumatol 20:456, 1993.

12. Weiss, DS, Kirsner, R, and Eaglstein, WH: Electrical stimulation and wound healing. Arch Dermatol 126:222, 1990.

13. Lee, RC, Canaday, DJ, and Doong, H: A review of the biophysical basis for the clinical application of electric fields in soft tissue repair. J Burn Care and Rehabil 14:319, 1993.

14. Mustoe, TA, et al: Accelerated healing of incisional wounds in rats induced by transforming growth factor-beta. Science 237:1333, 1987.

15. Brown, GL, et al: Enhancement of wound healing by topical treatment with epidermal growth factor. N Engl J Med 321:76, 1989.

16. Hunt, JK and LaVan, FB: Enhancement of wound healing by growth factors. N Engl J Med 321:111, 1989.

17. Robertson, WS: Digby's receipts. Ann Med Hist 7:216, 1925.

18. Smith, KW, Oden, PW, and Blaulock, WK: A comparison of gold leaf and other occlusive therapy. Arch Dermatol 96:703, 1967.

19. Burr, HS, Taffel, M, and Harvey, SC: An electrometric study of the healing wound in man. Yale J Biol Med 12:483, 1940.

20. Becker, RO: The bioelectric factors in amphibian limb regeneration. J Bone Joint Surg 43:643, 1961.

21. Smith, SD: Induction of partial limb regeneration in Rana pipiens by galvanic stimulation of the nerve supply. Anat Rec 158:89, 1967.

22. Becker, RO, Spadero, JA: Electrical stimulation of partial limb regeneration in mammals. Bull NY Acad Med 48:627, 1972.

23. Wolcott, LE, et al: Accelerated healing of skin ulcers by electrotherapy. South Med J 62:795, 1969.

24. Reich, JD, Tarjan, PP: Electrical stimulation of skin. Int J Dermatol 29:395, 1990.

25. Barker, AT, Joffe, LF, and Vanable, JW: The glabrous epidermis of cavies contains a powerful battery. Am J Physiol 242:358, 1982.

26. Nordenstrom, BE: Biologically Closed Electric Circuits: Clinical, Experimental and Theoretical Evidence for an Additional Circulatory System. Nordic Medical Publishers, Stockholm, 1983, p 122.

27. Becker, RO: The sign of the miracle. In Becker, RO and Selden, G. (eds): The Body Electric. William Morrow, New York, 1985, p 138.

28. Bourgignon, GJ and Bourgignon, LYW: Electrical stimulation of protein and DNA synthesis in human fibroblasts. FASEB 1:398, 1987.

29. Rowley, BA, et al: The influences of electrical current on an infecting microorganism in wounds. Ann NY Acad Sc 238:543, 1974.

30. Barranco, SD, et al: In vitro effect of weak direct currents on Staphylococcus aureus. Clin Orthop Rel Res 100:250, 1974.

31. Fakhri, O and Amin, M: The effect of low voltage electric therapy on the healing of resistant skin burns. J Burn Care Rehabil 8:15, 1987.

32. Weiss, DS, Eaglstein, WH, and Falanga, V: Exogenous electrical current can reduce the formation of hypertrophic scars. J Dermatol Surg Oncol 15:1272, 1989.

33. Hecker, B, Carron, H, and Schwartz, D: Pulsed galvanic stimulation: Effects of current frequency and polarity on blood flow in healthy subjects. Arch Phys Med Rehabil 66:369, 1985.

34. Sawyer, PN and Deutch, B: Use of electrical currents to delay intravascular thrombosis in experimental animals. Am J Physiol 187:473, 1956.

35. Brown, M and Gogia, P: Effects of high voltage stimulation on cutaneous wound healing in rabbits. Phys Ther 67:662, 1987.

36. Stromberg, BV: Effects of electrical currents on wound contraction. Ann Plast Surg 2:121, 1988.

37. Gault, WR and Gatens, PF: Use of low intensity direct current in management of ischemic skin ulcers. Phys Ther 56:265, 1975.

38. Carley, PJ and Wainapel, SF: Electrotherapy for acceleration of wound healing: Low intensity direct current. Arch Phys Med Rehabil 66:443, 1985.

39. Akerts, AT and Gabrielson, AL: The effect of high-voltage galvanic stimulation on the rate of healing of decubitus ulcers. Biomed Sci Instrum 20:99, 1984.

40. Alon, G, Azaria, M, and Stein, H: Diabetic ulcer healing using high voltage TENS. Phys Ther 66:755, 1986.

41. Kloth, L and Feedar, J: Acceleration of wound healing with high voltage, monophasic, pulsed current. Phys Ther 68:503, 1988.

42. Unger, PG and Raimastry, S: A controlled study of the effect of high voltage pulsed current (HVPC) on wound healing. Phys Ther 71:S119, 1991.

43. Gentzkow, GD, et al: Improved healing of pressure ulcers using Dermapulse, a new electrical stimulation device. Wounds 3:158, 1991.

44. Kloth, LC: Electrical stimulation in tissue repair. In McCulloch, JM, Kloth, LC, and Feedar, JA (eds): Wound Healing: Alternatives in Management, ed 2. FA Davis, Philadelphia, 1995.

45. Young, GH: Electric impulse therapy aids wound healing. Modern Vet Pract 47:60, 1966.

46. Assimacopoulos, D: Low intensity negative electric current in the treatment of ulcers of the leg due to chronic venous insufficiency. Am J Surg 115:683, 1968.

47. Dunn, MG: Wound healing using a collagen matrix: Effect of DC electrical stimulation. J Biomed Matter Res 22:191, 1988.

48. Alvarez, OM, et al: The healing of superficial skin wounds is stimulated by external electrical current. J Invest Dermatol 81:144, 1983.

49. Politis, MJ, Zanakis, MF, and Miller, JE: Enhanced survival of full thickness skin grafts following the application of D.C. electrical fields. Plast Reconstr Surg 84:267, 1989.

50. Carey, LC and Lepley, D: Effect of continuous direct electric current on healing wounds. J Surg Res 7:122, 1967.

51. Brown, M: Polarity effects on wound healing using electric stimulation in rabbits. Arch Phys Med Rehabil 70:624, 1989.

52. Brown, M, McDonnell, MK, and Menton, DN: Electrical stimulation effects on cutaneous wound healing in rabbits. Phys Ther 68:955, 1988.

53. Mertz, PM, et al: Electrical stimulation: Acceleration of soft tissue repair by varying the polarity. Wounds 5:153, 1993.

54. Bolton, L, Foleno, B, and Means, B: The effect of direct current stimulation on microorganisms in healing wounds. Trans Bioelectric Repair Growth Soc 1:70, 1981.

55. Alvarez, OM, Rozin, J, and Wiseman, D: Moist environment for healing: Matching the dressing to the wound. Wounds 1:35, 1989.

56. Brand, PW: The Effects of Pressure in Human Tissues. Rehabilitation Services Administration, United States Department of Health and Human Services, Washington, DC, 1977.

57. Feedar, JA and Kloth, LC: Conservative management of chronic wounds. In Kloth, LC, McCulloch, JM, and Feedar, JA (eds): Wound Healing: Alternatives in Management. FA Davis, Philadelphia, 1990, p 221.

58. Andersom, V: Over-the-counter topical antibiotic products. Date on safety and efficacy. Int J Dermatol 15(suppl):1, 1976.

59. Gentzkow, GD: Electrical stimulation for dermal wound healing. Wounds 4:227, 1992.

60. McCulloch, JM, Kloth, LC, and Feedar, JA (eds): Wound Healing: Alternatives in Management, ed 2. FA Davis, Philadelphia, 1995.

61. Bourgignon, GT, et al: Occlusive wound dressings suitable for use with electrical stimulation. Wounds 3:127, 1991.

62. Leduc, S: Introduction of medicinal substances into the depth of tissues by electrical current. Ann Electrobiol 3:545, 1900.

63. Leduc, S: Electric ions and their use in medicine. Rebman, London, 1908.

64. Shriber, WJ: A Manual of Electrotherapy, ed 4. Lea & Febiger, Philadelphia, 1975.

65. Yoshida, NY and Roberts, MS: Structure transport relationships in transdermal iontophoresis. Adv Drug Del Dev 9:239, 1992.

66. Banga, AK and Chien, YW: Iontophoretic delivery of drugs: Fundamentals, developments and biomedical applications. J Contr Release 7:1, 1988.

67. Phipps, JB and Gregory, JR: Transdermal ion migration. Adv Drug Del Dev 9:137, 1992.

68. Hasson, SM, et al: Dexamethasone iontophoretic effect on delayed muscle soreness and muscle function. Can J Spt Sc 17:8, 1992.

69. Singh, J and Roberts, MS: Transdermal delivery of drugs by iontophoresis: A review. Drug Design Deliv 4:1, 1989.

70. Cullander, C: What are the pathways of iontophoretic current flow through mammalian skin? Adv Drug Del Dev 9:119, 1992.

71. Kahn, J: Iontophoresis. In Principles and Practice of Electrotherapy. Churchill Livingstone, New York, 1987, p 119.

72. Tamburrini, LR, DiMonte, M, and Sfreddo, P: Iontophoresis of corticosteroids in senile osteo-arthropathy treatment. J Gerontol Abstract no.4, 1987.

73. Banta, CA: A prospective non-randomized study of iontophoresis. J Occup Med 36:166, 1994.

74. Bertolucci, LE: Introduction of anti-inflammatory drugs by iontophoresis: Double-blind study. J Orthop Sports Phys Ther 4:103, 1982.

75. Harris, PR: Iontophoresis: Clinical research in musculoskeletal inflammatory conditions. J Orthop Sports Phys Ther 4:109, 1982.

76. Delacerda, FG: A comparative study of three methods of treatment for shoulder girdle myofascial syndrome. J Orthop Sports Phys Ther 4:51, 1982.

77. Russo, J, et al: Lidocaine anaesthesia: Comparison of iontophoresis, injection and swabbing. Am J Hosp Pharm 37:843, 1980.

78. Sela, M, et al: Maxillofacial prosthetics and iontophoresis in management of burned ears. J Prosthet Dent 53:226, 1983.

79. Echols, DF, Norris, CH, and Tabb, HG: Anaesthesia of the arc by iontophoresis of lidocaine. Arch Otolaryngol 101:418, 1975.

80. Gangarosa, LP: Iontophoresis in Dental Practice. Quintessense , Chicago, 1983.

81. Elgart, ML and Fuchs, G: Tapwater iontophoresis in the treatment of hyperhydrosis. Int J Dermatol 26:194, 1987.

82. Hobson, RL: Treatment of hyperhydrosia. Arch Dermatol 123:883, 1987.

83. Shelley, WB, Horvath, PN, and Weidman, FPL: Experimental malaria in man. Production of sweat retention anhidrosis and vesicles by means of iontophoresis. J Invest Dermatol 11:275, 1948.

84. Cornwall, MW: Zinc iontophoresis to treat ischemic skin ulcers. Phys Ther 61:359, 1981.

85. Haggard, HW, Strauss, MJ, and Greenberg, IA: Fungus infections of hand and feet treated by copper iontophoresis. JAMA 112:1229, 1939.

86. Satyanand, A, Saxena, AK, and Agarwal, A: Silver iontophoresis in chronic osteomyelitis. J Indian Med Assoc 84:134, 1986.

87. Srinivasan, V, et al: Transdermal iontophoretic drug delivery: Mechanistic analysis and application to polypeptide delivery. J Pharmacol Sci 78:370, 1989.

88. Costello, CT and Jeske, AH: Iontophoresis: Applications in transdermal medication delivery. Phys Ther 75:554, 1995.

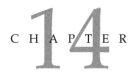

Pain Management With Electrical Stimulation

Kathleen M. Kenna, PT

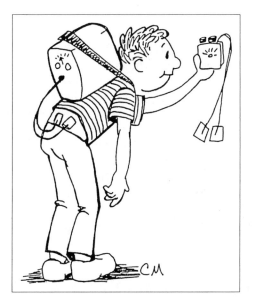

CHAPTER OBJECTIVES:

- Review the general principles of pain management.
- Discuss the physiology of pain, outlining sensory and pain fiber characteristics.
- Discuss the concepts of sensory analgesia and endogenous opiate liberation.
- Outline the procedures for the utilization of electrical stimulation to promote analgesia.
- Discuss the clinical decision making involved for determining the appropriate parameters for electrical stimulation.
- Discuss appropriate documentation for the use of electrical stimulation to promote analgesia.

CHAPTER OUTLINE

The symptom of pain commonly brings people to seek therapeutic intervention. The clinician has many types of physical agents to choose from to manage the patient's underlying pathology, symptoms, and associated dysfunctions effectively. Thermal and mechanical agents have been presented in Section 2 of this text as tools to address a variety of patient problems. In this chapter, the use of electrical stimulation as a method of pain management is presented. The following areas are addressed: (1) general principles of pain management with the use of electrical stimulation; (2) treatment rationale and method; (3) treatment expectations and progression; and (4) appropriate documentation.

Remember, pain management is only one aspect of the complete care of the patient. Depending upon the additional rehabilitation needs of the individual, other therapeutic interventions will be utilized.[1–3] Electrical stimulation, as with any other modality, is to be implemented to help achieve functional goals for a patient. For example, to facilitate greater comfort and improve pulmonary function following a thoracotomy, a patient may use electrical stimulation for postoperative pain management.[4]

GENERAL PRINCIPLES OF PAIN MANAGEMENT

TERMINOLOGY

The use of appropriate terminology is helpful when discussing pain management. *Analgesia* is defined as the absence of pain or noxious stimulation; the absence of the sensibility to pain; or the relief of pain without a loss of consciousness.[5] *Anesthesia* is defined as a loss of sensation, usually by damage to a nerve or receptor, that is, numbness; or the loss of the ability to feel pain caused by the administration of drugs or medical interventions.[5] Therapeutic intervention with the use of electrical stimulation can provide an analgesic effect. This occurs through a number of postulated neurophysiologic mechanisms.[2,3]

Pain management involves controlling the perception and/or sensation of pain. Management of pain allows the patient to better control his or her discomfort. This can lead to improved function. Electrical stimulation is a physical agent that can be used as one tool for pain control.[1–3]

Medications are also recommended or prescribed to help alleviate pain symptoms. The analgesics include nonnarcotic medications as well as narcotic drugs. Examples of nonnarcotic drugs are aspirin and nonsteroidal anti-inflammatory drugs (NSAIDs). Narcotic analgesics include codeine and morphine. Each class of drug affects the body in a different way to alter the experience of pain. Nonnarcotic pain medications act by selectively affecting the hypothalamus of the brain. At the site of injury, the synthesis of prostaglandins is inhibited and bradykinin is prevented from stimulating pain receptors. NSAIDs interrupt the inflammatory response by making cell membranes less permeable and inhibiting prostaglandin synthesis. Thus, the symptoms of inflammation are reduced. Narcotic analgesics are used to alleviate severe pain. The mechanism of action affects the central nervous system to decrease anxiety and the response to pain. The drugs do not affect the peripheral nerves and receptors, so the pain stimulus is still present. In effect, the patient does not respond to the stimulus because of the depression of the central nervous system.[6]

The adverse effects of this group of medications include gastrointestinal irritation, toxicity, mental confusion, drowsiness, and hypersensitivity. Narcotic analgesics, in addition to those previously mentioned, can produce tolerance and physical addiction to the drug. In many cases, the use of electrical stimulation for pain control has decreased the need for the use of analgesic medications.[6]

Electrical stimulation is believed to produce analgesic effects through the stimulation of the peripheral and central nervous system. Electrical stimulation devices are both clinical as well as portable models (see Chapter 15) that the patient can use at appropriate times during the day as needed. The portable units are generally the size of a "beeper" and run on rechargeable batteries. The portability of the electrical stimulators allows the patient greater autonomy in his or her own care as well as the option for use of extended periods of stimulation. When the unit and electrodes are used appropriately, side effects are minimal. There is a chance for a chemical burn at the stimulation site, hypersensitivity reactions to the stimulation, or allergic reactions to the adhesives used to hold an electrode in place.[7,8]

PHYSIOLOGY REVIEW

Pain Fiber Types and Central Pathways

Pain sensation is elicited by a noxious stimulus that is the result of excitation of the various sensory receptors and free nerve endings of the skin and internal structures. The nerve fiber types that are the mediators of pain impulses in the central nervous system are the A-delta and C fibers. A-β fibers transmit discriminative touch stimuli from the skin. A-delta fibers are sensitive to crude touch, pain, and temperature. C fibers are the afferent fibers coming from pain receptors.[9]

Once a pain receptor is stimulated, the nerve fiber transmits a signal to the dorsal horn of the spinal cord. A few ascending and descending fibers branch off to form Lissauer's tract and communicate with neighboring spinal segments. The main fiber continues in the dorsal horn to make connections with neurons of the lamina I, II, III, IV, and V. Lamina III is also known as the substantia gelatinosa. Synaptic connections are then made with neurons, giving rise to the lateral spinothalamic tract. These neurons cross over to the opposite side of the spinal cord at the ventral white commissure. The fibers of the lateral spinothalamic tract ascend the spinal cord and enter the brainstem, where some fibers send branches to the reticular formation. Other fibers continue to the thalamus where they form synapses with neurons that ascend to the primary and secondary somatosensory cortex. The fibers that have been projected to the reticular formation then synapse with other fibers that relay pain information to the thalamus, hypothalamus, and limbic system. The end result of all these connections is the perception of pain.[1,9] (For more information, refer to Chapter 1.)

Normal Responses to Trauma

The body responds to trauma by an acute inflammatory response. The symptoms associated with the inflammation are a warning to the individual, indicating tissue damage. The symptoms experienced are the cardinal signs of inflammation— pain, redness, increased tissue temperature, and swelling. Vascular changes occur with an inflammatory response that allow fluid and cells to exude from the blood vessels that promote clot formation, phagocytosis, fibroblastic activity, and the beginning of the formation of new capillary beds. The fluid exudate in the extravascular space results in swelling. Increased tissue temperature and redness are the result of the vasodilation of the blood vessels, allowing more blood to pass through the area and increasing metabolism. Pain is the result of stimulation of the pain receptors and free nerve endings of A-delta and C fibers by the chemicals present at the site and the mechanical pressure of the swelling.

The pain associated with an injury can also result in decreased function of the injured body part. Range of motion may be limited because of increased pain with motion because of added stress at the site of injury. Also, muscle contraction produces pain because of the "tension" created at the injury site by the contraction. Pain usually leads to muscle spasm, which causes more pain. The end result is the pain-spasm cycle.[10] The prolonged spasm of a muscle can lead to ischemia of the tissue because of compression of the blood vessels. The ischemia can also lead to pain. The combination of the pain and resultant muscle spasm is an inability to use the body part without pain.

Chronic pain can be considered pain that lasts more than 3 months.[1] Chronic pain can lead to a long-term loss of function as well as impose many psychosocial stresses on the pain patient and his or her friends and family. The mechanism by which acute pain is similar to or different from chronic pain is not fully understood. The extent that pain is perceived and responded to may be a function of the influences of biologic, psychosocial, behavioral, and neurohormonal and neurochemical factors.[1-3,11-13]

Sensory Analgesia

Sensory analgesia can be produced by causing a "tingling" sensation. The stimulation may be activity of A-β nerve fibers. The sensation produced may affect the "gating" mechanism at the spinal cord level, so pain impulses are not transmitted to the higher centers.[14,15] In effect, the patient experiences a tolerable stimulus that blocks pain impulses. Electrode placements can be directly over the painful site, along the corresponding dermatome, along the cutaneous nerve distribution of the painful area, or along the area superficial to the nerve trunk supplying the painful site. Parameters of stimulation are a rate of greater than 50 pulses per second (pps) to 125 pps, a pulse duration of 60 to 100 μs, and an amplitude to produce a strong tingling sensation. Duration of treatment initially can be up to an hour to assess the therapeutic effect.[16] Depending upon its effectiveness, this form of stimulation can be used up to 24 hours per day. Pain relief usually occurs during the time the stimulus is applied.

Endogenous Opiate Liberation

Theoretically, stimulation of the endogenous opiate system can also lead to pain relief. Electrical stimulators capable of rates of 1 to 5 pps, a pulse duration greater than 200 μs, and an intensity to create a muscle twitch may generate pain relief through this mechanism. The duration of treatment is 30 to 45 minutes. Electrode placements include motor points that may also be acupuncture points or trigger points.[17] (See Chapter 16 for more information regarding electrode placement.)

Stimulation of the A-delta and C fibers by the parameters described may affect the production of endorphins and enkephalin release that mimic the action of narcotic drugs to promote decreased perception of pain. Pain reduction usually lasts longer with this form of electrical stimulation than the application to produce sensory analgesia. This form of electrical stimulation is often used for the treatment of intense or chronic pain.[2,3,11]

Other Considerations

When utilizing electrical stimulation for promoting pain reduction, other factors need to be considered. The patient's attitude toward the use of electrical stimulation is important in the successful use of the modality. Explanations of the intended purpose and mechanism of affecting the pain experience need to be presented to the patient in appropriate, understandable terminology. Also, the expected results of treatment need to be discussed. Do not set the patient up for failure by trying to attain unrealistic goals. If a patient has heard of a form of electrical stimulation or has been treated with this modality in the past, find out more details about what the modality was, how it was used, and how effective it was. If the patient is biased toward the success of the treatment, build upon the experience and how the treatment has effectively been used on other patients with similar conditions. If electrical stimulation is utilized, the patient should be informed that there are a great variety of treatment parameters and electrode placements that can lead to a successful treatment outcome. If the stimulation was used in the past for sensory analgesia, emphasize the effectiveness of endogenous opiate stimulation or vice versa. If the patient indicates a certain type of electrode placement, discuss other options that can be utilized. Most importantly, the practitioner needs to discuss expected results of the use of electrical stimulation by developing realistic goals. If a patient is of the attitude that electrical stimulation does not help or they had a bad experience with the modality, the practitioner may choose another technique for pain control (see Treatment Expectations).

Narcotic pain medications produce analgesia by decreasing the perception of pain.[6] The release of endogenous opiates by electrical stimulation produces pain relief through the same mechanism. If electrical stimulation is effective in alleviating pain, a decrease in the amount of prescribed medication may be indicated. This should be discussed with the physician who prescribed the medication.

Alcohol consumption by the patient needs to be considered by the clinician. Alcohol is considered a sedative-hypnotic agent. The effects of dose-dependent central nervous system depression from alcohol produce analgesia.[6] Judgment is also impaired with alcohol consumption; therefore, home use of an electrical stimulator may not be recommended for patients who have a tendency to abuse alcohol by consuming large quantities on a regular basis. Intensity may have to be significantly increased in order to be perceived by the patient. In either case, safety of the patient becomes an issue. The clinician is to be prudent in informing the patient of this information.

The use of exercise is also a consideration when utilizing electrical stimulation for pain relief. Patients will be able to detect shape A-delta pain if an exercise is being done beyond the recommended range of motion or at an excessive level that could be causing tissue damage. Protective pain mechanisms remain intact when sensory analgesia is produced via electrical stimulation. Depending on the diagnosis of the patient, the desired response to treatment, and the perception of pain, electrical stimulation can be used to facilitate exercise by decreasing pain perception. Specific guidelines need to be reinforced for a home exercise program that is also being done by a patient who is using a portable electrical stimulation device.

POTENTIAL TREATMENTS AND HOW TO ACHIEVE SUCCESS

CLINICAL DECISION MAKING

Many electrical stimulation devices exist that allow several treatment options. These include, but are not limited to, interferential current, high-voltage pulsed current units, and low-voltage units. The details of the various types of devices are presented in Chapter 15. Look at the parameters a given machine is capable of producing in order to determine if its use is appropriate for treatment. The purpose of this section is to develop a process by which the clinician can determine the most appropriate forms of electrical stimulation treatments for a patient.

In order to provide effective treatment, the clinician goes through a decision-making process that concludes in treatment alternatives for the patient. Through thorough examination and assessment, the clinician may identify the source of a patient's pain symptoms. Past medical history and the history of the present condition assists the clinician in identifying contraindications and precautions relevant to the use of electrical stimulation. A summary of contraindications and precautions is presented in Table 14–1. In the presence of contraindications, a different pain-reducing modality that imposes less risk to the patient should be selected. If precautions are present, the patient should be monitored closely for signs of adverse reactions to treatment. If electrical stimulation is the chosen treatment, parameters are further delineated by identifying the type of pain present, the location of the pain, the characteristics of the pain, and the other rehabilitative needs of the patient. The findings influence treatment parameters, options for electrode placement, and goal setting. A decision-making paradigm is presented in Figure 14–1.

The portability of some electrical stimulation units allows for home use of the device, thus providing the patient treatment opportunities as needed for pain relief. The patient needs sufficient joint range of motion and dexterity to apply electrodes, plug in wires, and operate the controls. If the patient is not physically capable of using the machine, the individual may have another person at home that can apply the electrodes and adjust the controls as needed. The patient should also

Table 14–1   Contraindications and Precautions with the Use of Electrical Stimulation for Pain Management

---

Contraindications

Demand type cardiac pacemaker

Carotid sinus, stimulation over the area may result in a hypotensive incident

Directly over the eye

Epilepsy

Malignancies (see below)

Loss of or decreased sensation

Precautions

Patients with known cardiac disease or arrhythmias should be closely monitored for signs of adverse effects.

Directly over an open wound.

Directly over the lumbar paraspinals and abdominal area during pregnancy, except during labor and delivery in uncomplicated pregnancies.

For patients with diagnosed malignancies that have been diagnosed as terminal, it may be utilized for pain control with informed consent of the patient.

In addition the electrical stimulator is for external use only and should be kept out of the reach of children.

---

have the ability to understand the appropriate use of the machine. Clinicians should be able to explain the purpose and use of the device in understandable terms. The patient should also be instructed to monitor skin condition and respond accordingly.

Some form of written and/or pictorial home instruction material outlining the safe use of the unit should be provided. All important information concerning the safe and appropriate use of the unit should be included. This form should include, but is not limited to, the following information:

1. Purpose of the unit
2. Settings of the controls (pulse duration, pulse rate)
3. Some form of pain assessment chart to monitor results
4. Electrode placement site charts
5. Battery insertion instructions
6. Electrode care and instructions for use
7. The name and phone number of the clinician or another resource person to answer questions
8. A list of "do's and don'ts" regarding the use of the device
9. Potential trouble shooting tips for the unit
10. Instructions on appropriate skin care

A sample form is shown in Figure 14–2.

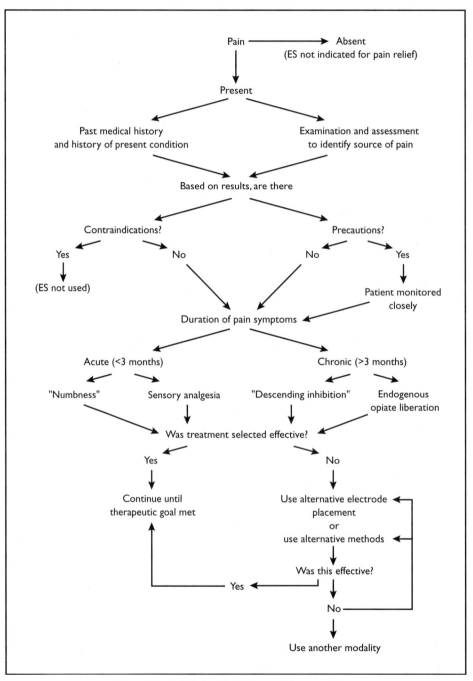

Figure 14–1. Clinical decision-making paradigm.

TENS
Home Instruction Form

Your clinician will determine the electrode placement sites and method of stimulation that will provide the most effective degree of pain control with the shortest treatment time. Your cooperation is essential to this process.

Complete the chart below recording your pain ratings as requested. If you have any questions call your clinician.

1	2	3	4	5	6	7	8	9	10
No pain									Maximal pain

pre-TENS rating	Treatment time	post-TENS rating	Relief time	Comments

Setting up the TENS unit . . .

The following descriptions will assist you in setting the controls on the TENS unit. Do not experiment with the settings unless instructed to do so by the clinician.

I Conventional

Pulse Duration: (PD, width) — Preset to the lowest setting

Frequency: (Hz, PPS, rate) — Preset to the highest setting

Amplitude: (intensity) — Increase to a comfortable level of tingling. Increase if it "fades."

Treatment time: — Leave it ON until you do not feel pain. Do not leave it turned ON for more than 60 minutes without turning if OFF to see how it feels.

II Acupuncturelike

Pulse Duration: (PD, width) — Preset to the highest setting

Frequency: (Hz, PPS, rate) — Preset to the lowest setting

Amplitude: (intensity) — Increase until muscle "thumping" occurs

Treatment time: — 25 to 30 minutes while resting.

III Brief Intense

Pulse Duration: (width) — Preset to the highest setting

Frequency: (Hz, PPS, rate) — Preset to the highest setting

Amplitude: (intensity) — Increase to the strongest level tolerable.

Treatment time: — 5 to 30 minutes as instructed

Electrode Placement Sites

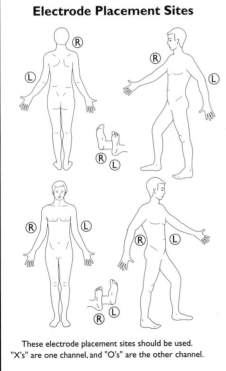

These electrode placement sites should be used. "X's" are one channel, and "O's" are the other channel.

TENS Reminders . . .

1. Do not wear the TENS unit while bathing, showering, or sleeping. Remove the electrodes and replace them after the activity.
2. The TENS unit may be worn at all other times, and turned ON whenever you are experiencing pain. There is no limit to the number of times (treatments) per day.
3. The TENS unit should be turned OFF when not in use, to insure a longer battery life.
4. If your TENS unit has rechargeable batteries, the extra set should be plugged into the recharger to ensure the availability of charged batteries at all times.
5. Carefully inspect the electrodes before applying them. Make sure that there is no metal or bare rubber showing through the side of the electrode that touches your skin. If the electrodes do break down, replace them.
6. If you need more electrodes, or new lead wires, call the TENS distributor.

Notes:

Important #'s:

Date: _____ Model: _____ Serial # _____

Clinician: _____

TENS Distributor: _____

Figure 14–2. Sample written and pictorial home instruction material. *(Diagram courtesy of Barbara Behrens, BS, PTA)*

TREATMENT METHODS

RATIONALE FOR ELECTRODE PLACEMENT

Chapter 16 discusses electrode placement sites for a number of treatment applications in detail. This section will deal specifically with electrode placement site selection for analgesia.

Optimal stimulation sites for electrodes are those that will facilitate goal accomplishment through the delivery of current.[18-20] If the skin resistance is too high, the target tissue may not be reached at a comfortable level of current. Motor points, trigger points, and acupuncture points all represent electrically active and identifiable points that enhance the potential flow of current into the target tissue.

Motor points are the anatomic location where the peripheral nerve enters the muscle. The amount of electrical current necessary to elicit a motor response from a muscle will be less over the motor point than other areas of the muscle. Placement of an electrode over this area facilitates a motor response of the underlying muscle belly with a lower-intensity setting than if this site was not selected. Whenever the desired response involves a motor response or muscle contraction, motor points should be selected for use.[17]

Trigger points are those areas that exhibit hypersensitivity to both pressure and electrical stimulation. Palpation of these sites causes pain to radiate away from the site.[21,22] Trigger points have a decreased resistance to electrical energy. There is a direct correlation between the location of trigger points and motor points.[21] Selection of a trigger point for electrical stimulation would tend to yield better results than not selecting one, since these points represent an area of decreased resistance.

Acupuncture points represent another type of point that has been described for use with electrical stimulation devices. These points are located over the entire surface of the body and have been mapped out for centuries. Acupuncture points may lie over muscle or connective tissue. They are also electrically active, exhibiting a decreased resistance to the flow of electrical current.[22] If the desired response to the electrical stimulation is a diffuse sensory analgesia, then acupuncture points may afford the greatest availability of sites for electrode placements.

Diffuse sensory analgesia can be readily accomplished through the use of two channels of electrodes for a total of four electrodes. These two channels can be set up in a criss-cross pattern. This pattern will promote an increase in sensation throughout the area with less discrimination of actual location of individual electrodes, as long as the electrodes surround the painful region. This setup will be enhanced with the use of acupuncture points.

The rationale for electrode placement is based on the type of response the clinician is trying to elicit through electrical stimulation. If a muscle twitch is desired, motor points are the placement of choice. If sensory analgesia is desired, the use of acupuncture points is warranted. The utilization of stimulation points does not guarantee the desired amount of stimulation. The appropriate parameters must be employed to create the desired analgesic effect.

Treatment methods for pain relief to be produced by electrical stimulation fall into four categories. Each method theoretically produces pain relief by a different neurophysiologic effect generated by the use of different parameters of the electrical stimulation device. All methods have been demonstrated to be effective forms of treatment when used appropriately.[4,11,15,23-28]

PRODUCING ANALGESIA FOR A PAINFUL PROCEDURE

Some manual techniques may be painful for a patient when the technique is being performed. It is possible to produce analgesia via "a strong tingling sensation" to ease the discomfort of the procedure through the use of electrical stimulation. Parameters for this technique are summarized in Table 14–2. Effective carryover of pain relief is brief, because once the stimulation is turned off, normal sensation returns very rapidly.

PRODUCING SENSORY-LEVEL ANALGESIA

Sensory analgesia is suggested to activate the "gating" mechanism in the spinal cord. This reduces pain impulses from reaching the brain to be processed.[29] Appropriate parameters and treatment indications are described in Table 14–3. Effective carryover is pain relief that persists after the stimulation is no longer present.

NOXIOUS STIMULATION TO PRODUCE ANALGESIA

Electrical stimulation, which is theorized to induce "descending inhibition," utilizes a noxious form of stimulation to help control pain. The painful stimulus activates the smaller pain fibers, which then make connections in the brainstem retic-

Table 14–2   Parameters for Producing Analgesia During a Painful Procedure[34]

Frequency:	150 + pulses per second
Pulse Duration:	Greater than 150 μs
Intensity:	A strong tingling sensation to tolerance. *Note:* a nonrhythmical muscle contraction may be produced at this intensity
Electrode Placement Sites:	Along involved dermatome, two points where the nerve is superficial
Treatment Time:	5 minutes prior to initiation of the painful technique, 15–30 minutes total time.
Indications:[2,34]	Acute pain, pain associated with wound debridement, pain associated with transverse friction massage, pain associated with aggressive stretching techniques, pain associated with aggressive joint mobilization techniques

Table 14–3   Parameters for Producing Sensory-Level Analgesia[17,35]

Frequency:	75–150 pulses per second
Pulse duration:	Less than 200 μs
Intensity:	Strong, but comfortable tingling sensation
Electrode Placement Sites:	Surrounding the site of pain
Indications:[17,35]	Acute pain conditions, chronic pain conditions

ular formation. Information is then conducted to the midbrain to an area called the periaqueductal gray matter. This area of the brain activates a descending pathway that inhibits pain at the spinal cord level.[20] Analgesia occurs quickly with this form of stimulation and effective carryover can last a few minutes to a few hours. Treatment parameters and indications are presented in Table 14–4. A disadvantage of this form of stimulation is that the patient must experience noxious stimuli to produce the desired effect.

ENDOGENOUS OPIATE LIBERATION

Low-rate electrical stimulation can potentially produce analgesia through the liberation of endogenous opiates. Parameters for pain relief by this method and indications are summarized in Table 14–5. The onset of pain relief may occur by the end of a treatment session or several hours later with potentially long-term carryover of pain relief.

TREATMENT EXPECTATIONS

When utilizing electrical stimulation as a tool in a pain management program, realistic goals must be considered. Goal determination is based upon evaluative findings, the nature of the disabling condition, the previous activity level of the pa-

Table 14–4 **Parameters for Producing "Hyperstimulation Analgesia"[20,35]**

Frequency:	1–4 pulses per second
Pulse Duration:	≥1 ms
Intensity:	Highest tolerable level of noxious stimulation
Electrode Placement Sites:	Active electrode is a small diameter probe that is placed over a point with decreased resistance to the flow of current. It may be an acupuncture point, trigger point, or motor point. The dispersive electrode can be held by the patient or placed on the skin at a point distal to the site of stimulation
Treatment Time:	30 seconds per point
Indications:	Acute or chronic pain syndromes

Table 14–5 **Parameters for Endogenous Opiate Liberation[36]**

Frequency:	1–5 pulses per second
Pulse Duration:	200–300 μs
Intensity:	Muscle twitch
Electrode Placement Sites:	Motor points
Treatment Time:	30–45 minutes
Indications:	Chronic pain syndromes

tient, the patient's psychosocial condition, and the prognosis of recovery. The goals established will also vary depending on the stage of the healing process and the nature of the pain—acute versus chronic. If a patient is not "invested in" or motivated toward his or her own recovery, the efforts of a clinician may have limited success.

A patient who is experiencing acute pain experiences decreased pain intensity and pain patterns as a result of the resolution of the inflammatory response and the healing process. During the acute phase, patients may experience pain at rest as well as with any movement.[10] The use of electrical stimulation can facilitate the healing process because of physiologic responses to the modality. Once pain decreases, the patient may also experience a decrease in the intensity of muscle guarding. The use of electrical stimulation can be utilized to help break up the pain-spasm-pain cycle. Goals for a patient during the acute phase of the inflammatory response and the healing process include decreasing the intensity of pain at rest and with movement. This response, if elicited by the use of electrical stimulation, may occur within the treatment time of 20 to 30 minutes. The desired response with other patients may only be elicited while the patient is using an electrical stimulation device. In that case, the patient may be a good candidate for a portable device to be used at times outside the clinical setting.

As the healing process enters the subacute phase, pain may be experienced at the end range of motion.[10] Pain at rest has usually resolved by this time. This process tends to occur from 7 to 21 days after the onset of injury, but may last up to 6 weeks. Tendons and ligaments may take several weeks to go through this initial healing phase. The severity of injury will also determine the duration of the subacute phase. The use of electrical stimulation may continue to be a treatment option for the patient; however, the underlying purpose for its use will change. The purpose now becomes directed toward controlling the pain that is created as a result of other therapeutic interventions that stress the tissue at end range of motion. The patient may have little discomfort prior to treatment, but the gentle therapeutic techniques utilized to enhance range of motion may cause an increase in pain perception. Electrical stimulation may then be used as a posttreatment modality. In this situation, the goal would be to bring the pain level back to a pretreatment level.

When the healing process has reached the maturation and remodeling phase, therapeutic interventions tend to become more aggressive to promote the patient's functional abilities. Progressive stretching, strengthening, and functional activities are commonly the emphasis of treatment.[10] Therapeutic techniques at this phase are intended to stress the immature collagen fibrils laid down in the subacute phase to develop stronger chemical bonds and to orient fibers in a direction that is conducive to function. This process lasts for an additional 8 to 14 weeks after the initial injury. The denser the connective tissue is, the longer the process. During this phase of healing, pain may be experienced at the end range of motion when overpressure is applied to shortened or weakened structures.[10] Electrical stimulation can be utilized for the purpose of treating pain created by the therapeutic intervention with the intent to bring pain levels back to pretreatment levels.

The purpose of the use of electrical stimulation during the normal course of the healing of an acute injury is a transition from managing pain at rest, to posttreatment pain reduction. Each patient's response will vary; therefore, the goals formulated are to be individualized for the patient and adjusted accordingly. If pain is at a tolerable level, not interfering with recovery, or can be controlled by other physical agents effectively, the use of electrical stimulation may be discontinued.

Individuals with chronic pain conditions may also benefit from the utilization of electrical stimulation. The expectation of eliminating pain symptoms may be unrealistic for the majority of patients; thus, the goal of electrical stimulation is to control pain to allow for better function. Recent studies indicate that between 50% and 80% of chronic pain patient's will experience a decrease in pain through the appropriate utilization of electrical stimulation.[2,3,11,12,15,24–26]

Electrical stimulation may be effective for at least three different purposes in treating a chronic pain patient. Electrical stimulation can be used to decrease the intensity of the pain the patient is experiencing at rest. It can decrease the pain associated with the therapeutic techniques utilized to enhance muscle flexibility and functional activity during and after treatment. Finally, it can also help treat acute "flare-ups" or exacerbations in pain symptoms.

Treatment goals for the use of electrical stimulation with chronic pain patients may emphasize functional ability while keeping pain symptoms at a manageable level. The goal may be an effective reduction in pain that allows the patient to walk for longer periods of time or that provides greater comfort for a person to do work-related tasks. The patient should also be able to use a home electrical stimulation unit effectively to manage his or her pain symptoms.

The complete treatment of a chronic pain patient is a multifaceted approach involving many medical disciplines and is beyond the scope of this text. Developing relaxation skills; improving coping skills; and increasing flexibility, strength, and endurance will further enhance patient recovery. The use of electrical stimulation is only one tool used to help these patients.

Although results of studies show that electrical stimulation does not provide 100% success for pain relief,[11,12,15,23–27] clinicians have used this modality to help reduce pain symptoms. Combining the appropriate parameters and electrode placements with the principles of the healing process and the appropriate communication approach to the patient provides the treatment that has a high potential for success. Pain may not be eliminated, but it may be controlled enough to facilitate a more comfortable recovery, facilitate other goals of treatment, and restore functional ability as a result of pain control.

DOCUMENTATION OF TREATMENTS WITH ELECTRICAL STIMULATION

The documentation of treatment parameters and patient responses are essential to the practice of determining the efficacy of any treatment. The treatment parameters that one clinician utilizes should be reproducible by another. Documentation is the key for accomplishing consistency in treatment between practitioners. When utilizing a subjective, objective, assessment, plan (SOAP) note format for documentation, different aspects of the pain management should be noted throughout different headings of documentation.

Objective (O) information for the documentation of pain management includes the pain drawings of the patient or the use of the visual analog scale (VAS) for pain intensity. Measurable aspects of the patient's condition and the treatment rendered would be reported in this section. Parameters used with electrical stimulation must be indicated. Documentation should include the type of electrical stimulation used, the mode of delivery, pulse duration (PD), frequency (F), rise and fall time (if used), treatment area, electrode placement sites, duration of treatment, and intensity.

SUMMARY

The use of electrical stimulation as a physical agent for the treatment of pain symptoms is multifaceted. The clinician should have a thorough understanding of the neurophysiologic basis of pain modulation and the variety of methods to achieve pain reduction with electrical stimulation. Treatment applications are based on this knowledge as well as the results of a thorough evaluation of the patient. Any modification of parameters is based on treatment outcome. This chapter presented a review of the underlying tenets of pain modulation and a variety of methods to achieve pain reduction. The paradigm of clinical decision making provides the practitioner with a framework of the process for treatment selection or modification to achieve the desired goals of electrical stimulation as an instrument for pain reduction.

DISCUSSION QUESTIONS

1. What forms of electrical stimulation can be used to treat the pain associated with the performance of a painful manual technique such as a deep tissue massage? What parameters would you use and why?

2. Explain the neurophysiologic mechanisms of the effects of electrical stimulation in terms that a patient would understand.

3. A patient is diagnosed with phantom limb pain. What information would you need to know about this patient in order to recommend a form of electrical stimulation for treatment of this syndrome?

4. What are the advantages and disadvantages of electrical stimulation for analgesia as compared to others that reduce pain perception?

5. Describe three possible forms of electrical stimulation treatments for an individual with a chronic pain syndrome.

REFERENCES

1. Cailliet, R: Pain: Mechanisms and Management. FA Davis, Philadelphia PA, 1993.

2. Wells, PE, Frampton, V, and Bowsher, D: Pain Management by Physical Therapy. Appleton & Lange, Norwalk, CT, 1988.

3. Tollison, CD, Satterthwaite JR, and Tollison, JW: Handbook of Pain Management, ed 2. Williams & Wilkins, Baltimore, 1994.

4. Ho, A, et al: Effectiveness of transcutaneous electrical nerve stimulation in relieving pain following thoracotomy, Physiotherapy 73:33, 1987.

5. Taber's Cyclopedic Medical Dictionary, ed 17. FA Davis, Philadelphia, 1993, pp 91, 100.

6. Hitner, H and Nagle, BT: Basic Pharmacology for Health Occupations. Glencoe Publishing, Mission Hills, CA, 1987, pp 70–71, 102–107, 112–116.

7. Bolton, L: TENS electrode irritation. J Am Acad Dermatol 8:134, 1983.

8. Zugarman, C: Dermatitis from transcutaneous electrical nerve stimulation. J Am Acad Dermatol 6:936, 1982.

9. Gilman, S and Newman, SW: Manter and Gatz's Essentials of Clinical Neuroanatomy and Neurophysiology, ed 8. FA Davis, Philadelphia, 1992, pp 56–59.

10. Hooshmand, H: Chronic Pain: Clinical Reflex Sympathetic Dystrophy Prevention and Management. CRC Press, Boca Raton, FL, 1993, pp 40–41.

11. Mullins P: Management of common chronic pain problems in the hand. Phys Ther 69:1059, 1989.

12. Manchikanti L: Chronic pain management. Physician's Assistant, 16:39, 1992.

13. Lamb, S and Barbaro, NM: Neurosurgical approaches to the management of chronic pain syndromes. Orthopaed Nursing, 6:23, 1987.

14. Melzack, R and Wal, P: Pain mechanisms: A new theory. Science 150:971, 1965.

15. Leo, KC, et al: Effect of transcutaneous electrical nerve stimulation characteristics on clinical pain. Phys Ther 66:200, 1986.

16. Mannheimer, JS and Lampe, GN: Clinical Transcutaneous Electrical Nerve Stimulation. FA Davis, Philadelphia, 1984, p 211.

17. Gersh, MR: Transcutaneous electrical nerve stimulation for management of pain and sensory pathology. In Gersh, MR (ed): Electrotherapy in Rehabilitation. FA Davis, Philadelphia, 1992, p 175.

18. Berlant, SR: Method of determining optimal stimulation sites for transcutaneous electrical nerve stimulation. Phys Ther 64:924, 1984.

19. Travell, J and Rinzler, SH: The myofascial genesis of pain. Postgrad Med 11:425–435, 1952.

20. Melzack, R: Myofascial trigger points: Relation to acupuncture and mechanisms of pain. Arch Phys Med Rehabil 62:114, 1981.

21. Melzack, R, Stilwell, DM, and Fox, EJ: Trigger points and acupuncture points for pain: Correlations and implications. Pain 3:3, 1977.

22. Mannheimer, JS and Lampe, GN: Clinical Transcutaneous Electrical Nerve Stimulation. FA Davis, Philadelphia, 1984, pp 267–268.

23. Mailis, A, et al: Chest wall pain after aortocoronary bypass using internal mammary artery graft: A new pain syndrome? Heart Lung Crit Care 18:553, 1989.

24. Denning, ML: Retrospective review of long-term transcutaneous nerve stimulation in the management of chronic back pain. Physiotherapy 74:149, 1988.

25. Smith, CR, et al: TNS and osteo-arthritic pain. Physiotherapy 69:266, 1983.

26. Reuss, R and Meyer, SC: The use of TENS in the management of cancer pain. Clin Manag 5:26, 1985.

27. Grim, LC and Morey, SH: Transcutaneous electrical nerve stimulation for relief of parturition pain. Phys Ther 65:337, 1985.

28.   Issenman, J, Nolan, MF, Rowley, J, and Hobby, R: Transcutaneous electrical nerve stimulation for pain control after spinal fusion with Harrington rods: A clinical report. Phys Ther 65:1517, 1985.

29.   Lampe, GN and Mannheimer, JS: Stimulation characteristics of TENS. In Mannheimer, JS: Clinical Transcutaneous Electrical Nerve Stimulation. FA Davis, Philadelphia, 1984, pp 212–213.

30.   Urban, BJ: Treatment of chronic pain with nerve blocks and stimulation. Gen Hosp Psychiatry 6:43, 1984.

31.   Jurf, JB and Nirschl, AL: Acute postoperative pain management: A comprehensive review and update. Crit Care Nursing Q, 16:8, 1993.

32.   Hargreaves, A and Lander, J: Use of transcutaneous electrical nerve stimulation for post-operative pain. Nursing Res 38:159, 1989.

33.   Fried, T, et al: Transcutaneous electrical nerve stimulation: Its role in the control of chronic pain. Arch Phys Med Rehabil 65:228, 1984.

34.   Lampe, GN and Mannheimer, JS: Stimulation characteristics of TENS. In Mannheimer, JS: Clinical Transcutaneous Electrical Nerve Stimulation. FA Davis, Philadelphia, 1984, p 210.

35.   Castel, JC: Seminar Notes, Electrotherapy and Ultrasound Update, New York, November 1994.

36.   Lampe, GN and Mannheimer, JS: Stimulation characteristics of TENS. In Mannheimer, JS: Clinical Transcutaneous Electrical Nerve Stimulation. FA Davis, Philadelphia, 1984, p 211.

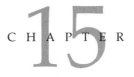

Electrical Stimulation Devices and Equipment

Barbara J. Behrens, BS, PTA

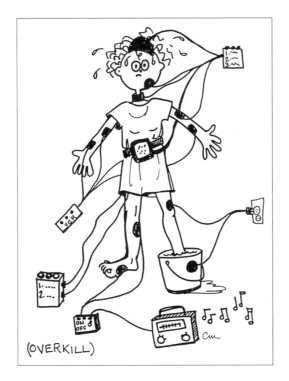

(OVERKILL)

CHAPTER OBJECTIVES

- Define the different types of electrical stimulators utilized in clinical practice (TENS, FES, NMES, HVPC, IFC, EMG, etc.).

- Differentiate between devices and parameters for therapeutic goals.

- Outline the process for determining which device is appropriate to accomplish a therapeutic treatment goal.

CHAPTER OUTLINE

WHERE DO THOSE NAMES COME FROM?

Many electrical stimulation devices have been named for their inventor, waveform, or electrical characteristics. A great deal of experimentation took place regarding observed electrically induced responses. The experimenters' names were then associated with their individual work or findings, and eventually either devices, waveforms, or current characteristics. This methodology for naming stimulators still persists to some degree today. Individuals such as Luigi Galvani, Alessandro Volta, and Michael Faraday were some of the first "experimenters" to have their names associated with their studies and resultant current characteristics or waveforms (Table 15–1).

"Faradic" stimulation initially referred to anything other than direct current stimulation, which also led to a great deal of confusion. Stimulators measure their output intensity in a variety of forms: amperage or voltage, dependent upon the stimulator. Clinicians are reminded to look at the specific treatment goals and define the treatment parameters by those characteristics, not "the originator" of the waveform, to keep documentation consistent and less confusing.

DEVICES FOR THERAPEUTIC ELECTRICAL STIMULATION

This section will deal with the devices used for therapeutic electrical stimulation. These devices are meant for use only by or under the direct supervision of licensed clinicians. They may be clinical models or portable models. Clinical models have historically had more flexibility in terms of parameters and output intensity, and consequently were larger in size than portable models. However, as technology has been advancing, the differences between the available features of the two types of stimulators have been diminishing (Fig. 15–1).

CLINICAL AND PORTABLE MODELS

Clinical models for electrical stimulation are designed to be utilized in the clinic for the management of a wide variety of clinical signs and symptoms. They may

Table 15–1 **Electrical Current Namesakes**

Luigi Galvani—Galvanic Current

Luigi Galvani published reports of his findings with electrical stimulation of nerve and resultant muscle contraction. His name is now associated with a unidirectional static flow of current: galvanic current. Galvanism in general also refers to the result of an applied electrical charge or net charge.

Alessandro Volta—Voltage

The term *voltage* refers to the potential or stored charge. It has the potential to do work. It provides the driving force to facilitate the flow of electrical energy. 1 volt is the unit of electrical pressure needed for 1 ampere of current to pass through 1 ohm of resistance (see Chap. 9). It is named for Alessandro Volta, who initially quantified this unit.

Michael Faraday—Faradic Current

One of the first individuals to explore the use of a modified form of current was Michael Faraday, who discovered electromagnetic induction and developed an electromagnetic machine in the early 1800s. The waveform that was produced was called *faradic* by medical practitioners of that era. It was actually a polyphasic, asymmetrical unbalanced waveform.[1]

---

be utilized to reduce pain, edema, muscle spasm or promote muscle re-education or strengthening. Electrical stimulation represents a therapeutic intervention for a variety of clinical symptoms as well as an unattended treatment technique.

Portable stimulators are designed either to be used by the patient at home, by the clinician who is treating patients in their homes, in the training room, or in other nontraditional "clinic" environments. Until recently, portable stimulators were simply transcutaneous electrical nerve stimulators (TENS) and neuromuscular electrical stimulation (NMES) devices. The family of devices has increased to include interferential current (IFC), high-voltage pulsed current (HVPC), and iontophoresis devices consistent with new advances in technology.

"ALPHABET SOUP" TRANSLATIONS

Devices are sometimes identified by their initials, e.g., NMES for neuromuscular electrical stimulation. Communication regarding electrical stimulation devices and techniques has created a veritable "alphabet soup" of devices. The acronym labels will be translated throughout this chapter. As technology has advanced, so has the number of available stimulators marketed to clinicians. The ever-present problem that emerged is one of differentiation of the capabilities of each machine. Each of the stimulators was developed in the footsteps of another stimulator, and had its own acronym, either for its application or for its current characteristics. Clinicians need to be able to differentiate between TENS, an IFC, a HVPC, an NMES unit, and an FES unit identifying the similarities, as well as the differences.

TENS: Transcutaneous Electrical Nerve Stimulation

The acronym TENS is most commonly associated with portable stimulators that the patient can utilize whenever they experience pain or discomfort and they are

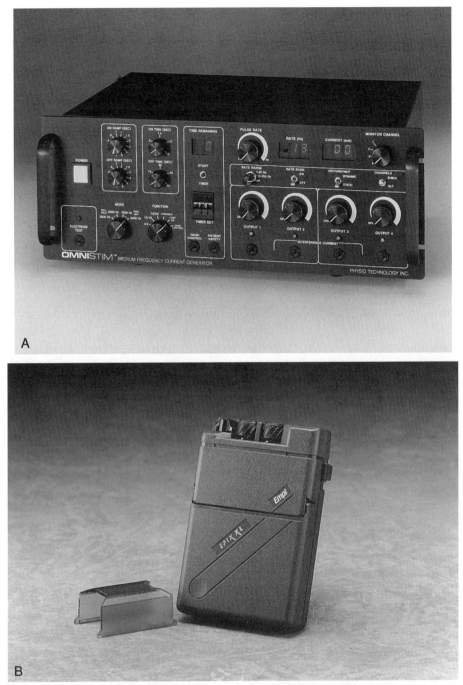

Figure 15–1. The potential difference in size and capabilities of portable stimulators and clinical models. *(A)* The OmniStim portable stimulator. *(Courtesy of PTI, Topeka KS.) (B)* Portable TENS unit. *(Courtesy of EMPI, Minneapolis, MN.)* Both units provide the necessary parameters for the accomplishment of therapeutic treatment goals, but the clinical model has the advantage of being able to stimulate larger muscle groups because of the greater output potential. The smaller unit has the advantage over the larger unit in that it can be worn underneath a patient's clothing throughout the day for pain management.

not in the clinic. Classically, TENS units have been comparable in size to a cassette tape. They are battery-operated stimulators that are capable of providing sensory or motor-level stimulation for pain management.

TENS refers to the stimulation of nerve fibers from surface electrodes to effect a change in the underlying innervated tissue. It can be utilized for a variety of applications, including all those applications of electrical stimulation employed as therapeutic interventions. TENS is widely utilized as a therapeutic modality for pain management.

As a technique, TENS accurately describes all of the electrical stimulation devices that will be covered in this chapter. However, when clinicians refer to TENS, they are usually referring to the portable stimulators used independently by patients for pain management.

A TENS unit provides patients with a method of relieving their own pain whenever it occurs. TENS units should be evaluated for use in the clinical environment, where appropriate monitoring can take place; electrical parameters, electrode interfaces, and placement sites can be assessed. This provides the clinician with the opportunity to assess the ability of the patient to utilize the TENS unit independently and appropriately, prior to home use of the device.[2]

Description of a TENS Unit   TENS units usually have adjustable frequencies, pulse durations, intensities, and often some type of modulation. Modulation options available range from frequency, pulse duration, and amplitude modulation to a combination of the three parameters. TENS units are usually employed as a form of sensory analgesia. They are predominantly set up for analgesia to relieve muscle guarding that occurs from the perception of pain.

TENS units usually utilize a 9-V battery that may or may not be rechargeable. They usually have two channels, each with two electrodes, for a total of four electrodes and two leads per device. The lead wires are small-diameter coated wires that plug into "jacks" or "ports" on either the top or side of the device depending upon the manufacturer. The other end of the lead wires has either "pins" that are small-diameter rounded metal tips for insertion into the electrodes or "snaps" for snap electrodes. Most TENS devices have a "belt clip" so that they can be worn by the patient while he or she is performing daily activities (Fig. 15–2).

Optimally, if a TENS unit has been ordered for a patient, it has been evaluated in the clinic for this patient, and they will be returning to the clinic for periodic reevaluation of the continued effectiveness of the unit. Some insurance carriers recommend that these units be rented for at least a month to determine whether or not continued use of the device will be necessary. Purchase decisions are reached by the combined efforts of the clinician, the patient, and the insurance adjustor.

TENS devices are regulated, requiring a physician's prescription prior to home use. Use of the devices can be recommended to the physician by the clinician, but for reimbursement reasons, a prescription for its use must be written by a physician. Regulations may vary by state or by region (Fig. 15–3).

NMES: Neuromuscular Electrical Stimulation

NMES units are utilized for the reduction of muscle spasm, muscle strengthening, and potentially for edema reduction via muscle pumping. These devices may be either clinical or portable.

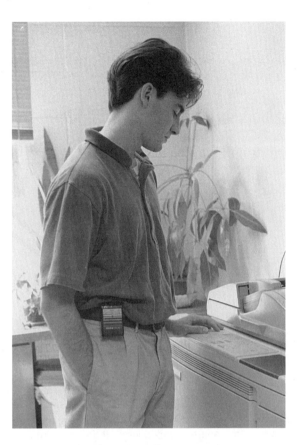

Figure 15–2. Patient wearing TENS unit.

Target Tissue for NMES   NMES devices are not named for their inventor or for their waveform characteristics. NMES devices deliver electrical stimulation across the skin the same way that TENS devices do, but the treatment goal is a motor response rather than a sensory analgesia response.

Description of a NMES Unit   Most clinical NMES stimulators utilize surface electrodes that are placed with one electrode over the motor point of the muscle to be stimulated and the other electrode either somewhere else on the muscle or over the spinal nerve root. The desired response of the stimulation is a motor response, which is easiest to accomplish through the use of motor points. Parameters necessary to produce a motor response are based on the strength–duration curve values for motor fibers and whether or not the muscle is innervated. Motor fibers usually require longer pulse durations to generate an action potential than a sensory fiber.

Adjustable parameters for NMES units may include: frequency, pulse duration, intensity, on time, off time, and on-off ramps. These units may have as many as four independent channels of stimulation, each with two electrodes (Fig. 15–4). Parameters that distinguish an NMES unit from an electrical stimulator designed to promote analgesia, e.g., TENS, rather than motor responses are on and off times or ramps and longer pulse durations. NMES applications of electrical stimulation involve the contraction of a muscle, and some form of relaxation time that will typically be adjustable, allowing the accomplishment of different goals. Contraction

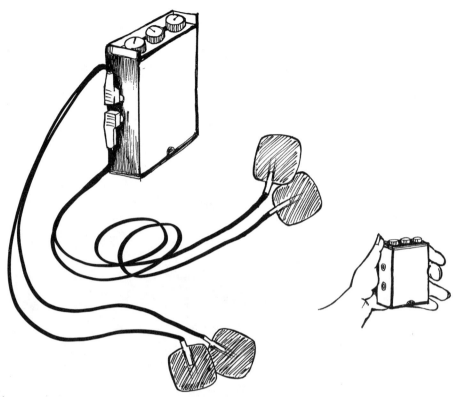

Figure 15–3. A TENS unit with two channels, four electrodes, two separate intensity controls, and a common frequency control. It fits easily into the palm of an adult hand.

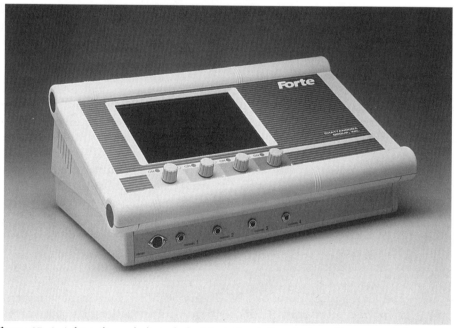

Figure 15–4. A four-channel clinical electrical stimulation device. *(Courtesy of Chattanooga Group Inc., Hixson, TN.)*

times with short relaxation times will promote muscle fatigue quickly. These will be inefficient for muscle-strengthening protocols, since they will fatigue the muscle quickly, but will be indicated for spasm-reduction protocols. Muscle pumping for the accomplishment of edema reduction has been utilized by clinicians who have sought to use electrically induced muscle contraction and an elevated position, to pump edema physically out of distal extremities.

NMES applications utilize surface electrodes placed over the motor point of muscles, intensity, and pulse-duration levels sufficient to produce a motor response, and rest times to allow or not allow the muscle to recoup a nutrient base sufficient for additional contractions. Other names have been associated with NMES devices, such as FES, HVPC, LVPC, IFC, and Russian stimulators; all will be discussed in this chapter.

FES: Functional Electrical Stimulation

FES units are often portable stimulators that are designed to be worn by the patient for the purpose of augmenting voluntary muscle contraction to perform a functional activity. FES application of a clinical NMES unit may be utilized via implanted electrodes for the purpose of accomplishing significant motor recruitment for activities such as standing or gait for the spinal cord patient. Most commonly, when a clinician refers to FES, he or she is referring to portable models of electrical stimulation for motor responses related to function.

Treatment Goals for FES   FES units would be considered TENS devices since they rely on surface electrode placement (except in the scenario listed above for implanted electrodes and clinical stimulation units). FES units may be utilized during gait training for the patient who experiences foot drop. These units can also be used to help increase or maintain tone in the shoulder following a cerebral vascular accident (CVA). These two cases represent examples of "orthotic replacement" by a portable stimulator. Rather than wearing an orthotic device to maintain dorsiflexion of the ankle during heel strike, the patient wears an FES to *assist* in heel strike by initiating a contraction of the dorsiflexors.

Shoulder subluxations and flaccid paralysis following a CVA can be managed during the day with an arm sling or muscle stimulation of the deltoid to reapproximate the humoral head in the glenohumoral joint. The FES unit would then *assist* in maintaining approximation to promote function of the upper extremity.

The application of an FES unit is geared toward muscle function of an innervated muscle; therefore, the adjustable parameters on these units tend to be biased toward muscle stimulation. Adjustable parameters include frequency, pulse duration, intensity, on-off times, and on-off ramps. Single-channel units or dual-channel units are available. FES units may have a treatment timer, but it is not essential. The units are intended to be worn during activity; therefore they utilize batteries and small-diameter lead wires. Battery operation gives patients the advantage of independence from a wall outlet. Small lead wires attach to electrodes that are approximately 2 inches square. They are usually self-adhering or reusable, potentially to be worn for several hours daily. The electrode size will be dependent upon the muscles being stimulated with strip electrodes for longer, narrower muscles and small square electrodes for smaller muscles. Refer to Chapter 16 for more specific information on electrodes. If the unit is being utilized as a dorsiflexion assist, then there might also be a "heel-strike switch" attachment that fits in the patient's shoe. This type of switch will activate the stimulation once the heel hits the floor. The active electrodes would have been placed on the tibialis anterior, which would dorsiflex the ankle on demand rather than on a timed cycle. Some clinical units for use during gait training have incorporated multiple channels of stimulation[4,5] (Fig. 15–5).

Some patients who benefit in the clinical setting from the use of an FES unit would potentially benefit from using the FES daily and independently. These units are prescribed by a physician for "home use" if the determination is made that the patient is cognizant enough to understand how to use the device, or if they have a "significant other" who will be able to assist them. If FES is found to be a viable alternative for the patient, then they may either rent or purchase the stimulator. Insurance companies may recommend that the stimulators be rented for at least one month prior to purchase. Some patients may need the unit for a few weeks, and others may need it for longer periods of time where purchase would be more cost efficient.

FES can be accomplished with an NMES device; however, the name FES refers to the functional goal of the electrical stimulation. The function is related to a motor response. Electrode placement sites will incorporate motor points. One of the goals of the device is functional independence outside of the clinic. NMES devices may also be utilized to promote a muscle contraction, but the NMES is being utilized to promote muscle strength for the performance of activities outside of the clinic. However, NMES is also utilized in the management of edema or to promote an increase in circulation to an area,[5] which are not specific functionally related goals. FES is usually applied transcutaneously, so it is also a form of TENS. Table 15–2 outlines the similarities and differences among the devices described thus far, NMES, TENS, and FES.

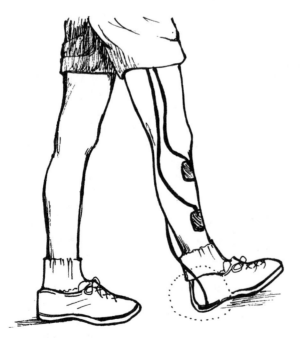

Figure 15–5. Patient using an FES to assist in dorsiflexion during the swing phase of gate. The electrodes are placed on the tibialis anterior. There is a heel switch in the patient's shoe, and the unit itself is worn at the patient's belt.

Table 15–2 **Electrical Stimulation Device Parameters: Similarities and Differences**

	Frequency	Pulse Duration	On/Off	Electrode Placement	Goals (Primary)
NMES	1–50 Hz or pps	200–300 μs	Adjustable	MP	Motor control, strength, 1 spasm, 1 edema
FES	1–50 Hz or pps	200–300 μs	Adjustable	MP	Motor control, functional activities, gait
TENS	1–120 Hz or pps	30–250 μs	N/A	AP, MP, TP	1 pain

Abbreviations: AP= acupuncture point; TP = trigger point; MP = motor point.

HVPC: High-Voltage Pulsed Current

HVPC, which has been marketed since the early 1970s, was named for its output parameters, which allowed voltage output levels of up to 500 V. This method of current delivery was possible because of the specifics of the waveform, which was a twin-peak or twin-spike waveform. The twin spike has a short pulse duration and a high peak current; both in such combination provide a comfortable stimulus. The devices were named after electrical galvanism (originally called high-voltage pulsed galvanic), which was actually not reflected in the waveform. Galvanic waveforms implied that the waveform was monophasic and uninterrupted. These devices produced an interrupted, not continuous, waveform.

Treatment Goals and Parameters for HVPC HVPC stimulators are utilized for a variety of therapeutic applications, including pain reduction, muscle spasm reduction, edema reduction, and muscle re-education. Surface stimulation is used, and therefore HVPC generators are also considered TENS techniques. When the therapeutic goal includes a motor response, they could also be referred to as NMES devices. Because of the wide variety of applications, HVPC devices have many adjustable parameters. The frequency (of the twin-spike waveform), pulse duration (of the twin-spike waveform) or interpulse interval (of the twin spikes), the intensity (monitored in volts), polarity, and there may be on-off times, on-off ramps and a balance control are features of most of these generators. The balance control enables the clinician to "weight" the delivery of current to the electrodes differently. It makes it possible for current density in one of the two electrodes to be "relatively" higher than the other electrode by shifting the output to either selected electrode, red or black.

HVPC Unit Descriptions These are single-channel units with one large dispersive electrode and two equally sized electrodes that represent the other "bifurcated" lead from the channel. The dispersive electrode is applied to any large surface area capable of accommodating the electrode and the other two electrodes are placed in the treatment area. Actual current flow will be from each of the two electrodes to the dispersive electrode representing one channel of stimulation. Because of the size relationship of the electrodes, the patient perceives sensation under the two smaller electrodes and usually no sensation under the larger dispersive electrode. If sensation is desired under all of the electrodes, then the size of the "dispersive" is reduced so that it is the equivalent size of the two electrodes. Reducing the size of this dispersive electrode will equal out the current densities of all of the electrodes so that sensation can be equally perceived under all of the electrodes. Alterations in conductivity of the underlying tissue can be the source of uneven sensation levels. This can be addressed by utilizing the balance control, which will shift the greater percentage of output to whichever electrode is selected.

HVPC stimulators represent probably one of the most common stimulators to be found in the clinical environment today. Current research has led to a resurgence of interest in the devices for edema reduction and wound care.[7-10] Table 15–3 outlines the parameters of an HVPC unit depicted in Figure 15–6.

IFC: Interferential Current

IFC devices are those that utilize more than one electrical generator; therefore, they have more than one channel of stimulation. The electrodes from the channels are set up in a "criss-cross" pattern so that the output from each of the channels can potentially "interfere" with the output of the other channel of electrodes. The interference then takes place within the patient, resulting in different pulse characteristics than those that were generated by the stimulator.

Interference generators are also utilized for a wide variety of treatment applications that include pain management, edema reduction, and muscle spasm reduction. The devices rely on the application setup of their electrodes to accomplish the stated goals and to differentiate them from the other stimulators that can be utilized to accomplish the same goals.

Interference is described as the mutual action of waves of light, sound, or electrical energy upon each other, where the resultant effect may be cumulative, adding to each other, or may cancel each other out. There are two separate sources of the same type of energy. They have the ability to interact with each other in a predictable manner.

Table 15–3 **HVPC Parameters**

Waveform	Twin Spike
Pulse Duration	Fixed, 5–10 μs with a 75-μs interpulse interval (time between the first and second spike). Some units allow adjustment of the interpulse interval. Increasing the interval would lower the average charge, since it would be delivered over a longer time period.
Frequency	Adjustable from 1 to 120 in twin pulses
Output	0–500 V
Polarity	Active electrodes adjustable + or −
Reciprocating	Ability to adjust timing sequence so that one electrode would be on while the other electrode is off, or have both electrodes on simultaneously.

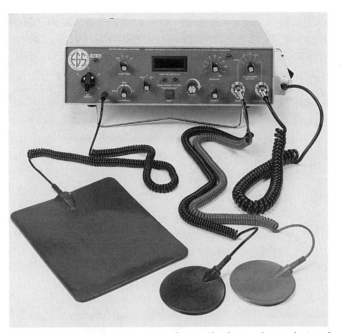

Figure 15–6. High-voltage pulsed-current stimulator. The large electrode is referred to as the dispersive electrode because of its large size in comparison to the two smaller electrodes on the right. The unit is a single-channel stimulator with one of the leads bifurcated to provide two electrodes from one lead. *(Courtesy of Electro-Med Health Industries, North Miami, FL.)*

Physical Examples of Interference   Sound has the ability to travel and interfere with other sounds, and it represents a different physical example of the interference phenomenon. Singing a round, that is, a song that has been written so that two versions of it may be sung slightly out of synchronization with each other and the sound is still pleasing to the ear, is another example of interference. One group will start singing and then another joins in, but starting at the beginning. The resulting sound is melodious, but the words become unrecognizable in the room where both groups are singing. Each individual group will be singing the same words, but when combined and out of synch, it is difficult to distinguish or understand them. The volume of the sound in between the two groups will be periodically louder, or summative, as both groups are singing. The combination of sounds is an example of interference.

Electrical Generators that Produce IFC   Electrical stimulation devices are capable of producing current waveforms that can "interfere" with each other in the body. This is typically accomplished with the following: two or more electrical generators, sinusoidal waveforms, frequencies above 1000 Hz.

Types of IFC   Interference electrical stimulators have been in use throughout the world since the 1950s.[11] Technologic advances have facilitated the emergence of different forms of interference, namely, frequency difference and amplitude summation or "full-field" interference. Both forms of IFC are applied with intersecting electrode pathways, and both have the ability to produce a stimulatory field within the tissue that is different than the perceived surface sensation. The next section will describe both the similarities and the differences of the types of interferential stimulation.

Frequency Difference Interferential The first form of interference current described was "frequency difference" interferential current. One generator would produce an output frequency of 4000 Hz, and another generator from the same stimulator would produce a frequency of 4100 Hz. The electrodes from the two channels would be set up so that they intersected each other. Since periodically the two waveforms would summate and periodically they would cancel each other out, they would produce a "beat" or resultant frequency that was equal to their difference. If the channels produced 4000 Hz and 4100 Hz, then the resultant would be 100 bps. The unit produced a sinusoidal waveform, which mathematically would "line up" to cause summation of the intensities (Fig. 15–7).

The sensation perceived by the patient would be the sensation from the "beat frequency." The individual channels would produce little to no sensation or numbness because of the carrier frequency of the channels. Analgesia may occur under the electrodes and within the tissue where the current pathways intersect. Treatment parameters are based on the desired beat or interference frequency. If a motor response was desired, then the selected difference would be 35 to 50 bps, just as it would for a generator that was not an interference generator. This form of interferential current relies on the fact that periodically, the generators will be out of phase with each other. The sensation is predictable and will be perceived within the tissue with little or no sensation occurring underneath the electrodes themselves. The "target tissue" or treatment area will be located somewhere within the paths of the two intersecting channels of electrodes. Electrical current travels in a path that reflects the path of least resistance, so it will be based upon the electrical conductivity of the underlying tissue.

Full-Field Interferential The next generation of interference stimulation involved two generators, but this time, rather than relying on them being out of phase by delivering different carrier frequencies, they are in phase. Both generators are producing the same thing at the same time. This can be illustrated by en-

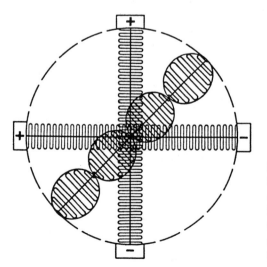

Figure 15–7. Frequency difference IFC. One of the generators (channels) is producing 4000 Hz, and the other generator is producing 4004 Hz. Since the generators are out of phase with each other, a frequency difference of 4 Hz occurs where the current pathways intersect each other.

visioning a room full of individuals saying the same thing at the same time. The resulting sounds would be very different than if the individuals were carrying on separate conversations. The result is understandable, predictable, and at an amplified volume. The room is the environment where the sounds interfere by summating. Electrical stimulation devices that have two generators that are in phase are described as "amplitude-summation IFC devices" or "full-field IFC".

Amplitude-summation IFC relies on the phase relationship of the two generators. Both generators are doing the same thing at the same time, so that the resulting current in the tissue will be at an increased amplitude. Both generators may be interrupted, producing pulsed bursts of current or uninterrupted current. If the channels are pulsed bursts, then the patient will feel the pulse burst rate underneath the electrodes *and* where they intersect in the tissue. The selection of a parameter for treatment would still be based on the desired effect. If a motor response was the goal, then a pulsed burst rate of 35 to 50 bps should be selected, just as it would for any other form of stimulation where the desired result was a motor response (Fig. 15–8).

Dynamic Versus Static IFC   Localization of tissue for IFC is more diffuse than for other forms of electrical stimulation, since it relies on the interference vector for stimulation rather than the electrodes themselves. It may be delivered in a static, nonmoving manner, or in a dynamic manner where the perception of current changes. Just as there are different types of IFC, there are different ways to produce this movement pattern perception. The result of a moving "vector" is a larger sensory field or greater area of target tissue coverage.

IFC in Summary   IFC refers to the application of more than one channel of electrodes to a given area to produce the desired effect. There are different types of interferential current that have varied characteristics based on the electrical generators and how they are set up. It may be possible to predict a static stimulation field within the tissue that is actually perpendicular to the setup of the electrodes. Use of IFC may produce either a continually changing sensation or a constant sensation, depending on the generator.

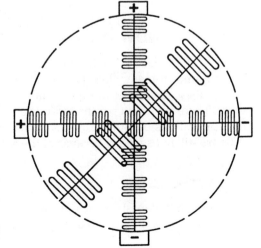

Figure 15–8. This illustration depicts amplitude summation IFC or full-field IFC. Both of the channels have a carrier frequency that is pulse burst in phase with the other generator. The amplitude of the resultant "third line of current" is equivalent to the sum of the two individual channels.

IFC generators can be utilized to accomplish a wide variety of therapeutic goals. Specific goal accomplishment will be dependent upon the chosen parameters and electrode placement sites, just as it would with any other electrical stimulation device.

Special Safety Considerations with IFC Patient safety is an important consideration with the application of all forms of electrical stimulation. Because of the way in which it is delivered to the patient, IFC has some additional precautions. IFC produces a resultant line of current within the patient where the current pathways intersect. IFC should not be set up so that the intersecting pathways would have the potential for crossing the thoracic cavity. IFC is contraindicated transthoracically. There is also a high potential for electrode interfaces to "dry out" during the treatment time with IFC. Relatively high current densities are utilized with IFC as compared to other stimulators. Additional care should be taken to ensure that the electrode interface remains moist throughout the treatment time. If the electrode interface "dries out," there is a potential risk of skin irritation.

"RUSSIAN TECHNIQUE" ELECTRICAL STIMULATION

The term *Russian technique* was introduced following the 1976 Olympics, and the successes of the Soviet wrestling team. Team physicians reported training programs that utilized electrical stimulation for strength augmentation.[12] Because of the political climate of the time, few details were released regarding electrical parameters or treatment protocols.

The Russian technique has become associated with the use of a sinusoidal stimulator that produces 2500-Hz pulse burst at 50 bps, with an on time of 10 seconds and an off time of 50 seconds. These parameters have been preset into various electrical stimulators for the purpose of facilitating strength gains. The parameter set may initially appear unique; however, it is consistent with the typical frequency range to accomplish a tetanic contraction, 35 to 50 Hz. It just utilizes a carrier frequency to accomplish the current delivery (see Chap. 12 for more detail on strength augmentation with electrical stimulation).

PUTTING IT ALL TOGETHER: HOW DO YOU CHOOSE AND WHY?

TENS, NMES, FES, IFC, high-voltage and "Russian" electrical stimulation devices can be found in many clinics today. Recent advances in technology have made many of these modalities more affordable for clinicians, and easier to use than ever before. There are preset parameters on some devices and fixed parameters for specific applications on other devices. Some of the devices introduced in the early 1970s are still in use today because of the reliability and durability built into them.

WHAT TO CHOOSE?

One problem that exists is the question of what to choose? The electrical stimulation device that was purchased in 1978, and has been faithfully utilized on a daily basis, is not necessarily less desirable than a new "high tech" device purchased today. The age of the device should not be the determining factor in whether or not to use a piece of equipment that has been properly maintained. The true determining factor should be the desired outcome of the use of the device. Can the goal be effectively and efficiently accomplished? The answer comes from the *parameters* that are necessary to accomplish the desired goal and the availability of those parameters on a given device.

Many clinics have a wide variety of stimulators to choose from that have been purchased over as many as 20 years. Those older devices that are still utilized are used because they contain the necessary parameters to accomplish treatment goals. New technology incorporating those parameters that work clinically should not replace the older devices, it should supplement the number of devices that a clinic utilizes. When selecting a device, the goal should be the accomplishment of the therapeutic treatment not to try out a new toy. Simply stated, which device has the parameters that are necessary to accomplish the specific treatment goal for a given patient?

Perhaps another factor that is commonly overlooked in clinics today is the durability of some of the electrical stimulation devices. Part of the success in the use of electrical stimulation is the reliability of a device to perform as expected. Many clinics have electrical stimulators that were purchased over 10 years ago and are still in use today because they work! In this respect the technology must keep pace with the demands that have been placed on the modalities, as their use has continued to become more common.

There has been a resurgence of interest in manufacturing electrical stimulation devices. This is exemplified by stimulators that combine IFC, HVPC, Russian, and TENS in one unit. The same treatment goals of pain relief, edema reduction, prevention of muscle atrophy and promotion of joint mobility can be accomplished with each of the "modalities," but the choices are within the unit rather than just in the clinic among a variety of units.

Why Choose a Specific Stimulator?

Parameter sets and electrode placement sites are the keys to success to accomplish clinical goals with electrical stimulation, not necessarily the technology. Clinicians need to look critically at the real available parameters of a stimulator and make the determination of the potential applications for the device based on that knowledge, not on the claims that the manufacturer of the device may make. These parameter sets need to match up with the clinical goals. They can be found by reading the specification page of the users' manual for the device. Manufacturers should not be the innovators for parameters; clinicians should determine what is needed for the manufacturers to supply.

Terminology and Pseudoterminology

Throughout this text a wide variety of techniques and devices have been identified and described. A concerted effort has been made toward explaining each of the devices in understandable terminology and translating the origins of some of the pseudoterms that are commonly in use in clinics today. Each of the devices described is capable of accomplishing a variety of therapeutic treatment goals. Documentation of the stated goals rather than the device will facilitate an end to the confusion of "the box" or "the unit," since the goals are accomplished with parameters, and whatever box contains the parameters can be utilized for the treatment. This will also facilitate a more consistent form of communication for the purposes of the establishment of new protocols that are parameter based, not box based. If the box selected has the parameters, it can be utilized; if it does not contain the parameters, it cannot be utilized. *Parameters and treatment goals represent appropriate terminology that should be observed and documented.* Pseudoterminology is represented by the type of box or waveform utilized and should not be specifically referred to in the documentation.

ONE MORE ACRONYM. . .EMG

EMG is an acronym for electromyography. A muscle contraction is the result of electrical activity summing from the action potential of the motor units. It is a measurable event of the motor unit action potential, and it can be recorded via surface electrodes or needle insertion electrode probes. There are predictable responses that a normal muscle should produce when eliciting a contraction. Variances from the normal response occur with neuromuscular disorders.

The electrical activity of the muscle at rest during a contraction can be utilized to provide both the clinician and the patient with a sense of precisely what is taking place within the muscle. It can be used to supply information regarding function if the patient is unable to express or volitionally alter the condition of the electrical activity of the muscle being monitored.[13] When the EMG is utilized to provide information regarding the level of activity occurring, it is referred to as biofeedback.[14]

BIOFEEDBACK

Biofeedback can take many forms. It is a method of providing the patient with information such as joint movement, pressure, muscle activity, skin temperature, heart rate, blood pressure, or other physiologic information so that the patient can learn how to potentially impact them.[15] EMG biofeedback is a tool that can be utilized to provide the patient with information regarding the activity of the muscles in a given area. It can also be used to allow patients to monitor specific muscles as they perform a given activity to see whether or not they have been successful in altering the state of those muscles.[14,16,17] It is similar in concept to the use of a very sophisticated mirror. When trying on clothing, one seeks a mirror for feedback to see how the clothing looks when it is on. When trying to alter the condition of a muscle, the EMG tracing provides the picture of what it looks like.

EMG AND MUSCLE STIMULATION

Technology offers many exciting opportunities for the clinical environment and the accomplishment of therapeutic treatment goals. One example of this is the potential benefits presented with the combination of EMG signals and a threshold triggering device for electrical stimulation. This pairing of two devices would allow the clinician to set a baseline for motor unit firing to trigger a muscle to contract. Patients with neurologic impairment who have difficulty eliciting an appropriate motor response may find this method of information discrimination beneficial. Patients with chronic hemiplegia represent one of the potential target populations for this type of device.[3]

SUMMARY

This chapter has dealt with a wide variety of electrical stimulation devices. It has covered the origins of many of the terms and names for pieces of electrical equipment that are currently in use in the clinical environment today. There are texts specifically devoted to each of the "boxes" discussed, and this chapter is not meant to be representative of all of the information currently available.

Biofeedback is a science all to itself with volumes published regarding the clinical applications for therapeutic goal accomplishment. The intent here is to provide the clinician with some baseline information. Further research into any of the topics will provide the reader with multiple perceptions, clinical research protocols, and potential applications for each modality.

Perhaps the most important aspect of this chapter is the example of the confusion that accompanies modalities when they are associated with such a wide variety of acronyms. There needs to be uniformity of terminology and a more concerted effort to maintain the integrity of terminology through documentation. In 10 years, a chapter such as this one should theoretically be unnecessary if all clinicians report their results based on the parameters utilized and treatment goals rather than on the type of box.

DISCUSSION QUESTIONS

1. What are the differences and similarities between IFC and TENS?

2. Why is it accurate to say that an FES unit is a TENS device, but a TENS device is not necessarily an FES unit?

3. What are the determining factors in whether or not an electrical stimulation device is selected for a given patient?

4. Of what significance would the availability of adjustable parameters be for NMES devices, or should they be preset without the potential for adjustment?

5. If your treatment goal for a patient included muscle stimulation for the prevention of muscle atrophy, how would you select the most appropriate stimulator from the following list of stimulators? TENS, NMES, IFC, FES, Russian stimulator. What would you need to know about the devices?

6. Describe in terminology that a patient would understand, the effects of interference current.

7. What are the potential benefits of the two described types of IFC?

Appendix: Electrical Stimulation Devices

The following companies have contributed materials for the preparation of this chapter. Their participation is greatly appreciated, and the reader is encouraged to seek out this type of information to make decisions regarding devices for use in their practice of clinical environment.

Manufacturer Operations Manuals and/or Product Specification Sheets

Chattanooga Group Inc.   615-870-2281
    4717 Adams Road
    PO Box 489
    Hixson, TN 37343-0489

Dynatronics   800-874-6251
    7030 Park Centre Drive
    Salt Lake City, UT 84121

Electro-Med Health Industries   305-892-2866
    11601 Biscayne Blvd. Suite 200-A
    North Miami, FL 33181-3151

Empi, Inc.   612-636-6600
    1275 Grey Fox Road
    St. Paul, MN 55112-6989

Mettler Electronics Corp.   714-533-2221
    1333 So. Claudina Street
    Anaheim, CA 92805

PTI   800-255-3554
    P.O. Box 19005
    Topeka, KS 66619-0005

Rich-Mar Corp.   800-762-4665
    PO Box 879
    Inola, OK 74036

REFERENCES

1. Benton, LA, et al: Functional Electrical Stimulation—A Practical Clinical Guide, ed 2. Rancho Los Amigos Rehabilitation Engineering Center, Downey California, 1981, pp 1–10.

2. Mannheimer, JS and Lampe, GN: Clinical Transcutaneous Electrical Nerve Stimulation. FA Davis, Philadelphia, 1984.

3. Kraft, GH, Fitts, SS, and Hammond, MC: Techniques to improve function of the arm and hand in chronic hemiplegia. Arch Phys Med Rehabil 73:220, 1992.

4. Bogataj, U, et al: Restoration of gait during two to three weeks of therapy with multi-channel electrical stimulation. Phys Ther 69:319, 1989.

5. Ferguson, ACB and Granat, MH: Evaluation of functional electrical stimulation for an incomplete spinal cord injured patient. Physiotherapy 78:253, 1992.

6. Twist, DJ: Acrocyanosis in a spinal cord injured patient—effects of computer-controlled neuromuscular electrical stimulation: A case report. Phys Ther 70:45, 1990.

7. Mendel, FC, Wylegala, JA, and Fish, DR: Influence of high voltage pulsed current on edema formation following impact injury in rats. Phys Ther 72/9:668, 1992.

8. Mendel, FC, et al: High voltage pulsed current using surface electrodes: Effect on acute ankle edema formation after hyperflexion injury in frogs. J Orthop Sports Phys Ther 16:140, 1992.

9. Fish, DR, Mendel, FC, and Gottstein-Yerke, LM: Effect of anodal high voltage pulsed current on edema formation in frog hind limbs. Phys Ther 71:724, 1991.

10. Fitzgerald, GK and Newsome, D: Treatment of a large infected thoracic spine wound using high voltage pulsed monophasic current: Phys Ther 73:355, 1993.

11. Deller, AG: Physical principles of interferential therapy. In Savage, B (ed): Interferential Therapy. Faber and Faber, Boston, 1984, p 15.

12. Low, J and Reed, A: Electrotherapy Explained, Principles and Practice. Butterworth Heinemann, London, 1992, pp 84–85.

13. Portney, L: Electromyography and nerve conduction velocity tests. In O'Sullvan, SB and Schmitz TJ (eds): Physical Rehabilitation: Assessment and Treatment, ed 2. FA Davis, Philadelphia, 1988, pp 159–190.

14. Headley, B: EMG and postural dysfunction. Clin Manag 10:14 1990.

15. Krebs, DE: Biofeedback. In O'Sullivan, SB and Schmitz, TJ (eds): Physical Rehabilitation: Assessment and Treatment, ed 2. FA Davis, Philadelphia, 1988, pp 629–645.

16. Headley, B: EMG and low back pain. Clin Manag 10:18, 1990.

17. Headley, B: EMG and myofascial pain. Clin Manag 10:43, 1990.

SUGGESTED READINGS

Report by the Electrophysiology Standards Committee of the Section on Clinical Electrophysiology of the American Physical Therapy Association: Electrotherapeutic Terminology in Physical Therapy. Published by the Section on Clinical Electrophysiology and the American Physical Therapy Association. 1990.

De Domenico G: Interferential Stimulation: A Monograph. Chattanooga Group Inc., 1988.

Nikolova L: Treatment with Interferential Current. Churchill Livingstone Publishers, New York, 1987.

Savage, B: Interferential Therapy. Faber & Faber Publishers, Boston, 1984.

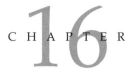

Electrodes: Materials, Care, and Placement Sites for the Accomplishment of Therapeutic Treatment Goals

Barbara J. Behrens, BS, PTA
Wayne Smith, PT

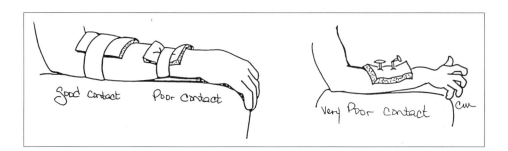

CHAPTER OBJECTIVES

- Describe the components and care of the electrode interface.
- Discuss the treatment goals potentially accomplished with electrical stimulation.
- Outline the process of electrode selection and placement.
- Discuss the similarities and differences in types of electrode placement sites.
- Outline the importance of careful placement selection to accomplish a treatment goal.

CHAPTER OUTLINE

Clinical electrical stimulation involves the passing of current through the skin via electrodes. An electrode is used to either deliver electric current or record electrical activity of muscle. The delivery of current is accomplished through a system of electrically conductive elements. This includes the lead wire, the electrode, a conductive substance referred to as the electrode interface, and the patient. Each of these components will affect the amount of electrical charge delivered to the patient. The influence of each of the components will either facilitate the flow of current, if the resistance is low, or inhibit the flow of current if the resistance within the system is too high. Refer to Chapter 10 for a review of resistance and current flow.

Electrodes represent the "instrument" for current delivery from an electrical stimulation generator. Leads connect the electrodes to the stimulator. Each lead has both a jack and a pin to interconnect the electrode to the lead and the lead to the stimulator. Each of these components will be discussed in terms of the structures themselves, their possible configurations, and appropriate handling techniques.

Electrodes vary in shape, size, and flexibility, to fit the needs of the therapeutic application of the electrical current to the patient. An electrode is made of an electrically conductive material that is housed in a nonelectrically conductive material. The purpose of the housing material is to inhibit the delivery of electrical energy to either the patient or the clinician if either should touch the back of the electrode.

TYPES OF ELECTRODES

METAL PLATE ELECTRODES

Electrodes serve as an interface between the stimulation unit and biologic tissues. In order to achieve this, the conductivity of the electrode must be given consideration. Early electrodes were composed of metals plates such as tin, steel, aluminum, and zinc, which are good electrical conductors for therapeutic stimulation. The electrode was usually contained within a rubber casing with only one surface exposed to the patient. The interface between the metal electrode and skin was accomplished through a sponge or felt pad moistened with water. This served to reduce the skin–electrode impedance, since water is a good conductor of electricity. Distilled water should not be used; it contains no free ions, and therefore would not be electrically conductive (Fig. 16-1).

Disadvantages of metal plate electrode systems include:

1. Metal plates may not be flexible enough to maintain adequate contact with certain body parts.
2. These electrodes may be difficult to secure comfortably to the patient.
3. There are few sizes of these electrodes, making specific treatment goals for smaller treatment areas difficult to accomplish.

CARBON-IMPREGNATED RUBBER ELECTRODES

Electrodes composed of rubber, silicon, and polymer have mostly replaced the older metal plate electrodes. Carbon-impregnated silicon rubber electrodes are commonly utilized in many clinics. They are backed with a nonconductive material to prevent unintentional current delivery. These electrodes are available in many shapes and sizes, and they can be trimmed or fitted to different locations of the body (Fig. 16–2).

Carbon-impregnated silicon rubber electrodes should be replaced when necessary. They degrade over time, resulting in nonuniformity of current delivery, or the presence of "hot spots." Hot spots represent those areas of the electrode that continue to maintain their conductivity while other areas of the surface no longer conduct electrical energy. The result is analogous to ten cars trying to merge onto an uncrowded highway versus those same ten cars trying to merge onto a crowded highway. The ten cars will still get on the highway, but if time was a factor, the amount of resistance that they would face in meeting their goal would be significantly higher when the traffic was heavy, or the window to merge was

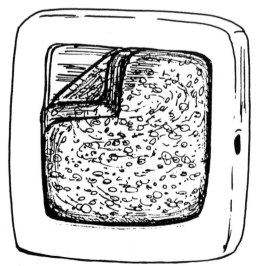

Figure 16–1. Metal plate electrode. The metal surface of the electrode is covered by a sponge that would be soaked in water. The left-hand corner of the sponge is folded back to reveal the metal plate. The electrode is encased in a nonelectrically conductive rubber cover.

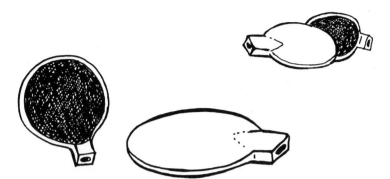

Figure 16–2. Several sizes of carbon-impregnated rubber electrodes. The dark surface is the conductive surface that would be covered with either a wet sponge or electrically conductive medium, and then placed on the skin. The lighter-colored back of the electrode is nonelectrically conductive so that it can be easily handled.

smaller. Hot spots represent an increase in current concentration or current density within the electrode area, which could result in skin irritation. Patients who complain that they feel a biting or stinging sensation when receiving therapeutic current, are probably describing an electrode with uneven conductivity. It is time to replace the electrode, or at least have it checked with an ohmmeter for resistance to determine whether or not use of the electrode should be continued. Carbon rubber electrodes should be rinsed off and dried after each use. Replace these electrodes every twelve months to ensure good conductivity.

SELF-ADHERING SINGLE-USE OR REUSABLE ELECTRODES

Self-adhering single-use or reusable electrodes are composed of other flexible conductors such as foil or metal mesh, conductive Karaya, or synthetic gel layered with an adhesive surface. The advantage of these electrodes is convenience of application. No strapping or taping is necessary to secure the electrodes to the patient.

Clinicians should carefully read the manufacturer's suggestions before utilizing these electrodes. Because of the potential for cross-contamination, use of a package of electrodes for each patient is prudent. The package can be marked with the patient's name and identification number so that they will only be utilized for a given patient.

CONSIDERATIONS FOR ELECTRODE SELECTION

There are advantages and disadvantages with each type of electrode, including self-adhering electrodes. Often, the impedance of these electrodes is significantly higher than other electrode systems, resulting in reductions in potential current outputs of the stimulation device.[1] These limitations may make it difficult or impossible to accomplish the desired clinical goal with a given stimulator, if the output of the stimulator is not sufficient to overcome the resistance of the electrodes.

The resistance of the electrode, which is listed in ohms, should be as low as possible when significant motor levels of stimulation are required. If the desired

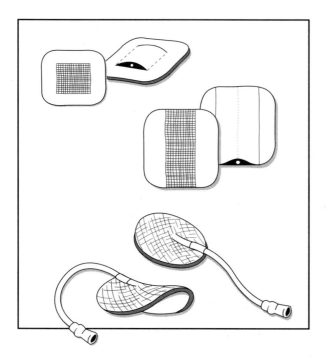

Figure 16–3. Several different sizes of self-adhering electrodes that have a mesh of electrically conductive material woven into them. This illustration depicts other self-adhering electrodes with smaller conductive surface areas and also illustrates the flexibility of the mesh electrodes. The mesh electrodes easily conform to irregular body surfaces.

effect is a comfortable nonmotor level of stimulation, the impedance value of the electrodes is not as critical to success. If the impedance value of the electrodes is high, then the stimulator will need to overcome that value before the current is delivered to the patient. This may result in higher output levels of stimulation, which may be uncomfortable to the patient. The package of the electrodes may indicate the ohms of resistance, which will be lower with larger electrodes and higher with smaller electrodes.

The method of current delivery into the electrode will also impact the uniformity of the current delivery from the electrode. Some self-adhering electrodes have a metal wire than inserts into the center of a conductive-adhesive or adherent surface. The current delivery at the point of attachment of the wire to the surface will be relatively higher than the current delivery to the periphery of that electrode. This may result in hot spots. Optimally, the conductive surface of the electrode will have "uniform" conductivity. This potential for uniformity of conductivity is enhanced through foil or mesh surfaces within the electrode to spread out the delivered current (Fig. 16–3).

ELECTRODE SIZE AND CURRENT DENSITY

Current density describes the amount of current concentrated under an electrode. It is a measure of the quantity of charged ions moving through a specific cross-sectional area of body tissue.

Electrode surface area is inversely related to total current flow. The same total current flow passing through large and small electrodes would result in lower current density at the larger electrode. The total current would be distributed over a larger surface area. Conversely, the smaller electrode would be delivering a high-current density because of its smaller surface area. Therapeutic electrical stimulation involves the active or stimulating electrode, the one that exhibits the greater current density, and the dispersive or inactive electrode, which delivers less current density. Electrodes should be appropriately sized for the desired result. If, for example, the treatment goal involved a motor response of one of the forearm muscles, an electrode that was 3 inches in diameter would produce a great amount of "overflow" of current into the surrounding muscles. It would be more appropriate to utilize a small electrode that more closely approximates the size of the target tissue, such as a 1½-inch diameter electrode. The reverse is also true. If the treatment goal involved a tetanic contraction of the rectus femoris, then the electrode size that would afford the greatest comfort would probably be 3 inches in diameter or greater. Smaller electrodes may provide too great a current density, but not enough current flow to elicit a tetanic contraction (Fig. 16–4).

COUPLING MEDIA AND ATTACHMENT

Surface-stimulating electrodes require the use of a coupling medium. This medium can be water via soaked sponges, Karaya gum, or electrically conductive gel. The coupling medium reduces the impedance at the interface between the electrode and the skin. This results in less current amplitude needed to produce the desired effects of stimulation.[2,3]

The pliability of the electrode to conform to the body part is necessary. Rigid metal electrodes do not conform well to certain anatomic regions. Poor conformity can also result in hot-spot delivery of the electrical energy. In this case the hot spot is a factor of not having all of the conductive surface of the electrode in contact with the patient's skin. Patient responses indicative of this would be noticeable after several minutes of treatment: the patient moved, they now feel a prickling sensation (hot spot), and they are afraid to move back to the original position. To remedy this, the concentration of the energy will diminish if the patient returns to the original position, since the uniformity of the contact between the electrode and the

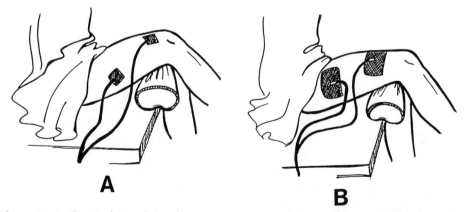

Figure 16–4. Electrical stimulation for a motor response of the quadriceps. *(A)* The electrodes are too small for the size of the muscle to be stimulated. The current density of these electrodes would be too high for enough stimulation to cause a motor response. *(B)* The electrodes are more appropriately matched to the size of the target tissue of the quadriceps.

patient will have been restored. It is often difficult to convince a patient that if they lean back on the electrode that is causing the prickling sensation, that the degree of prickling will subside. Explanations for the phenomenon can reduce the patient's anxiety regarding the electrical stimulation and potentially offset increased muscle guarding as a result of that fear.

Caution should be exercised to make sure that the electrode interface has not dried out during the treatment. If the surface has in fact dried out during the course of the treatment, repositioning the patient will not remedy their complaint. Rehydration of the electrode may. This is yet another reason to check on a patient after treatment with electrical stimulation has been initiated.

The electrode should conform to the anatomic region to obtain optimal stimulation. Electrode attachment methods to maximize surface contact include the use of straps, tape, vacuum pumps, and self-adhesives.

STRAPS OR TAPE FOR THE ATTACHMENT OF ELECTRODES

Straps have been commercially manufactured to be easy to use, inexpensive, and versatile. Many of the commercially available straps have rubber-backed stretch "eyed" surfaces, with one end of the reversed side of the strap covered with "hooks." These straps should be utilized to secure either the carbon-impregnated rubber electrodes or the metal-plate electrodes. Proper utilization involves strapping circumferentially around the limb with enough pressure to maintain good uniform contact between the electrode and the patient's skin. The pressure should be centered so that the electrode remains flat against the surface of the skin. Once the strap is secured, it should be checked for positioning that may have changed slightly once the strap has been stretched. Straps come in a variety of lengths for different areas of the body and different strapping configurations (Fig. 16–5).

Tape can also be utilized to attach electrodes to the patient and has several distinct disadvantages. For example, it can be costly and patients may be allergic to the adhesive. If the electrodes are not properly cleaned after use, the adhesive may collect on the conductive surface of the electrode. This decreases both the conductive surface area and increases the potential for skin irritation.

VACUUM ELECTRODE ATTACHMENT SYSTEMS

Vacuum pump systems for electrode attachment utilize suction cups that are placed over the sponge and metal-plate electrodes. Air is pumped through the system so that a suction force is created to hold the electrode tight to the skin surface. Pulsed suction may increase the sensory stimulation of the treatment, and may allow a better transport of tissue fluids via the increase in local circulation that is visible following removal of the suction electrodes.[4,5] The skin may appear to have a slight erythema following the removal of the suction electrodes. If the erythema persists, then the level of the pressure may have been too high. Suction pumps have variable pressure settings and pulsed suction options, so that the suction is more tolerable to the patient (Fig. 16–6).

This form of attachment lends itself well to irregular surfaces that would be difficult to strap electrodes to, but has some disadvantages as well. Vacuum pumps conduct the electrical stimulation through the water-soaked sponges

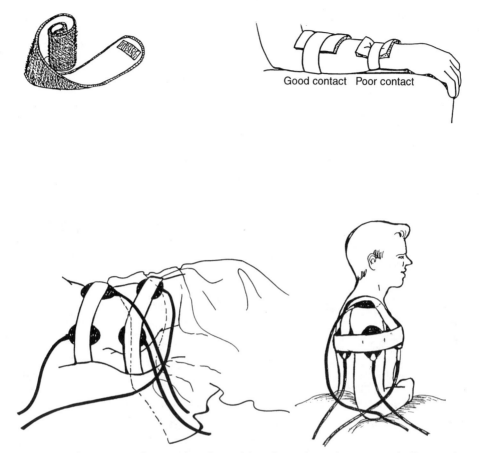

Figure 16–5. The straps used to attach carbon rubber electrodes with sponges. The forearm has an example of good contact of the electrode. Poor contact between the electrode and the skin surface would result in an uneven distribution of the current and would potentially be uncomfortable for a patient. Uses for different-length straps are also illustrated for a shoulder and a hip.

through hollow metal leads. Water may collect in the leads themselves, resulting in internal corrosion of the leads and decreased conductivity of the leads. Suction cups may cause damage to superficial blood vessels of persons who bruise easily.

LEADS

Leads provide a conductive path for current flow. Electrical stimulators will always have a pair of leads emerging from them. They are the intermediary between the generator and electrodes. The electrodes are connected to the electrical stimulation generator by lead wires. A lead wire has several parts: the point of exit from the stimulator, the wire itself, and the point of attachment to the electrode, known as the tip. The point of exit is referred to as the "jack," which if it contains two leads is referred to as a "stereo jack".

The jack plugs into the stimulator, and is typically encased in hard plastic.

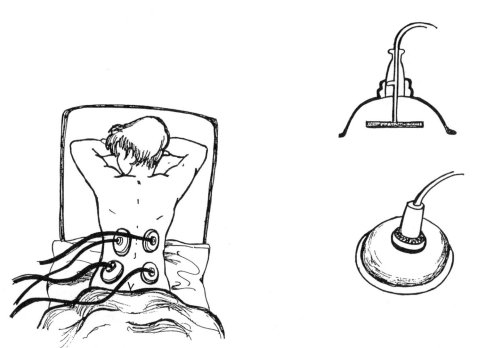

Figure 16–6. Vacuum pump electrodes. The metal plate of the electrode is covered by a sponge that fits inside of the rubber suction cup. A lower back is set up with the suction electrodes. The lead wires for a suction system need to carry airflow, electrical current, and the water that will be pulled through the hoses and leads from the wet sponges. There are many points in this system that have potential for corrosion that would raise the resistance of the leads to the flow of the current.

The jack is the portion of the lead that is meant to be handled, and it is constructed to maintain its integrity even with multiple plugging and unplugging of the lead into the stimulator. In order for the lead to be able to deliver electrical energy, the jack must be securely plugged into the stimulator so that there is no metal showing between the jack and its plug or receptacle. Each lead wire will usually have two electrodes attached to it by a metal tip that inserts into the electrode. There are different types of electrode–lead wire configurations, such as the pin tip lead and the banana tip lead, which are attempts to standardize the lead electrode interface and ease the attachment of the electrode to the lead for the clinician (Fig. 16–7). Regardless of the type of tip, it is prone to corrosion and should be cleaned regularly. Scheduled maintenance of the tips should prevent potential problems with current delivery. Steel wool can be utilized to clean a tip. Gentle rubbing with the steel wool should restore the shiny metal surface of the tip.

The tip can only assist in the delivery of electrical energy if it is in contact with the conductive surface of the electrode. There is a small housing that surrounds the tip opening within every electrode. The tip must be pushed as far as possible into the opening so that it does come in contact with the conductive surface of the electrode. There should be no metal showing between the plastic-coated pin housing and the electrode. Failure to insert the electrode properly will

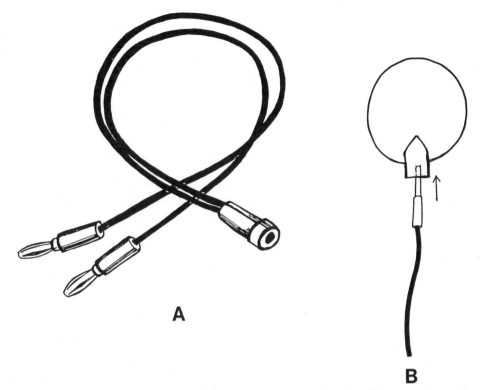

A

B

Figure 16–7. *(A)* "Banana" tip. *(B)* "Pin" tip. Banana tips are adjustable. If the tip no longer fits tightly in an electrode, then the sides of the tip may be spread apart slightly. The pin tip is a smaller diameter than the banana tip. In the illustration, the tip must be fully inserted into the electrode so that the metal pin tip touches the conductive surface of the electrode. Failure to insert the pin into the electrode fully will result in poor current delivery to the electrode.

result in poor clinical results because current cannot be delivered to the patient (Fig. 16–7).

Many stimulators have multiple lead wires that have one stereo jack with two leads and pins for two electrodes. If the desired result is to cover a larger area and there are not any additional channels of electrodes available, then each lead may be "split" through the use of a bifurcator. A bifurcator is an attachment that fits on the pin of the lead wire and has two smaller leads coming off of it. Use of a bifurcator will split the output from that lead into the two electrodes attached to it. It will therefore decrease the total amount of current flow through each independent electrode. It represents the opposite of a hot spot. If a patient perceives too much sensation underneath one of the electrodes from a channel, then either the size of the electrode can be increased or a bifurcator can be used, which would then split the output delivered to that electrode.

Neither lead should be considered a "ground," but part of the electrical circuit. Each stimulation device will have its own set of peculiarities with respect to the management of leads. Examples of the channel setups and lead management can be found in Table 16–1. Potential causes and remedies for patient complaints of prickling or itching sensations underneath the electrodes are listed in Table 16–2.

Table 16–1 **Examples of Electrode and Channel Configurations for Different Types of Stimulators**

Portable stimulators for home use	Pair of single leads for each channel for a total of four electrodes, two channels
Clinical models	Stereo jack leads each with two tips for electrodes. May have one, two, four, or more channels, each with two electrodes
High-voltage pulsed-current generators	Commonly single channel stimulators that have one large electrode (the dispersive) from one lead wire and a pair of leads from the stimulator to two electrodes. The system is a single-channel system where the terminal end of one of the leads was bifurcated within the stimulator. The result is a generator with three electrodes. There are two smaller electrodes from one lead, and the dispersive from a single lead wire. The dispersive electrode surface area is much larger than the surface area of the other two electrodes combined. This size differential will result in sensation being perceived underneath the smaller electrodes, and no sensation being perceived underneath the larger electrode. The dispersive is usually applied proximal to the treatment area covering a large soft tissue area capable of maintaining good uniform contact with the electrode.

TRANSCUTANEOUS AND PERCUTANEOUS ELECTRODES

Electrodes that are applied to the surface of the skin are termed *transcutaneous electrodes*. Transcutaneous refers to the delivery of electrical energy or recording of electrical energy across the skin. *Percutaneous electrodes* are inserted into the skin. Percutneous electrodes are commonly utilized for invasive EMG procedures, or they may also be utilized for the application of electrical stimulation for patients

Table 16–2 **Itching or Prickling Sensations Under an Electrode, Possible Problems and Remedies**

1. The patient might have moved, so that the electrodes are no longer in full contact with the entire surface of the electrode.
2. The electrode interface may have dried out, decreasing the conductive surface area of the electrode.
3. The electrode may have worn out, resulting in multiple hot spots caused by increased levels of resistance over large areas of its surface. Skin oils can collect on the surface and dry out the interface.

who are paraparetic or quadriparetic. Of the two types of electrodes, transcutaneous electrodes are more common in therapeutic delivery of electrical stimulation.

TERMINOLOGY FOR CONFIGURATIONS OF ELECTRODE SETUPS

Electrodes can be oriented in monopolar, bipolar, and quadripolar manner.[6–9] Placement across body tissues can be longitudinal, such as when stimulating quadriceps muscles of the thigh to facilitate a stronger contraction, or they may be criss-crossed, as when administering electrical stimulation treatment for pain management.

MONOPOLAR APPLICATION OF ELECTRODES

The monopolar technique involves a single electrode from a channel, usually smaller in size, placed over the target area called the *active electrode.* The greatest stimulation perception will be in the target tissue area. The larger dispersive electrode or second electrode is placed at a distance from the target electrode to complete the circuit. Its placement is usually over the nerve root supplying the target treatment area. The size differential between the electrodes ensures a greater current concentration in the treatment area[6–11] (Fig. 16–8).

BIPOLAR ELECTRODE SETUP

The bipolar electrode technique requires two electrodes from one channel within the target treatment area. They are usually of equal dimension and shape.[7,11] Current flow through tissue is usually confined to the problem area. When using the bipolar placement, the patient will experience an excitatory response and/or sensation under both electrodes.[8,9] One can be smaller if the intention is a more effective activation of excitable tissues.[7–9,11] This would be an appropriate electrode setup for eliciting a motor response. One of the electrodes will be placed over the motor point, and the other electrode, which may be slightly larger, will be placed somewhere else over the muscle belly. Occasionally a clinician may bifurcate the leads when a situation requires a larger target area, such as dealing with a combination of back and lower extremity radicular pain[12] (Fig. 16–8). Bipolar techniques are well suited for stimulation of a large muscle.[6–10] Monopolar techniques are better suited for stimulation over a trigger point or a wound.[7,9]

QUADRIPOLAR ELECTRODE PLACEMENT

The quadripolar method of electrode application involves electrodes from two or more channels, each lead with two electrodes. The electrodes can be positioned in a variety of configurations. Quadripolar electrode placement occurs with an interferential device; however, it also occurs when there are four electrodes within the treatment area, regardless of the type of stimulator utilized to deliver the current.

Quadripolar electrode setups are often utilized to deliver the electrical stimulation to a larger area, for example, pain management techniques that rely on sensory stimulation of larger fibers for analgesia.

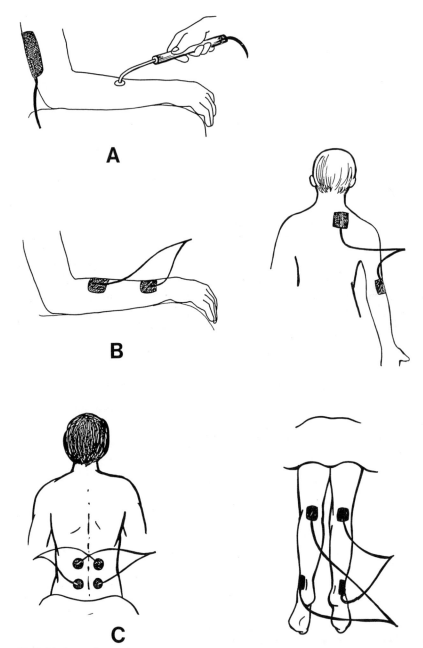

Figure 16–8. Various electrode setups. *(A)* Monopolar electrode placement setups with only one electrode from the channel in the target of treatment area. *(B)* A bipolar electrode setup, with both electrodes from the same channel in the target or treatment area. *(C)* A quadripolar treatment setup in the low back and a dual bipolar setup for the lower extremity.

CARE OF ELECTRODES

Since electrodes represent the point of delivery of therapeutic electrical stimulation, the proper care for and cleansing of electrodes is essential. The impedance of carbon-impregnated silicon rubber electrodes can be significantly altered if the surface is allowed to dry or cake with gel. Carbon-impregnated silicon rubber electrodes can easily be cleaned in mild soap and warm water to remove gels. Cracking or "polished" appearance of the electrode surface may indicate that the surface is no longer uniformly conductive. This may result in the formation of spots of high current density on the electrode and poor current delivery. Harsh disinfectants can damage both carbon rubber and metal electrodes. Excessive alcohol use can cause carbon rubber electrodes to lose conductivity. An early sign of electrode wear is a stinging sensation under the electrodes. If there are cracks or uneven surfaces, the electrodes may need to be replaced.

If not cleaned on a regular basis, sponges soaked with water may be a source of potential cross-contamination from patient to patient. Germicidal soaps can be utilized to rinse through the electrodes prior to their application on a patient. Soap residue must be removed because soap acts as an insulator to the passage of electrical energy.

ELECTRODE PLACEMENT GUIDELINES

Electrical stimulation can be utilized to accomplish a variety of therapeutic goals. These goals revolve around the patient's specific response to the electrical stimulation, sensory "tingling" analgesia, or a motor response.

RATIONALE FOR ELECTRODE PLACEMENT SITES

Successful use of electrical stimulation is dependent upon several components, including appropriate selection of the stimulator, the electrodes, the parameters, and the placement of the electrodes. Each may ultimately contribute to the success or failure of the treatment. Selection of the device will be dependent upon the parameters necessary to accomplish the identified clinical goal (see Chapter 15). The electrodes and their interface with the patient are an important component of the success of the application of electrical stimulation. Placement of the electrodes is equally important.

Electricity follows the path of least resistance, so it is advantageous to know low resistance areas along the surface of the skin. Sites for electrode placement may be referred to as motor points, trigger points, and acupuncture points.

Motor Points

Motor points are the anatomic location where the motor nerve enters the muscle. It is also referred to as the myoneural junction. At the location of the motor point, the amount of electrical current necessary to elicit a motor response from a muscle will be less than for other areas along the muscle. These areas have a decreased resistance to the flow of current and are located in the center of the muscle belly. Motor point maps serve as a reference tools for specific point locations for different muscle groups.

Whenever the desired clinical response is to elicit a muscle contraction, motor points should be selected for use as electrode placement sites. If a motor response is the desired response, frequency, pulse duration, and intensity settings must also be appropriate. A frequency and pulse duration sufficient to produce a twitch or a tetanic contraction must be selected. Failure to look at each parameter and select the appropriate sites will result in ineffective treatment. Intensity must be high enough to elicit a tetanic contraction. Each of the parameters is important.

Trigger Points

Trigger points are those areas that exhibit hypersensitivity to both pressure and electrical stimulation. They cause pain to radiate away from the site with palpation.[13,14] The patterns of the radiating pain have been mapped out for the purpose of assisting clinicians in the location of the possible soft tissue component to the referred pain pattern (Fig. 16–9). These points may fall over the muscle belly or connective tissue. Trigger points can be located with an ohmmeter, an instrument utilized to measure resistance levels. Trigger points have a decreased resistance to the flow of electricity.

Trigger points may or may not be located directly over motor points, but there is a high degree of correlation among the points being found at exactly the same site.[15] Selection of a trigger point for electrical stimulation would tend to yield better results than not selecting one, since these points do represent areas of decreased resistance. If palpation of a point elicits referred pain, it is a good place to try as an electrode placement site. If the desired result is a motor response and the trigger point happens to be a motor point also, then it may be a better site than other options in the area. If, however, the trigger point is located over connective tissue and is not also a motor point, then a treatment goal related to motor responses would not be successful if the trigger point was utilized.

Acupuncture Points

Acupuncture points represent another type of point that has been described for use with electrical stimulation devices. These points are located over the entire surface of the body and have been mapped out for centuries. Acupuncture points may lie over muscle, fascia, or connective tissue. They too are electrically active, exhibiting a decreased resistance to the flow of electrical energy.[16]

The locations of acupuncture points have been identified with an unusual form of reference, the meridian. There are twelve paired meridians and two unpaired meridians of acupuncture points on the human body. Acupuncture principles date back thousands of years into Chinese history, and the points are but a small portion of the principles of acupuncture as they relate to Chinese culture and medicine. The meridian names do, however, serve as a reference point for ease of locating the points, just as street names serve as a point of reference in finding an address. There may or may not be any relationship between stimulating a given point and finding a response in its namesake organ. The same phenomenon exists with the names of streets; Vine Street in Philadelphia is not now known for having vines, but it is an identifiable location. Points are also numbered along a meridian, which further serves as an "address" along the "street." Once the general locations of the meridians are known, the meridian naming system serves as an efficient way of referring to a specific point. For example, the large intestine (LI) meridian is located on the posterolateral aspect of the upper extremity, with numbering starting in the hand. It is easier to refer to LI 4 than to say "in the middle of the web space of the back of the hand, with the thumb and index finger outstretched."

Acupuncture Point Location: "The Body Inch." A body inch is the measure of the distance across the widest part of the thumb or the distance between the two inter-

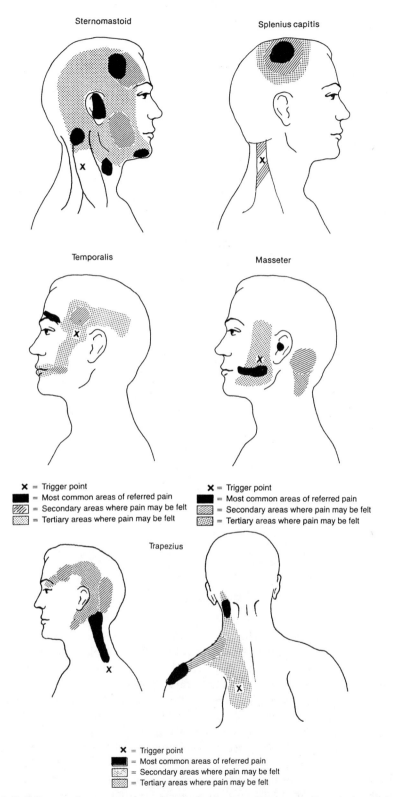

Figure 16–9. Trigger points cause the referral of pain to a distal area. Knowledge of the pattern is helpful for determining the origin of the discomfort. (*From Rothstein, JM, Roy, SH, and Wolf, SL: The Rehabilitation Specialist's Handbook. FA Davis, Philadelphia, 1991, pp 171–174, with permission.*)

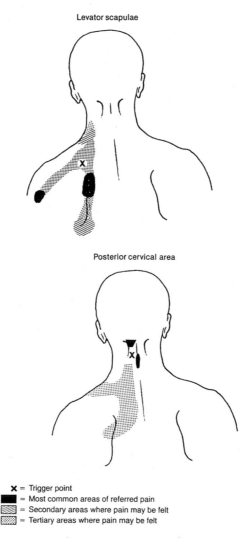

Levator scapulae

Posterior cervical area

X = Trigger point
█ = Most common areas of referred pain
▨ = Secondary areas where pain may be felt
▨ = Tertiary areas where pain may be felt

Figure 16–9. Continued

phalangeal creases of the long finger, with the IP and DIP joints flexed.[17] The width of the extended four fingers of the hand is known as 3 inches. Acupuncture point locations are described in terms of body inches so that they can be readily located based on the individual, not on an arbitrary system of measure, such as a ruler. Every individual has his or her own body inch, which is consistent for his or her body. For example, an individual who is 6 feet tall will have significantly different body inches than an individual who is 4 feet tall (Fig. 16–10).

Clinicians who try to identify acupuncture point locations on their patients will first need to compare their body inch to that of the patient. This is easily done by comparing the size of the hands. If your body inch is larger than the patient's, then point locations will be found by subtracting distance from the description. Acupuncture points are often sensitive to palpation, so they are distinctly identifiable with either palpation or an ohmmeter.

The system of naming the points initially appears cumbersome to clinicians

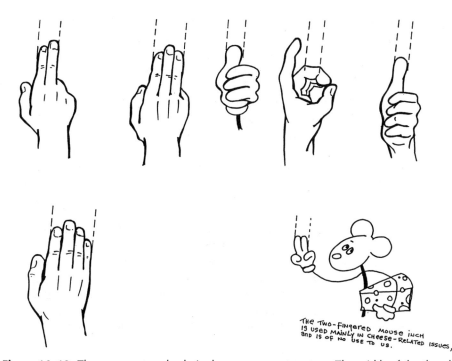

Figure 16–10. The acupuncture body inch measurement system. The width of the thumb is equal to 1 body inch. The width of the hand is equal to 3 body inches. The width of the first two fingers is 1½ body inches.

until the terminology is utilized regularly. The point location description system is enhanced by the palpation skills and knowledge of surface anatomy of the clinician.

Among the three types of points mentioned, that is, acupuncture, motor, and trigger points, there is a high degree of correlation.[15] This is mapped out in the following charts where acupuncture points are indicated by a small triangle, motor points are indicated with a small circle, and trigger points are identified by a small square. Many of the points on the charts are depicted by all three marks in exactly the same location.

Electrode placement sites for achieving sensory analgesia rely on the location of the discomfort and the anatomic cause for the discomfort. Electrical stimulation for the relief of pain usually involves the placement of electrodes around the area of pain. Selection of acupuncture points for these electrodes will provide an easier path for the current to enter the body. If the desired response from the stimulation is *not* a motor response, then acupuncture points that are *not* motor points should be selected. If the desired response from the electrical stimulation is a motor response, then acupuncture points that are motor points should be selected.

OPTIMAL STIMULATION SITES

Optimal stimulation sites for electrodes are those sites that will facilitate goal accomplishment. The most basic goal in the utilization of electrical stimulation is to have the electrical stimulation actually interface into the patient. If there is too much resistance at the skin, then the current will not be able to produce a favorable result simply because it could not reach the target tissue. Acupuncture points, trigger points, and motor points all represent electrically active and identifiable points that would not impede the flow of current into the body, but rather enhance the potential current flow into the body. It must then be determined if treatment goals involve a motor response.

Motor responses are achieved with motor points, with the other electrode from the channel either distally placed on the desired muscle (bipolar setup) or at the segmental level that innervates the muscle paraspinally (monopolar setup). If the desired response to the electrical stimulation is a diffuse sensory analgesia, then it is not necessary to use motor points. Acupuncture points would afford the greatest availability of sites for placement, with the assurance that there would be a greater potential for the current to enter the body. Diffuse sensory analgesia can be readily accomplished through the use of two channels of electrodes, for a total of four electrodes. These two channels can be in a criss-cross setup, which will promote an increase in sensation throughout the area, with less discrimination of actual location of the electrodes, as long as the electrodes surround the painful region. This quadrapolar setup will also be enhanced through the use of acupuncture points. Consult a chart and select points that fall just outside of the painful region, which can be acupuncture or trigger points. Motor points should only be used if the sensory analgesia is to be accomplished via a motor response.

HOW MANY CHANNELS OF ELECTRODES SHOULD BE USED?

Sensory analgesia via electrical stimulation was discussed in Chapter 14. In order for the level of stimulation to produce this sensory analgesia throughout the painful area, the entire painful area must be included within the stimulation field. If discomfort is well localized to a discrete area, then a single channel of electrodes may be adequate. If, however, the area of discomfort is not well localized, then two or more channels may be indicated.

SENSORY STIMULATION FOR ANALGESIA

A normal response to immediate trauma would be to rub the area. The act of rubbing would provide sensory stimulation in much the same way that this form of electrical stimulation would. You would rub the entire area at the site of the injury to provide as much sensory stimulation as possible to decrease the discomfort. The same principles for location and quantity would be true when utilizing a stimulator for sensory analgesia. The stimulation should occur throughout the injury site, wherever pain is perceived, and it should encompass the entire area to provide as much sensation as possible.[18] This may include criss-cross setups above and below the painful region, but most importantly, surrounding it.

This form of stimulation for pain management is often the first mode selected since it is typically well tolerated by patients, and if it is successful in accomplishing pain reduction, it tends to do so relatively quickly once the sensation is perceived throughout the injured area.[19]

MOTOR-LEVEL STIMULATION FOR ANALGESIA

Pain reduction via motor-level stimulation requires that there be visible motor responses in the treatment area. Since the desired response is a motor response, then motor points should be utilized, and the intensity should be strong enough to elicit a visible muscle contraction. This form of stimulation is not tolerated as well by patients and is therefore not the first choice for an acutely painful condition. It is also a mode of stimulation that may utilize distally related areas for central pain management. An example of this would be the setup of the electrodes for a patient who had been referred for therapy to help reduce his or her level of discomfort from a chronic low-back pain syndrome with radiating sciatic pain. Protocols for electrical stimulation for this type of patient would involve electrode placement at the distal extent of the sciatic nerve, and the desired response would be muscle twitching of the gastroc-soleus muscle group. The necessary visible muscle twitching is not tolerated well in the local region of the lower back, but it tends to be reasonably comfortable when administered to the more distally related muscle groups.[18,19]

Since the level of stimulation is not described as a comfortable tingling but rather a visible muscle twitching, and because the stimulation needs to provide a motor response, motor-level stimulation tends to be tolerated better by patients if the stimulation takes place in areas that are segmentally related but distal to the painful area. Myotomes represent anatomic mappings of muscles that are innervated by specific spinal nerve roots.[20] Correlation of the segmental level of discomfort with the anatomic myotomes for electrode placement sites provides the solution for pain management for some patients.

NOXIOUS STIMULATION FOR ANALGESIA (MOTOR AND NONMOTOR)

At first glance, noxious stimulation for the accomplishment of pain management may appear to be contradictory; however, it remains a viable alternative to more conventional forms of stimulation. Noxious stimulation involves the utilization of parameters that will selectively stimulate A-delta and C fibers, which are pain fibers. A motor response would be seen in conjunction with the noxious level of stimulation if the threshold for the motor fibers is exceeded before the threshold for the A-delta or C fiber is reached. Motor responses may also be seen in conjunction with point stimulation if the point being stimulated happens to be overlying the muscle belly and be a motor point. Refer to Chapters 2 and 11 for discussions of various fiber types and necessary minimal parameter requirements for their activation. Stimulation of these specific fiber types in locations that are once again distal or distant from the site of injury has been suggested to elicit the manufacture and release of endogenous opiates into the bloodstream.[21]

Noxious-level stimulation often utilizes a point locator system for identification of those areas along the surface of the skin that demonstrate a lower level of resistance to the passage of electrical energy than the surrounding tissue. One metal point is often one of the electrodes, and the other electrode from that channel (the dispersive) may be a modified electrode that is held in the palm of a hand. Both electrodes need to be in contact with the patient in order for the circuit to be complete.

EDEMA REDUCTION (MOTOR)

Edema, as discussed in Chapter 8, is an excessive amount of fluid within the body interstitial tissues. One mechanism for the reduction of edema is muscle contraction of the muscles in the edematous area. The pressure exerted on the lymphatic vessels may assist in the return of fluids and help decrease localized posttraumatic or chronic edema. This method is sometimes referred to as muscle pumping, and proper positioning and elevation of the limb will further assist in lymphatic return.

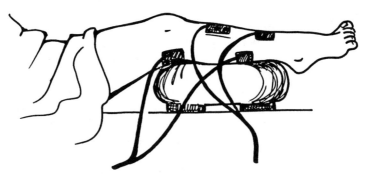

Figure 16–11. Electrode placement sites for edema reduction in the ankle via muscle pumping. One channel is set up on the gastrocnemius and the other channel is set up on the tibialis anterior. The channels are set to reciprocate with each other.

Muscle contraction in the surrounding muscle groups is the key to success with this form of stimulation. Motor points of the muscle that cross the involved area should be selected, and the intensity should be high enough to elicit a tetanic contraction of the muscles. Reciprocal stimulation of the agonist and then the antagonist for edema reduction of the ankle are illustrated in Figure 16–11.

MUSCLE ATROPHY AND MOTOR CONTROL (MOTOR)

Electrical stimulation for the prevention of muscle atrophy and the promotion of motor control was discussed in Chapter 12 and represents another potential utilization for electrical stimulation. Electrically eliciting a muscle contraction when volitional contraction control or strength is impaired is an exciting venue for the future of electrical stimulation. Electrode placement sites should incorporate bipolar setups on involved muscles, and intensity levels strong enough to elicit tetanic contractions.

Each of these stated treatment goals can be further categorized to indicate the potential mechanism of action as either a motor response to the electrical stimulation or a nonmotor response. Characterization of these outcomes into motor and nonmotor responses is helpful when determining the appropriate electrode placement sites and parameter requirements. Each goal that involves a muscle contraction either for a twitch response or a tetanic contraction would be considered a motor response. Each goal that is accomplished without a muscle contraction would be considered a nonmotor response.

Regardless of the mode of stimulation, the patient should be instructed in what constitutes a normal sensation response as well as an abormal sensation response to the treatment. This will help ensure that the patient is able to relax comfortably during the treatment and that he or she will seek assistance when needed.

SUMMARY

Electrode placement sites are based on the desired goals. Treatment parameters that require either a muscle twitch or tetanic contraction should employ motor points. A monopolar technique of stimulation would mean that one electrode would be placed over the motor point and the other electrode should be placed over an acupuncture point paraspinal to the segmental level of innervation of that muscle. A bipolar technique of stimulation would mean that one electrode would be placed over the motor point of the muscle, and the other electrode would be placed over a point distal to the motor point but still on the muscle being stimulated. Utilization of motor points does not guarantee that a motor response will occur. The response is intimately related to the electrical parameters as well as the placement sites. If a motor response is not desired, then motor points should not be utilized; acupunctures or trigger points should be used instead.

DISCUSSION QUESTIONS

1. Of what significance is the choice of electrodes for a given patient?

2. Of what significance is the choice of electrode placement sites, and why would it matter where electrodes are placed?

3. If the treatment goal was pain management via sensory analgesia, which would tend to produce more sensation, two or four electrodes? Why?

4. If the patient complained of a prickling sensation underneath one of the electrodes, what would be the potential causes and potential remedies?

5. Explain the significance of the use of acupuncture points for electrode placement sites so that a patient would understand your rationale.

REFERENCES:

1. Castel, JC: Seminar notes, "Electrotherapy and ultrasound update" New York, December 1994.

2. Nolan, MF: Conductive differences in electrodes used with transcutaneous electrical nerve stimulation devices. Phys Ther 71:746, 1991.

3. Lieber, RL and Kelly, MJ: Factors influencing quadriceps femoris torque using transcutaneous neuromuscular electrical stimulation. Phys Ther 71:715, 1991.

4. Nikolova, L: Treatment with Interferential Current. Churchill Livingstone, New York, 1987, p 9.

5. Savage, B: Interferential Therapy. Faber & Faber, Boston, 1984, pp 38–39.

6. Binder, SA: Application of low and high voltage electrotherapeutic current. In Wolf, SL (ed): Electrotherapy. Churchill Livingstone, New York, 1981, pp 17–20.

7. McCulloch, JM, Kloth, LC, and Feedar, JA (eds): Wound Healing: Alternatives in Management, ed 2. FA Davis, Philadelphia, 1995, p 84.

8. Myklebust, B and Robinson, AF: Instrumentation. In Snyder-Mackler, L and Robinson, AJ (eds): Clinical Electrophysiology, Electrotherapy and Electrophysiologic Testing. Williams & Wilkins, Baltimore, 1989, pp 31, 32, 40, 41.

9. Myklebust, B and Kloth, LC: Electrodiagnosis and electrotherapeutic instrumentation: Characteristics of recording and stimulation systems and the principles of safety. In Gersh, MR (ed): Electrotherapy in Rehabilitation. FA Davis, Philadelphia, 1992, pp 55–57.

10. Benton, LA, et al: Functional Electrical Stimulation—A Practical Clinical Guide, ed 2. Rancho Los Amigos Rehabilitation Engineering Center, Downey CA, 1981, pp 34–36.

11. Newton, R: Electrotherapeutic Treatment Selecting Appropriate Wave Form Characteristics. JA Preston Corporation, Clifton, NJ, 1984, pp 32–40.

12. Mannheimer, JS and Lampe, GN: Clinical Transcutaneous Electrical Nerve Stimulation. FA Davis, Philadelphia, PA. 1984, pp 23, 396, 416, 420.

13. Travell, J and Rinzler, SH: The myofascial genesis of pain. Postgrad Med 11:425, 1952.

14. Melzack, R: Myofascial trigger points: Relation to acupuncture and mechanisms of pain. Arch Phys Med Rehabil 62:114, 1981.

15. Melzack, R, Stillwell, DM, and Fox, EJ: Trigger points and acupuncture points for pain: Correlations and implications. Pain 3:3, 1977.

16. Mannheimer, JS and Lampe, GN: Clinical Transcutaneous Electrical Nerve Stimulation. FA Davis, Philadelphia, 1984, pp 267–268.

17. Chu, LSW, Yeh, SDJ, and Wood, DD: Acupuncture Manual: A Western Approach. Marcel Dekker, New York, 1979, pp 12–20.

18. Mannheimer, JS and Lampe, GN: Clinical Transcutaneous Electrical Nerve Stimulation. FA Davis, Philadelphia, 1984, p 285.

19. Mannheimer, JS and Lampe, GN: Clinical Transcutaneous Electrical Nerve Stimulation. FA Davis, Philadelphia, 1984, p 211.

20. Mannheimer, JS and Lampe, GN: Clinical Transcutaneous Electrical Nerve Stimulation. FA Davis, Philadelphia, 1984, pp 256–261.

21. Lapeer, GL: High-intensity transcutaneous nerve stimulation at the Hoku acupuncture point for relief of muscular headache pain. Craniomandib Pract 4:164, 1986.

SUGGESTED READINGS

1. Alfieri, V: Electrical treatment of spasticity. Scand J Rehabil Med 16:29, 1984.

2. Alon, G: In Nelson, RM and Currier, DP (eds): Clinical Electrotherapy. Appleton & Lange, Norwalk, CT, 1987, pp 65–72.

3. Baker, LL, et al: Electrical stimulation of wrist and fingers for hemiplegic patients. Phys Ther 59:1495, 1979.

4. Bettany, JA, Newsome, L, and Stralka, S: High voltage pulsed current-effect on edema formation after hyperflexion injury. Arch Phys Med Rehabil 71:677, 1990.

5. Caputo RM, Benson JT, and McClellan E: Intravaginal maximal electrical stimulation in the treatment of urinary incontinence. Reproductive Med 38:667, 1993.

6. Cosgrove, KA, et al: The electrical effect of two commonly used clinical stimulators on traumatic edema in rats, Phys Ther 72:227, 1992.

7. Currier, DP and Mann, R: Muscular strength developments by electrical stimulation in healthy individuals. Phys Ther 63:915, 1983.

8. Feedar, JA, et al: Chronic dermal ulcer healing enhanced with monophasic pulsed electrical stimulation, Phys Ther 71:639, 1991.

9. Feedar JA, Kloth, LC, and Gentzkow, GD: Chronic dermal ulcer healing enhanced with monophasic pulsed electrical stimulation. Phys Ther 71:639, 1991.

10. Fitzgerald, GK and Newsome, D: Treatment of a large infected thoracic spine wound using high voltage pulsed monphasic current. Phys Ther 73:355, 1993.

11. Gordon, T and Mao, J: Muscle atrophy and procedures for training after spinal cord injury. Phys Ther 74:50, 1994.

12. Griffin, JW, et al: Efficacy of high voltage pulsed current for healing of pressure ulcers in patients with spinal cord injury. Phys Ther 71:433, 1991.

13. Griffin, JW, et al: Reduction of chronic posttraumatic hand edema: A comparison of high voltage pulsed current, intermittent pneumatic compression, and placebo treatments. Phys Ther 70:279, 1990.

14. Halstead, LS, et al: Relief of spasticity in SCT men and women using rectal probe electrostimulation. Paraplegia 31:715, 1993.

15. Karnes, JL, Mendel, FC, and Fish, DR: Effects of low voltage pulsed current on edema formation in frog hind limbs following impact injury. Phys Ther 72:273, 1992.

16. Kloth, LC and Feedar, JA: Acceleration of wound healing with high voltage, monophasic, pulsed current. Phys Ther 68:503, 1988.

17. Laughman, RK, et al: Strength changes in the normal quadriceps femoris muscle as a result of electrical stimulation. Phys Ther 63: 1983.

18. Leo, KC, et al: Effect of transcutaneous electrical nerve stimulation characteristics on clinical pain. Phys Ther 66: 1986.

19. McIntosh, LJ, et al: Pelvic floor rehabilitation in the treatment of incontinence. Reproductive Med 38:662, 1993.

20. Melzack, R and Wall, DW: Pain mechanisms: A new theory. Science 150:971, 1965.

21. Michlovitz, SL, Smith W, and Watkins, M: Ice and high voltage pulsed stimulation in the treatment of acute ankle sprains. J Orthop Sports Phys Ther 68:301, 1988. Section on Clinical Electrophysiology American Physical Therapy Association: Electrotherapeutic Terminology in Physical Therapy:APTA, Alexandria, VA, 1988.

22. Selkowitz, DM: Improvement in isometric strength of the quardiceps femoris muscle after training with electrical stimulation. Phys Ther 65:186, 1985.

23. Taylor, K, et al: Effect of a single 30-minute treatment of high voltage pulsed current on edema formation in frog hind limbs. Phys Ther 72:63, 1992.

24. Wood, JM, et al: A multicenter study of the use of pulsed low intensity direct current for healing chronic stage II and III decubitus ulcers. Journal Invest Dermatol 98:, 1992.

Appendix: Optimal Stimulation Sites for TENS Electrodes

Key to Illustrations and Tables on Following Pages

▼	Acupuncture point	K. or k. . . .	kidney meridian
○	Motor point	LI. or li. . . .	large intestine
□	Trigger point	LU. r lu. . . .	lung
○	Cutaneous nerve	LV. or lv. . . .	liver
○	Peripheral nerve	P. or p. . . .	pericardium
		SI. or si. . . .	small intestine
BL. or bl. . . .	bladder meridian	SP. or sp. . . .	spleen
GB. or gb. . . .	gallbladder meridian	ST. or st. . . .	stomach
H. or h. . . .	heart meridian	TW. or tw. . . .	triple warmer

Researched and developed by Jeffrey S. Mannheimer, M.A., R.P.T., and Barbara J. Behrens, A.A.S.P.T.A. © 1980.
*From Mannheimer, JS and Lampe GN: Clinical Transcutaneous Electrical Nerve Stimulation. FA Davis, Philadelphia, 1984, pp 301, 306–307, 309–319, 324–325, with permission.

Spine and Occiput

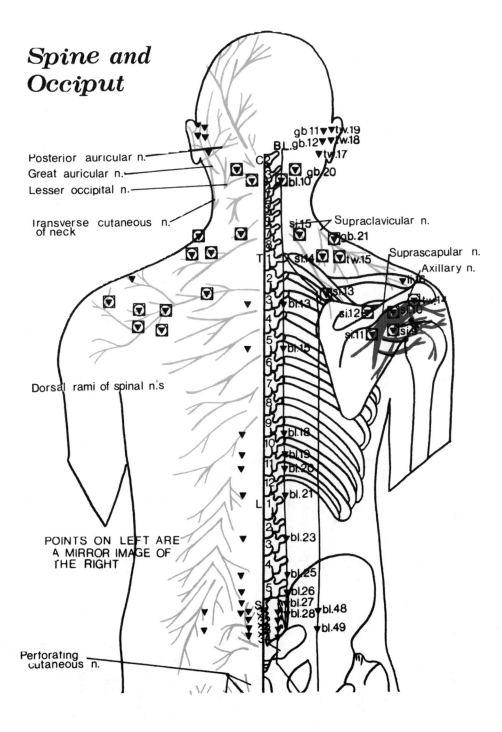

Posterior auricular n.

Great auricular n.

Lesser occipital n.

Transverse cutaneous n. of neck

gb 11 ▼▼tw.19
BL gb.12 ▼▼tw.18
▼tw.17
gb.20
bl.10
si.15   Supraclavicular n.
gb.21
Suprascapular n.
Axillary n.
si.14 tw.15
si.13
bl.13   si.12
si.11   si.10

Dorsal rami of spinal n.'s

bl.15

bl.18
bl.19
bl.20
bl.21

POINTS ON LEFT ARE
A MIRROR IMAGE OF
THE RIGHT

bl.23

bl.25
bl.26
bl.27
bl.28   bl.48
bl.49

Perforating cutaneous n.

C
T 1
2
3
4
5
6
7
8
9
10
11
12
L 1
2
3
4
5
S

Optimal Stimulation Sites for TENS Electrodes

Location	Occiput				
	Superficial Nerve Branch	Acupuncture Point	Motor Point	Trigger Point	Segmental Level
Posterior ear upper third (TW 19) same level but slightly moremedial on occiput (GB 11)	Great auricular, posterior branch communicates with lesser occipital, auricular branch of vagus, posterior auricular branch of facial. Transverse cutaneous nerve of neck	TW 19 GB 11 is just medial			Cranial C2–4
Posterior ear middle third (TW 18) same level but slightly more medial on occiput (GB 12)	Same as above	TW 18 GB 12 is just medial			Cranial C2–4
Behind ear in depresion between angle of mandible and mastoid process	Great auricular, posterior branch and lesser occipital	TW 17			C2–4
Suboccipital depression, between sternocleidomastoid (SCM) and upper trapezius	Greater and lesser occipital nerves	GB 20 B 10 is nearby, slightly medial and inferior	Splenius capitis (branches from C2–4) semispinalis capitis	Splenius capitis Semispinalis capitis	C2–3

The explanation of optimal stimulation sites for the shoulder girdle as seen on this view can be found on the view of posterolateral shoulder and dorsal region of the upper extremity.

Optimal Stimulation Sites for TENS Electrodes *(continued)*

Location	Superficial Nerve Branch	The Spine — Acupuncture Point	Motor Point	Trigger Point	Segmental Level
In depression between medial border of posterior superior iliac spine (PSIS) and 1st sacral spinous process	Dorsal ramus of L2	B 27			L2
2″ lateral to spinous process of S2	Dorsal ramus of L2	B 48	Gluteus maximus (upper motor pt) (inferior gluteal L5–S2)	Gluteus maximus	L2 L5–S2
2″ lateral to spinous process of S4	Dorsal rami of L2–3	B 49	Gluteus maximus (lower motor pt) (piriformis directly below) (inferior gluteal) (L5–S2)	Gluteus maximus (piriformis directly below)	L2–3 L5–S2
Directly over 1st sacral foramen	Dorsal ramus of S1	B 31			S1
Directly over 2nd sacral foramen	Dorsal ramus of S2	B 32			S2
Directly over 3rd sacral foramen	Dorsal ramus of S3	B 33			S3
Directly over 4th sacral foramen	Dorsal ramus of S4	B 34			S4

The twelve cutaneous branches of thoracic posterior primary rami become superficial adjacent to the spinous processes. They each have multiple cutaneous twigs. Havelacque considers the dorsal ramus of T2 to be the largest and most diffuse.[265]

The cutaneous disbribution of the dorsal ramus of T2 reaches up to the posterior aspect of the acromion, covering the mid-back (to the region of T5–6) and laterally to the superior region of the posterior axillary fold. A number of optimal stimulation sites are depicted as overlying this nerve.

Cutaneous branches of the dorsal rami of L1–3 descend as far as the posterior part of the iliac crest, skin of the buttock and almost to the greater trochanter of the femur (see lower extremity, lateral and posterior views).[1(p1033),93]

Anteromedial Shoulder and Volar Region of Upper Extremity

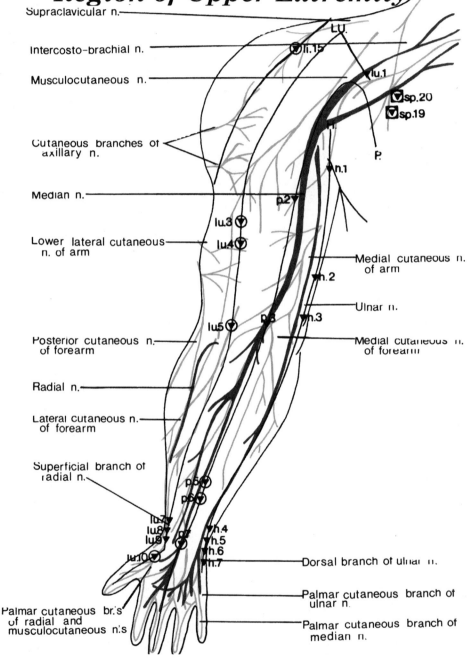

Supraclavicular n.

Intercosto-brachial n.

Musculocutaneous n.

Cutaneous branches of axillary n.

Median n.

Lower lateral cutaneous n. of arm

Posterior cutaneous n. of forearm

Radial n.

Lateral cutaneous n. of forearm

Superficial branch of radial n.

Palmar cutaneous br.'s of radial and musculocutaneous n.'s

LU.

li.15

lu.1

sp.20

sp.19

P.

n.1

p.2

lu.3

lu.4

Medial cutaneous n. of arm

n.2

Ulnar n.

n.3

p.3

lu.5

Medial cutaneous n. of forearm

p.5

p.6

lu.7

lu.8

lu.9

p.7

lu.10

h.4

h.5

h.6

h.7

Dorsal branch of ulnar n.

Palmar cutaneous branch of ulnar n.

Palmar cutaneous branch of median n.

Optimal Stimulation Sites for TENS Electrodes *(continued)*

	Anteromedial Shoulder and Volar Region of Upper Extremity					
Location	**Superficial Nerve Branch**	**Acupuncture Point**	**Motor Point**	**Trigger Point**	**Segmental Level**
Between first and second ribs, about 4″ lateral to sternum, medial to coracoid process	Musculocutaneous nerve	LU 1	Coracobrachialis is nearby (musculocutaneous) (C6)		C5–7
Radial side of biceps brachii 2″ below anterior axillary fold. 3″ below anterior axillary fold	Musculocutaneous nerve and its lower lateral cutaneous branch	LU 3 / LU 4	Biceps brachii (musculocutaneous) C5–6		C5–7
In antecubital fossa on crease at radial side of biceps tendon	Lateral cutaneous nerve of arm	LU 5	Brachialis (musculocutaneous) (C5–6)		C5–7
Just lateral to radial artery from 1st volar crease to just above radial styloid	Lateral cutaneous nerve of forearm communicating with superficial radial nerve	LU 7–9			C5–7 / C6–8
Volar surface of hand at midpoint of 1st metacarpal	Superficial branch of radial nerve and palmar cutaneous of median	LU 10	Abductor pollicis brevis (median) (C8–T1)		C6–8 / C5–T1

Optimal Stimulation Sites for TENS Electrodes (continued)

	Anteromedial Shoulder and Volar Region of Upper Extremity					
Location	Superficial Nerve Branch	Acupuncture Point	Motor Point	Trigger Point	Segmental Level	
Between heads of biceps brachii 2″ below anterior axillary fold with medial cutaneous	Musculocutaneous and intercostal brachial nerves, may communicate nerve of forearm	P 2			C5–7 T2	
Just medial to biceps tendon in ante-cubital fossa	Median nerve and anterior branch of medial cutane-ous nerve of forearm	P 3	Pronator teres (median) (C 6)		C5–T1 C8–T1	
Between tendons of flexor carpi radialis (FCR) and palmaris longus (PL) 2″ and 1 ½″ above volar crease respectively	Median and anterior branch of medial cutaneous nerve of forearm	P 5 P 6 is 1″ below			C5–T1 C8–T1	
Between tendons of FCR and PL at midpoint transverse volar wrist crease	Median and anterior branch of medial cutaneous nerve of forearm and palmar cutaneous branch of median	P 7			C5–T1 C8–T1	
Between ribs 2–3 and 3–4, midway between anter-ior axillary fold and sternum	Medial and intermedial supraclavicular nerves to 2nd rib, lateral cutaneous nerves of thorax (2–4), the 2nd nerve is the intercostal brachial nerve	SP 19–20	Pectoralis major (medial) and lateral anterior thoracic nerves)	Pectoralis major	C3–4 T2–4	

Optimal Stimulation Sites for TENS Electrodes *(continued)*

	Anteromedial Shoulder and Volar Region of Upper Extremity				
Location	Superficial Nerve Branch	Acupuncture Point	Motor Point	Trigger Point	Segmental Level
Medial to brachial artery in axilla	Ulnar nerve, intercosto-brachial, medial cutaneous nerve of arm and median nerve which is just lateral to artery	H 1			C7–T1 T2 C9–T1 C5–T1
In groove medial to lower ⅓ of biceps brachii medial to brachial artery	Median and medial cutaneous nerve of arm	H 2			C5–T1 C8–T1
Just superior to cubital tunnel by medial epicondyle	Medial cutaneous nerve of forearm	H 3			C8–T1
Ulnar aspect of wrist lateral to flexor carpi ulnaris (FCU) tendon from 1 ½″ above 1st volar wrist crease to pisiform bone	Ulnar nerve and its palmar cutaneous branch	H4–7			C7–T1
In depression anterior and inferior to acromion	Upper lateral cutaneous nerve branch of axillary	LI 15	Anterior deltoid (axillary) (C5–6)		C5–6

Posterolateral Shoulder and Dorsal Region of Upper Extremity

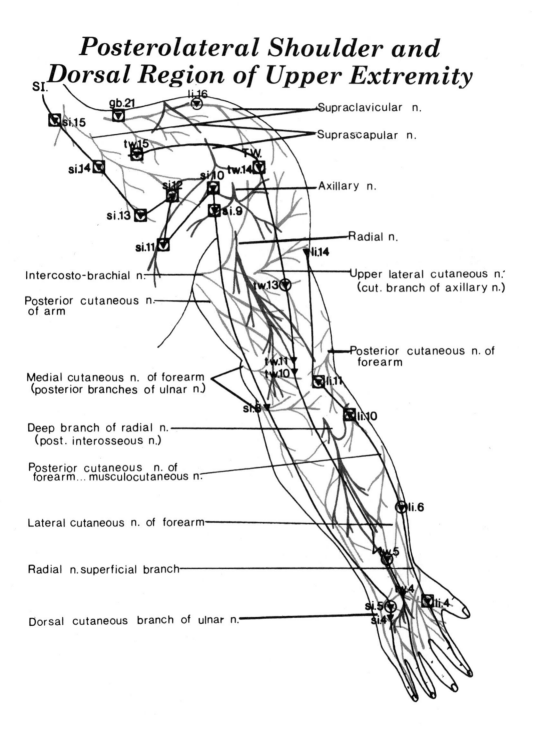

SI.

gb.21

li.16

si.15

tw.15

T.W.

si.14

tw.14

si.12

si.10

tw.13

si.13

si.9

si.11

li.14

tw.11
tw.10

li.11

si.8

li.10

li.6

tw.5

tw.4

si.5

li.4

si.4

Supraclavicular n.

Suprascapular n.

Axillary n.

Radial n.

Upper lateral cutaneous n.
(cut. branch of axillary n.)

Posterior cutaneous n. of
forearm

Intercosto-brachial n.

Posterior cutaneous n.
of arm

Medial cutaneous n. of forearm
(posterior branches of ulnar n.)

Deep branch of radial n.
(post. interosseous n.)

Posterior cutaneous n. of
forearm...musculocutaneous n.

Lateral cutaneous n. of forearm

Radial n. superficial branch

Dorsal cutaneous branch of ulnar n.

Optimal Stimulation Sites for TENS Electrodes *(continued)*

Posterolateral Shoulder and Dorsal Region of Upper Extremity					
Location	**Superficial Nerve Branch**	**Acupuncture Point**	**Motor Point**	**Trigger Point**	**Segmental Level**
1 ½″ lateral to spinous process of C7	Medial branch of supraclavicular	SI 15	Levaor scapulae (spinal accessory and dorsal scapular (C3–4)	Levator scapulae	Cranial C3–4
1 ½″ above superior angle of scapula at the level of the spinous process of T1	Lateral (posterior) branch of supraclavicular	SI 14 TW 15 is just lateral	Middle trapezius (spinal accessory (C3–4)	Middle trapezius	Cranial C3–4
Suprascapular fossa (medial end) 3″ lateral to spinous process of T2	Lateral (posterior) branch of supraclavicular and dorsal ramus of T2	SI 13	Middle trapezius (spinal accessory) (C3–4)	Middle trapezius	Cranial C3–4 T2
At midpoint of suprascapular fossa	Dorsal ramus of T2	SI 12	Spuraspinatus (suprascapular) (C5–6)	Supraspinatus	C5–6 T2
At midpoint of infrascapular fossa	Dorsal ramus of T2	SI 11	Infraspinatus (suprascapular) (C5–6)	Infraspinatus	C5–6 T2
Directly above posterior axillary fold. Just below spine of scapula	Dorsal ramus of T2 and axillary (posterior branch), which continues as the upper lateral cutaneous nerve of the arm	SI 10 (axillary)	Posterior deltoid (C5–6)	Posterior deltoid T2	C5–6
Directly below SI 10. Just superior to posterior axillary fold	Axillary and dorsal ramus of T2	SI 9	Teres major (subscapular) (C5–6)	Teres major	C5–6 T2
In groove between olecranon and medial epicondyle of humerus	Ulnar nerve and its medial cutaneous branches	SI 8			C7–T1

Optimal Stimulation Sites for TENS Electrodes *(continued)*

	Posterolateral Shoulder and Dorsal Region of Upper Extremity				
Location	**Superficial Nerve Branch**	**Acupuncture Point**	**Motor Point**	**Trigger Point**	**Segmental Level**
In depression between pisiform bone and ulnar styloid	Dorsal and palmar cutaneous ranches of ulnar nerve	SI 5			C7–T1
In depression between fifth metacarpal and triquetral	Dorsal and palmar cutaneous branches of ulnar nerve	SI 4	Palmaris brevis (median) (C8–T1)		C7–T1
On cephalad surface of upper trapezius directly above superior angle of of scapula	Supraclavicular	GB 21	Upper trapezius (spinalaccessory)	Upper trapezius	Cranial C3–4
In depression posterior and inferior to acromion and above greater tubercle of humerus with arm in anatomical position	Intercostal brachial, upper lateral cutaneous nerve—branch of axillary, and dorsal ramus of T2	TW 14	Posterior deltoid (axillary) (C5–6)		C5–6 T2
Just below deltoid insertion by lateral head of triceps	Upper lateral cutaneous nerve branch of axillary	TW 13	Lateral head of triceps (radial) (C7–8)		C5–6
In depression 1″ above olecranon with the elbow flexed to 90°	Posterior cutaneous nerve of arm (radial) medial cutaneous of forearm (ulnar posterior branches) posterior cutaneous nerve of forearm	TW 10, TW 11 is just above			C5–8 C8–T1 C5–8
Between radius and ulna on dorsal surface about 2″ proximal to transverse wrist crease	Posterior cutaneous nerve of forearm, branch of radial communications with lateral cutaneous nerve of forearm, branch of musculocutaneous	TW 5	Extensor indicis proprius (radial) (C7)		C5–8 C5–6

Optimal Stimulation Sites for TENS Electrodes (continued)

	Posterolateal Shoulder and Dorsal Region of Upper Extremity				
Location	**Superficial Nerve Branch**	**Acupuncture Point**	**Motor Point**	**Trigger Point**	**Segmental Level**
In depression on dorsum of hand between tendons of extensor digitorum communis (EDC) and extensor indicis proprius (EIP) just distal to transverse crease of wrist	Posterior cutaneous nerve of forearm (radial, superficial radial and dorsal cutaneous branch of ulnar nerve)	TW 4			C5–8 C6–8 C8–T1
In depression between acromio-clavicular (AC) joint and spine of scapula	Posterolateral branch of supraclavicular nerve	LI 16	Musculotendinous junction of supraspintus		C3–4
In depression anterior and inferior to acromion	Upper lateral cutaneous nerve branch of axillary	LI 15	Anterior deltoid (axillary) (C5–6)		C5–6
Lateral arm at deltoid insertion	Upper lateral cutaneous	LI 14			C5–6
Lateral end of cubital crease in depression with elbow flexed.	Posterior cutaneous nerve of forearm (medial), communicates with intercostal brachial nerve	LI 11	Brachioradialis (radial) (C5–6)	Brachioradialis	C5–8
Just below lateral epicondyle of humerus with forearm pronated	Superficial radial nerve superior to posterior interosseous nerve	LI 10	Extensor carpi radialis longus, supinator nearby (radial) (C6)	Extensor carpi radialis longus, supinator nearby	C6–8
8–10 cm above radial styloid with arm in anatomical position	Superficial radial and lateral cutaneous nerve of forearm	LI 6	Extensor pollicis brevis (radial) (C7)		C6–8 C5–6
Midpoint of radial aspect of second metacarpal	Superficial radial in communication with distal branches of musculocutaneous	LI 4	First dorsal interosseus (ulnar nerve)	First dorsal interosseus & adductor pollicis	C6–8 C5–7 C7–T1

Lower Extremity, Anterior View

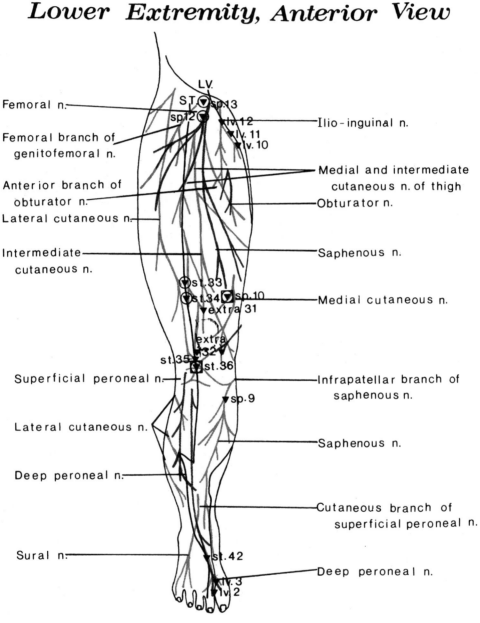

Femoral n.

Femoral branch of genitofemoral n.

Anterior branch of obturator n.

Lateral cutaneous n.

Intermediate cutaneous n.

Superficial peroneal n.

Lateral cutaneous n.

Deep peroneal n.

Sural n.

LV.
ST
sp.13
sp.12
lv.12
lv. 11
lv. 10

Ilio-inguinal n.

Medial and intermediate cutaneous n. of thigh

Obturator n.

Saphenous n.

st.33
st.34
sp.10
extra 31

Medial cutaneous n.

extra 32

st.35
st.36

Infrapatellar branch of saphenous n.

sp.9

Saphenous n.

Cutaneous branch of superficial peroneal n.

st.42

Deep peroneal n.

lv.3
lv.2

Optimal Stimulation Sites for TENS Electrodes *(continued)*

Lower Extremity, Anterior View

Location	Superficial Nerve Branch	Acupuncture Point	Motor Point	Trigger Point	Segmental Level
2″ lateral to superior border of symphysis pubis	Anterior cutaneous branches of iliohypogastric, ilio-inguinal and genitofemoral	LIV 10–12	Pectineus (femoral) (L2–4)		L1 L1 L1–2
Between 1st and 2nd metatarals just above web space junction on dorsum of foot	Deep peroneal nerve via its medial terminal and interosseous branches	LIV 2–3	1st dorsal interosseus (lateral plantar) (S1–2)		L4–5 S1–2
From inguinal ligament to femoral triangle lateral to femoral artery	Anterior branch of obturator communicating with medial cutaneous. Forms subsartorial plexus.	SP 12 SP 13	Iliopsoas (femoral) (L2–4)		L2–4 L2–4
2″ above medial aspect of patellar base	Medial cutaneous nerve of thigh and saphenous nerve (infrapatellar	SP 10	Vastus medialis (femoral) (L2–4)	Vastus medialis	L2–4 L2–3
Just below medial condyle of tibia, level with tibial tuberosity between satorius and gracilis	Saphenous nerve	SP 9			L3–4

Optimal Stimulation Sites for TENS Electrodes (continued)

Lower Extremity, Anterior View

Location	Superficial Nerve Branch	Acupuncture Point	Motor Point	Trigger Point	Segmental Level
Just superior to midpoint of patellar base	Intermediate cutaneous nerve of the thigh	Extra 31			L2–3
Medial to patellar tendon	Medial cutaneous nerve of thigh	Extra 32 (medial)			L2–3
In depression just below patella, lateral to tendon with knee flexed	Medial and lateral cutaneous nerve of thigh and infrapatellar branch of saphenous which form a patellar plexus	ST 35 Extra 32 (lateral)			L2–3 L3–4
2–3″ above lateral aspect of patellar base	Intermediate and lateral cutaneous nerve of thigh	ST 33–34	Vastus lateralis (femoral) (L2–4)		L2–4
In depression just below patella, lateral to tendon with knee flexed	Medial and lateral cutaneous nerve of thigh and infrapatellar branch of saphenous which form a patellar plexus	ST 35 Extra 32 (lateral)			L2–3 L3–4
2″ below inferior angle of patella, lateral to tibial crest.	Infrapatellar branch of saphenous	ST 36	Superior motor point of anterior tibialis (deep peroneal) (L4–5, S1)	Anterior tibialis	L3–4
Below malleoli at center of dorsum of foot, lateral to anerior tibialis tendon	Superficial peroneal	ST 42			L4–S2

Lower Extremity, Posterior View

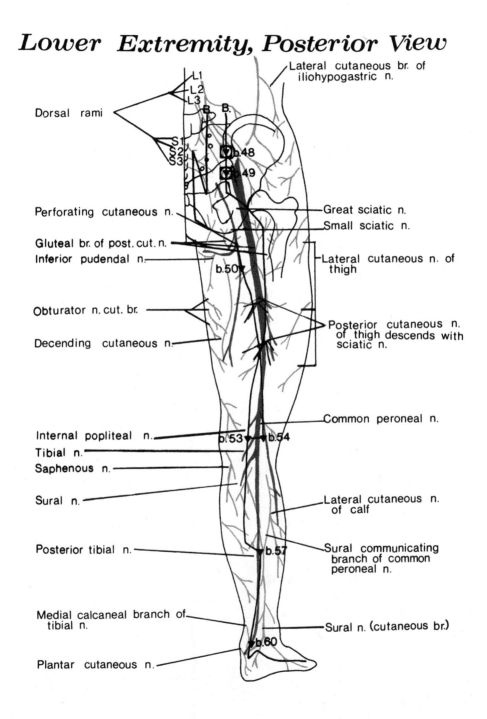

Lateral cutaneous br. of iliohypogastric n.

L1
L2
L3

Dorsal rami

B. B.

S1
S2
S3

b.48

b.49

Perforating cutaneous n.

Great sciatic n.
Small sciatic n.

Gluteal br. of post. cut. n.
Inferior pudendal n.

b.50

Lateral cutaneous n. of thigh

Obturator n. cut. br.

Posterior cutaneous n. of thigh descends with sciatic n.

Decending cutaneous n.

Common peroneal n.

Internal popliteal n.

b.53 b.54

Tibial n.
Saphenous n.

Sural n.

Lateral cutaneous n. of calf

Posterior tibial n.

b.57

Sural communicating branch of common peroneal n.

Medial calcaneal branch of tibial n.

Sural n. (cutaneous br.)

b.60

Plantar cutaneous n.

Optimal Stimulation Sites for TENS Electrodes (*continued*)

	Lower Extremity, Posterior View				
Location	**Superficial Nerve Branch**	**Acupuncture Point**	**Motor Point**	**Trigger Point**	**Segmental Level**
2″ lateral to spinous process of S2	Dorsal ramus L2	B 48	Gluteus maximus (upper motor pt) (inferior gluteal L5–S2)	Gluteus maximus	L2 L5–S2
2″ lateral to spinous process of S4	Dorsal rami L2–3	B 49	Gluteus maximus (lower motor pt) (piriformis directly below) (inferior gluteal L5–S2)	Gluteus maximus (piriformis directly below)	L2–3 L5–S2
At midpoint of junction between buttock and posterior thigh	Posterior cutaneous nerve of thigh, medial and lateral branches	B 50			S1–3
Popliteal fossa between biceps femoris and semitendinosus tendons	Posterior cutaneous nerve of thigh, medial and lateral branches	*B 54/40 *B 53/39 (lateral aspect of popliteal fossa medial to biceps femoris tendon)			S1–3
Midline of leg below heads of gastrocsoleus at junction of upper 2/3 and lower 1/3 of leg	Sural, communicating branch of lateral cutaneous nerve of calf (common peroneal)	B 57	Soleus (tibial nerve) S1–2	Soleus	L5–S2 L4–S2
Between lateral malleolus and heelcord	Dorsal lateral cutaneous nerve–end of sural	B 60			L4–S2

*Numerical systems differ according to texts.

B 53 & 54 Acupuncture Therapy[115]

B 39 & 40 An Outline of Chinese Acupuncture[116]

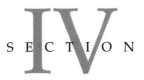

Comprehensive Approach
to Treatment

Modality Integration for the Accomplishment of Therapeutic Treatment Goals

Barbara J. Behrens, BS, PTA

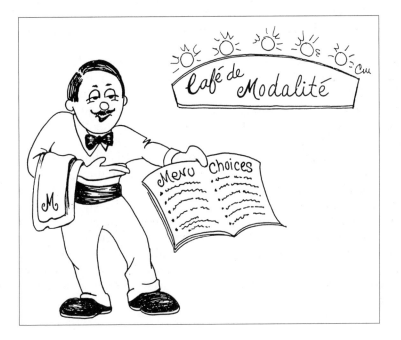

CHAPTER OBJECTIVES

- Review the physical agent modalities utilized in the clinic.
- Discuss the integration of the use of physical agent modalities.
- Discuss the importance of the participation of the health care team in accomplishing the treatment goals.
- Outline appropriate parameter guidelines for the documentation of physical agent modalities.
- Discuss the clinical decision making involved in the selection of the sequencing of several physical agents to accomplish a treatment goal.

Throughout this text, a wide variety of therapeutic modalities have been discussed for the treatment of physical signs and symptoms. Clinicians are responsible for safe and efficacious delivery of these modalities to accomplish therapeutic goals. Research efforts continue, raising more questions to challenge our dogmas of clinical practice.

Manufacturers of electromedical equipment have emerged as a strong allies of the clinician in the quest for the delivery of safer, more reliable, and more predictable treatments. The manufacturers have become a driving technologic force in the advancement of delivering safer, easier to use modalities for quality patient care. The technology, however advanced, cannot take away the responsibility for the selection of the proper techniques for a given patient to accomplish a specific goal. That responsibility lies with the clinician, who ultimately may need to modify the technique or alter the sequencing with other techniques so that optimal results can be achieved.

Therapeutic goal accomplishment will typically be based on several different factors that must be part or the integration process in the use of physical agents. Factors include treatment goals, time available for treatment, time since the injury, medical stability of the patient, and cognitive ability of the patient. In addition, what modalities are available to accomplish these goals? Patient compliance, family reinforcement, staff compliance, and technical support availability must not be overlooked.

TREATMENT GOALS WITH PHYSICAL AGENTS

The therapeutic goals generally are for (1) reduction of a symptom or (2) promotion of a response. Modalities may assist in the promotion of tissue healing,[1–4] increased blood flow into the injured area,[5,6] muscle strengthening,[7–9] tissue exensibility,[10–12] and pain relief.[13–16] These goals can often be interdependent. For example, a modality used for the reduction of pain may reduce the level of discomfort enough to decrease the protective muscle guarding in the area. If the guarding subsides, then the potential exists that the blood flow into or from the area will no longer be impeded by the spasm, and metabolite retention in the area will have a chance to diminish, resulting in less chemical irritation (from the metabolite retention), and ultimately less pain. Pain can also initially be considered a protective response warning the individual not to stress the injured area because it is damaged and no longer as strong as it had been. Pain perception may intensify because of the muscle guarding and its impact on metabolite retention in the injured tissue.

Many of the individual techniques presented throughout this text address the three sides of the pain triangle, but to different degrees (Fig. 17–1). Some techniques primarily target the pain, or the muscle spasm, and indirectly address the dysfunction. Others specifically target the dysfunction by promoting tissue healing and experience a resultant decrease in pain perception and muscle guarding as the area heals.[17] One important consideration in the selection of physical agents is the concept of causal factors. The mark of excellence in clinical practice is the attention paid to the cause-and-effect relationship, and acknowledgment of the importance of understanding the relationship. Clinicians treat the patient considering "the patient," and the normal courses of response to therapeutic interventions. Technicians treat the individual symptom, without regard for causal factors.

The clinician's approach in treating a patient experiencing discomfort involves the recognition of the discomfort and assessment of its impact on functional activities and the patient's life in general,[18,19] assessment of what might have contributed to the symptoms, and how to help the patient limit the potential for the return of the symptoms. The technician applies a modality indicated for the treatment of pain.

AVAILABLE TREATMENT TIME

Patients who have been referred for treatment are usually either inpatients, in a hospital setting, or outpatients, where they are well enough to be living at home and commuting to an outpatient facility for treatment or receiving care at home by a visiting clinician. Some outpatient facilities are housed in hospitals and some are freestanding. The time constraints and support mechanisms will vary significantly between these settings. Patients in an inpatient setting will have the reinforcement

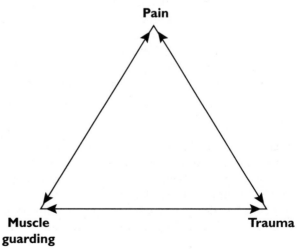

Figure 17–1. The pain triangle. Trauma causes both pain and muscle guarding. Pain can cause both muscle guarding and trauma. Muscle guarding can cause pain and trauma. It is important to address each side of the triangle when treating patients.

of the hospital nursing staff that a home-based patient may not have. Inpatients are typically transported to a department for treatment and transported back to their rooms following treatment. Patients who are living at home need to either transport themselves, make arrangements for their transportation to treatment, or seek resources for home visits for treatment.

An important consideration in the treatment with physical agents and therapeutic modalities is the patient. The accomplishment of therapeutic goals is important; what is probably less apparent is that the patient will also have a daily agenda that they need to follow. They will realistically not devote every waking hour to their recovery, nor be totally compliant with a therapy schedule that occupies more than an hour two to three times per week. Time management in the accomplishment of therapeutic goals must be a consideration. Treatment sessions with physical agents involve approximately 20 to 30 minutes and an additional 20 to 30 minutes of teaching, therapeutic exercise, and assessment. There are exceptions, based on the diagnosis and other related factors, but many treatment sessions involve approximately 1 hour.

During this time, the goals that have been established and negotiated with the patient need to be addressed. This is where true integration must take place. Many of the techniques that have been discussed will directly treat the primary complaints of the patient, and indirectly address the other complaints of the patient. It is not necessary or realistic to utilize every modality that could possibly be employed to treat a patient because of this overlapping of responses. Time management and technique assessment revolve around carefully limited choices to accomplish a goal, assessing the outcome of a given modality, and then the possibility of adding an additional modality to address the other symptoms unrelieved by one modality.

Use of every "unattended" modality for 20 to 30 minutes that could conceivably be done for edema or pain reduction could involve several hours of time with no more significant results than the careful selection of one of the modalities. If the treatment time becomes excessively long, the patient may actually experience more muscle guarding secondary to tension, with a potential increase in pain perception. Some treatment modalities for a given patient condition produce comparable results through the use of a completely different mechanism. The approach taken may be more reflective of the individuality of the patient and his or her responses to previous intervention techniques than a specific technique itself.[20] If, for example, a patient had read an article in a magazine that outlined the successes of the use of electrical stimulation for the relief of "muscle tension" via pain relief, they may respond better to electrical stimulation than to traction. Their beliefs may override the potential benefits of the selected modality.

Time Since Injury

Acute injuries typically have less of an impact on function. Mobility needs to be maintained and further injury prevented while the complaints of pain, inflammation, edema formation, and muscle guarding are addressed.[21] Traumatic injuries with substantial soft tissue involvement, such as fractures, neuropathies, and surgical interventions for repair or recovery of function, may be treated on an inpatient or on an outpatient basis. Patients with neurologic impairment represent a population that will typically require a more lengthy recovery time. Both the severely involved patient with multiple trauma and the patient with neurologic impairment will most often be seen for treatment initially in an acute care hospital setting and then be transferred to a rehabilitation facility for a more intensive approach to their recovery. Generally, the more devastating the injury in terms of tissue destruction or manipulation, the longer the recovery. In these instances, the patient may be seen by a clinician to address their physical complaints, often twice daily for several hours, in an inpatient setting. Even though the time period has increased, the focus on careful selection of modalities should not change. Since these patients have experienced a significant change in their functional ability, they will be involved in a broader-based therapeutic program. There will be a greater emphasis on therapeutic exercise and adaptive skills for functional independence or return to functional levels of performance, in addition to modality utilization to reduce symptoms and promote a return to function. Overall, time management and goal optimization in the utilization of therapeutic modalities should remain constant.

MEDICAL STABILITY OF THE PATIENT

Therapeutic interventions are performed to promote optimal recovery of the patient, not simply the symptom. Patients may have other complicating medical problems that will limit the potential choices of modalities that may be utilized. Suppose, for example, that a patient had been referred to physical therapy for the treatment of cervical strain and sprain, and the primary complaints included pain with a lack of motion in the cervical spine because of muscle tightness. The patient's medical history reveals that he or she is being treated for hemophilia. Although cervical traction may be a beneficial modality for the relaxation of the cervical musculature, it would not be indicated for a patient being treated for hemophilia because of the risk of microtearing of the muscle fibers or joint capsule. The approach may change to one of managing the pain with the intent that the muscle tightness will subside if the pain subsides. A TENS unit may be a better alternative for this patient, so that the pain relief would be the primary focus with an anticipated reduction in muscle guarding. The focus changes to address the primary complaint indirectly because of the medical condition of the patient.

Another example of an alteration in modality selection arising regarding medical stability or complicating factors would be the patient who is referred to therapy for lower-extremity edema. Upon assessment of the lower extremity, there are no palpable pedal pulses. Although one of the treatments that might have been employed for the management of the edema could have been intermittent compression, it would not be indicated if there were no palpable pedal pulses. The lack of pedal pulses would indicate a decreased blood supply to the lower extremity and may be indicative of further medical complications that would need to be evaluated by a physician.

COGNITIVE ABILITY OF THE PATIENT

Patient cognitive abilities or the involvement of significant others play a crucial role in the recovery process. Therapeutic interventions for the accomplishment of treatment goals involve the patient; the diagnosis; the treatment plan, including the modalities utilized; the exercise program; and the "home instructions" for the patient. If the focus of the therapy is the reduction of cervical muscle spasm, and the patient leaves therapy to go home and sit on a couch to watch television, then the recovery time will be longer.

PATIENT EXPECTATIONS

Another problem that exists is the perpetuation of a phrase among fitness fanatics and athletes of "no pain, no gain." It is important to realize that when administering a physical agent, the appropriate responses to the treatment should be explained to the patient, as well as the inappropriate responses to treatment. Let's use the example of an athlete who was referred to therapy for the treatment of a contusion to the quadriceps. Ultrasound had been recommended for the alteration of the scar tissue that had formed that is now limiting torque production. During the application of the ultrasound, the patient was thinking of the "no pain, no gain" philosophy and began to feel a prickling sensation leading to a burning sensation, and now thought to themselves, "OK, now it's really working, it's really beginning to burn now," without ever making a comment to the clinician delivering the treatment. The patient may have been experiencing a periosteal burn, which is potentially detrimental to the tissue. The patient should have been instructed to report any perceived sensation to the clinician during the delivery of the ultrasound. Instruction needs to be continuous, and the patient's ability to respond appropriately needs to be assessed to determine whether the selected modality will be safe for that patient.

THE MODALITIES AVAILABLE

Since there is a wide degree of overlap of many clinical modalities in the accomplishment of therapeutic goals, and since several of the modalities address primary complaints as well as secondary complaints, it is important to recognize what "tools" are available. Patients may plateau with their progress after repeated attempts with a given modality, and when appropriate alternate choices may be made. It is also feasible that when a patient arrives in the department for treatment, the specific modality that was utilized during the last treatment session is not available. Clinicians need to understand how to accomplish the goals using alternative methods if their first choice is unavailable.

Electrical stimulation devices represent one of the clearest examples of confusion among practicing clinicians. Chapter 15 presented the multitude of electrical stimulation devices that are currently in use today. Chapters 10, 11, and 12 discussed applications for electrical stimulation as a modality without specific mention of the device itself. Many of the electrical stimulation devices have been developed, based on the available technology for current delivery to the patient. Many of the same therapeutic goals can be accomplished with each of the electrical stimulators, dependent upon the electrical parameters of the stimulator. The accomplishment of the goal then is not dependent upon the specific box chosen, but on the knowledge of the parameters, electrode placement sites, and the specific characteristics of the stimulator. "Faradic" stimulators or asymmetrical alternating current stimulators were initially utilized to elicit a muscle contraction, to prevent muscle atrophy. They were also utilized to reduce muscle spasm and decrease pain. High-voltage or twin-spiked pulsed monophasic stimulators were also utilized to elicit a muscle contraction, reduce a muscle spasm, or decrease pain. IFC units and TENS units are also utilized for these purposes, dependent upon the electrical parameters of the devices. The key factor, then, is the knowledge of the stimulation parameters and the appropriate electrode placement sites, not the type of electrical stimulator.

SUPPORT FOR THERAPEUTIC INTERVENTIONS

Patient compliance is one aspect of support for the therapeutic intervention. Compliance on the part of the patient's family or significant other is also an important component. Suppose, for example, that a pediatric patient has been referred for therapy to assist in the reduction of the lateral curvature of his or her scoliosis. The patient has been referred for a trial usage of electrical stimulation on the concave side to fatigue the muscles, and on the convex side to strengthen the musculature. The physician is recommending that the stimulator be worn at night to potentially offset the need for corrective surgery. Once the patient is utilizing a portable stimulator, he or she complains of aches after the muscle fatigue cycle of stimulation. Noncompliant family members allow the child to sleep without the stimulator every other night. The response to the trial of stimulation is minimal after 2 months. In actuality, the stimulation regimen was not adhered to because of the parents. The course of therapeutic intervention was unsupported and was therefore unsuccessful.

Another example of the importance of patient compliance would be the elderly man with a diagnosis of herpes zoster, who is referred to therapy for pain management. In the clinical setting the patient is able to reduce his level of discomfort from a rating of 10 before the application of a TENS unit, to a level of 3 after 15 minutes of stimulation around the lesions on the lower lateral aspect of his chest. He lives alone and has difficulty applying the electrodes and fitting the lead wires for the unit in his clothing. After 1 week he returns the stimulator stating that it did not work, despite the documentation that he provides that states that initially his relief from the unit lasted 1 hour and the last entry on his log states that 4 hours of relief were realized after 15 minutes of stimulation time.

Another component of the success of any therapeutic intervention can be traced back to the reliability of the performance of a particular piece of equipment. If a patient is being treated for a specific condition, and multiple modalities have been tried with limited or no substantive success, except for one individual parameter set, it now becomes critical to the therapeutic intervention that the modality perform in a reproducible and predictable manner. The Food and Drug Administration (FDA) regulates the introduction of "new" therapeutic modalities into clinical practice and acts as a "watchdog" for unfounded claims and patient safety concerns. Manufacturers of electromedical devices must file documents with the FDA prior to the marketing of a modality. These documents (known as a 510K) must be kept on file by the manufacturer. Liability rests with the clinician and with the manufacturer if there is any form of technical difficulty that could potentially injure a patient (Table 17–1).

Table 17–1   **Clinical Considerations for Treating With Therapeutic Modalities**

---

1. What is the available treatment time?
   Inpatient versus outpatient
   How much time will it take? (more or less than 1 hour?)
2. How long has it been since the actual injury?
3. What is the medical stability of the patient?
4. What is the cognitive ability of the patient?
5. What expectations does the patient have about the treatment?
6. What modalities are available to accomplish the treatment goals in the time available for treatment?
7. What types of support for the treatment are available to the patient?

THERAPEUTIC MODALITIES INTEGRATION PRINCIPLES

Several types of modalities have been discussed in previous chapters: thermal agents, electrical agents, mechanical agents, and other techniques. There is a significant overlapping of clinical results from each of these modalities. Whether they are thermal or mechanical or electrical, each grouping has the ability to reduce the amount of discomfort that a patient may be experiencing.

This next section will attempt to point out those areas of clinical overlap, and suggest a method of modality selection based on the commonality of the therapeutic goals that can be potentially accomplished with a given modality. The questions that any clinician will need to address are what should you choose? When should it be chosen? What was the patient's response to treatment? Was the treatment goal accomplished? Should you follow the same sequence again? and How should the treatment be documented?

WHAT TO CHOOSE?

Indications: Primary and Secondary

The first step in deciding what modality or modalities to use lies in the indications for a given modality. What are the direct effects, and what are the secondary benefits of selecting a given modality? Is the modality primarily utilized to reduce edema; will it reduce pain indirectly because the decreased edema? By establishing a list of the primary and secondary indications of a given modality and comparing that list with the treatment goals for a patient, you can start to determine which modalities might be of benefit for that patient.

Safety Considerations: Precautions and Contraindications

After this initial list is compiled, look at each of the modalities selected and compare them with the medical condition of the patient. Determine whether or not there are any safety concerns, such as compromised sensation, or peripheral vascular disease that would eliminate any of the modalities as potential treatment options.

Equipment Availability

Next look at the availability of the potential modalities that you have selected. Typically, there are multiple pieces of equipment in any therapy department that can accomplish a multitude of goals, some better than others. Determine exactly what is available by looking at the necessary parameters for the protocol that you have selected. Do any of the pieces of equipment available meet the parameter requirements?

Reliability

Now, of the pieces of equipment available to you that are not contraindicated for your patient and that meet the appropriate parameters for you to accomplish your treatment goals, how many are reliable? When was the last inspection date from the biomedical engineering department? Inspect the equipment and its accessories to determine whether or not it is complete and operating properly before you apply it to a patient. Also make sure that if you are going to apply it to a patient that you are familiar with all of the controls and parameters and their settings for this unit.

Previous Patient Experience with the Selection Modality

One aspect that can easily be overlooked is the resource of the patient. Many patients who are receiving therapy have either been treated before for a similar condition or by someone else for another condition. The patient may have had either a positive or an adverse response to a therapeutic modality once before. Ask the patient whether or not they have had this type of treatment before, and whether or not they found it to be of benefit. Failure to use the patent as a resource may lead to treatment failure and potentially an increase in muscle guarding if they have had a negative experience in the past that they have not had a chance to discuss with a clinician.

What Does the Rest of the Plan of Care Include?

It is important to look at your choices in terms of efficient use of time and expected outcome. If you have selected a modality that will address only the primary complaints requiring 20 minutes to apply, and you identify that you will also need to utilize something else to address additional symptoms, can you combine two modalities and apply them simultaneously without compromising the therapeutic benefit of either one? This can be done with superficial heat, which can be applied during an electrical stimulation treatment. Both modalities can be applied simultaneously during a 20-minute treatment time.

If you have selected electrical stimulation for the reduction of muscle spasm and pain perception, can more than one form of electrical stimulation be applied if one form of stimulation is unsuccessful for both goals? There are a variety of different parameter sets for electrical stimulation. Electrical stimulation for the reduction of pain may involve sensory analgesia levels of intensity for 15 to 20 minutes, but chronic aching pain sensations may require noxious or motor levels of electrical stimulation delivered through a probe or handheld electrode system. The differentiation of the modality will lie in the parameters and desired physiologic response (Table 17–2).

Table 17–2 **How to Decide What to Choose**

---

1. What are the indications for the use of a particular modality?
   Primary indications
   Secondary indications
2. What are the safety considerations for the use of the modality?
   Precautions
   Contraindications
3. What equipment is available to accomplish the treatment goals?
   Does it have the necessary parameters?
4. How reliable is the selected equipment?
5. Has the patient been treated previusly with the selected modality?
6. What does the rest of the plan of care consist of?
7. Is the selected modality to be used to prepare the patient for something else?
8. What will follow the modality application?

Preparatory Treatment? Is your goal for the modality one that involves preparation for another activity within the Plan of Care? If the plan involves the reduction of muscle spasm with muscle stretching, and the modality selected is electrical stimulation, the treatment could potentially include the application of superficial heat to assist in the stretching activity to follow the electrical stimulation. If the plan involves increasing joint range of motion (ROM), and ultrasound is utilized to elevate tissue temperature, then the position of application should be adjusted to promote the stretching activity during the application of the ultrasound. This approach should assist in maximizing the effects of both the ultrasound and the stretching.[10]

Strong levels of electrical stimulation for the purpose of potentially increasing muscle strength may not be tolerated well by some patients. The clinician may want to consider applying ice massage to the skin that will underlie the electrodes. This may help to decrease the amount of discomfort and result in a greater response from the patient in terms of torque production.[22]

Follow-Up to an Activity or Treatment Approach? Treatment sessions may involve a wide variety of treatment techniques, some of which may result in some minor levels of discomfort to the patient. Therapeutic exercise may increase the amount of friction on the joint structures, which may result in some localized edema following the activity. Ice may be applied post exercise to reduce the localized inflammation that was just caused by the increased activity level of the injured area.[2] If the plan does involve the application of a modality to reduce inflammation after an activity, it is important for the clinician to explain the process to the patient so that the discomfort can be understood, and not offset fear of activity in the future.

When to Choose It? Patient Response to Treatment? Now that the modality has been selected, has been determined to be appropriate, is available for use, and is being used in combination with another modality in preparation for the next phase of the treatment session, how did the patient respond to your selection? Were there objective favorable responses to this approach? Objective and documentable responses were discussed in detail in Chapter 2. There should be an observable change in the condition of the patient in order for the application of this modality to be considered justified for future applications.

Functional Outcomes   Functional outcomes have emerged as one of the most important barometers for the continuation or termination of the use of a particular treatment approach. *Functional* is typically defined as something that has a useful purpose or special activity. It is designed, developed, and considered with reference to functioning. Function in this regard deals with the work to be performed by a person as a result of his or her trade, profession, position, or the like. In other words, functional refers to an individual's ability to perform an activity, an objective measure rather than a subjective measure of the individual's perception of his or her level of impairment. Outcome is defined as the result, consequence, or upshot of something. When the two words are linked, the definition becomes one of the results of a particular treatment approach with respect to the patient's ability to perform a specific task or set of tasks, as a result of the therapeutic intervention that has taken place.

If, for example, a patient had been referred for therapy after injuring himself or herself while lifting a heavy box at work, the patient's primary complaints may be paraspinal and radiating pain with muscle guarding and joint stiffness. Therapeutic intervention techniques that may be employed might include electrical stimulation, superficial heat, deep heat, traction, joint mobilization, and therapeutic exercises. After 2 weeks of treatment, the patient may still be complaining of pain in the lumbar area but now demonstrates an increase in mobility and increased endurance to therapeutic exercises, with documented isometric torque increases of 50% above the initial torque measurements. Objectively, the patient has improved but subjectively there has been little to no change. Based on current trends in reimbursment for therapeutic interventions, this patient is nearing the end of the course of therapy, and whatever modalities that have been used to date have probably contributed to the recovery, but now the course of treatment should be focused on improving the more objective aspects of function and not simply reducing reports of pain. The exception to this would be through the use of a portable stimulator to manage pain, which the patient would be instructed to use independently whenever pain interfered with the performance of an activity. At this point they should have discontinued the use of electrical stimulation in the clinic.

Did I Accomplish the Goals?   After utilizing a modality or set of modalities, it is important to revisit the original goals and whatever measures were utilized to establish them. If one of the original goals included muscle spasm reduction, and the assessment of the spasm involved palpation, pain scales, facial expression, performance of a functional activity, and tone assessment, then the same measures need to be re-employed. It is not enough to simply treat the identified goals with modalities or treatment protocols that have been utilized in that facility before for other patients who have had similar diagnoses or complaints. Clinicians must reassess after the application of each specific component of therapeutic intervention to determine whether or not the approach is having a positive impact on this patient. The question becomes one of "how will you know if you effected a change if you do not reassess, following the application of a given modality?" The reassessment should contain both subjective and objective measures of patient responses.

Reassessment is perhaps one of the most easily overlooked factors determining satisfaction for any clinician in the application of therapeutic interventions. If during the daily course of treatment the focus for the clinician pertains more to the number of patients and the amount of time available during the day, the focus of why they are doing what they are doing can become easily lost. The most obvious answer for why a particular modality has been selected for a patient is the indication presented by the patient. Whether or not the use of the given modality should be continued should be equally as obvious—simply, did it work? As clinicians become more involved in day-to-day routines, they may not be as able to answer the question of did the modality accomplish the goal unless they focus on outcome assessment (refer to Chapter 2 for more information regarding specific reassessment tools).

Would You Follow the Same Sequence Again?   This question is also linked to the outcome assessment of the course of care, but it pertains more specifically to the individual sequencing within the plan of care, with such questions as: "Should ice have been administered before or after the exercises?"; or "Should the stretching have taken place during the application of the ultrasound?" In order to state accurately whether or not the sequence of a set of given modalities for a patient is appropriate, the patient must be reassessed following the application of the modalities to determine whether or not they effected the desired change. If, for example, a patient had been referred to therapy with a cervical strain, and following an evaluation the therapist decided that for this patient, the plan of care would include: cervical traction, superficial heat, and deep heat with some stretching exercises and a home trial of a TENS unit to decrease pain and prevent the return of muscle guarding. The traction was applied first with a cervical hot pack placed on the cervical spine during the traction. The patient is then asked to sit up, is instructed in stretching exercises, and asked to dress and schedule an appointment later in the week.

The patient returns 2 days later and reports that he felt much worse after he left the first treatment than when he arrived. Should the course of treatment be stopped since the symptoms increased, or should the modalities be discontinued since they increased the patient's pain perceptions? It is impossible to answer either one of these questions accurately without looking more specifically into the course of events of the initial treatment. First of all, the traction and hot pack applications should have been followed by a reassessment of how the patient felt, and how much mobility was present. If the traction and superficial heat were sufficient to relieve the discomfort so that muscle guarding subsided, then maintenance of the mobility through the use of a home traction unit may have been a more appropriate recommendation. Perhaps the patient does not have a clear understanding of why things are being done and does not like the type of work that he does. Going to therapy represents an excuse from work, and the patient senses that clinicians in your facility will spend time with them listening to their complaints and trying to make them feel comfortable, based solely on their subjective complaints.

All of these factors contribute to whether or not the treatment sequence should be continued or repeated again as a potential option for other patients with similar complaints. Each patient represents an individual, with individual symptoms, perceptions of those symptoms, and a varied response to any therapeutic intervention dependent upon a wide variety of physiologic and psychologic characteristics. Successful therapeutic interventions rely heavily on acknowledgement of the differences, similarities and individual responses to treatment techniques employed in current day practice settings.

DOCUMENTATION

Documentation of any therapeutic intervention forms the historic basis of the success or failure of any technique. Documentation of any therapeutic treatment technique serves as the substantiation of the delivery of a treatment. In order for the documentation to be of use, it should contain all pertinent information regarding the treatment, so that the details of the treatment are evident to whoever reads it. This includes both subjective and objective findings regarding the patient, treatment approach, reassessment, and the plan for that patient.

SOAP NOTES

One format that is fairly common is the SOAP note format. SOAP is an acronym for subjective, objective, assessment, and plan. A SOAP note is a form of progress note to document both the treatment and the patient's responses to the treatment. This form of documentation is recorded in the patient's chart and becomes a permanent record of therapy for that patient. It is these progress notes that will answer the basic questions of how a patient responded to a given treatment technique when the chart is reviewed following the discharge of that patient from therapy. The chart should present a clear and concise record of exactly what was done and how the patient responded so that anyone reading the chart would understand exactly why the particular course of actions took place upon subsequent visits. Table 17–3 outlines the components of a SOAP note.

SUMMARY

A variety of treatment approaches have been discussed in detail throughout the text and reviewed briefly in this chapter. Each phase of the delivery of care must be looked at as a component of the overall care the patient is receiving in order to accomplish treatment goals. Appropriate delivery of patient care involves the participation of all of the members of the health care team and the patient. Without patient participation, the therapeutic intervention may be unsuccessful for that patient despite its documentation in the literature. There are many therapeutic tools that can be utilized to treat a specific condition; appropriate choices yield the best results for the patient. Clinical decision making regarding the selection and sequencing of therapeutic interventions is an ongoing process that must be documented in the patient's chart. Ultimately, the progress of the patient marks the success of the interventions.

DISCUSSION QUESTIONS

1. Give examples of the physical agent modalities presented that have common goals either as primary or secondary indications for them?

2. Why is there a distinction made regarding when a therapeutic modality is applied. Shouldn't the indications be universally constant regardless of sequencing? Why or why not?

3. In terminology that a patient would be able to comprehend, explain the relationship between pain and dysfunction.

Table 17–3 **SOAP Notes**

S=Subjective Subjective information refers to the information offered by the patient pertaining to how they "feel." Subjective information is influenced by personal biases and emotional background. It may encompass physical complaints and emotional or psychologic difficulties. The comments by the patient are typically entered into the patient record in quotation marks and identified by the phrase "the patient stated that . . ." Asking patients how they feel lets them report their perception of their current state, and can also orient the clinician as to what questions should be asked next.

O=Objective Objective information, unlike subjective information, is unbiased, impersonal, unprejudiced, and truly factual information. This is the portion of the documentation that includes all relative parameters of the treatment approach so that anyone reading the chart could precisely duplicate the treatment. Examples of objective entries for each modality are listed with the modality they pertain to:

Heat and Cold Modalities
  Treatment area as precisely as possible
  Treatment time
  Type of heat or cold
    hot pack, cold pack, ice pack, paraffin, shortwave diathermy, Fluidotherapy, cold, ice massage
  Parameters of treatment
    patient position, intensity (if applicable), duty factors (if applicable), treatment temperature (if applicable)
Ultrasound
  treatment area, e.g., right superior lateral epicondyle
  Patient position (if applicable, stretch or neutral)
  Treatment time
  Transducer size
  Coupling medium or technique (if other than acoustic gel or lotion)
  Type of ultrasound application
    frequency, duty factor, intensity (stated with either W/cm^2 or total power per ERA)
  Use of any pharmacologic agent? (if so, how was it applied?)
Ultraviolet
  Treatment Area
  MED calculation
  Patient position
  Distance from the source to the patient
  Incident angle of the light (if other than 90°)
  Model of the unit (if there is more than one unit in the department)
Laser
  Precise treatment area
  Treatment time
  Treatment technique (grid, sweep, etc.)
  Wavelength of the laser or active medium description (HeNe or GaAs)
  Tissue preparation if any
  Parameters
    continuous or pulsed
    power of the laser (1mW or greater)
Hydrotherapy
  Treatment area
  Treatment time
  Activities performed (if any)
    number or repetitions and stablization (if any)

Table 17–3   **SOAP Notes** (*Continued*)

devices utilized in the water (if any)
Type of hydrotherapy utilized
  tank or therapeutic pool
  transfer aides necessary ? (Hoyer or chair lift)
Temperature of the water
Agitation?
Turbulence? Pointed where?
Cleansing agents in the water? What and how much?
Traction
  Treatment area (cervical or lumbar)
  Treatment time
  Patient position
  Intermittent or continuous
    parameters: poundage, hold time, rest time, incremental
  Type of harness or straps: cervical halter or Saunders, etc.
CPM
  Treatment area
  Treatment time
  Patient position
  Type of device (brand name)
  Angle limitations of movement
  Speed of movement
Intermittent Compression
  Treatment area
  Treatment time
  Device utilized
  Settings: pressure, hold, rest, release pressure setting
  Patient positioning (if remarkable)
Electrical Stimulation
  Precise treatment area
  Treatment time
  Treatment goal (there may be several)
    electrode placement sites (per goal)
  Treatment parameters
    type of device
    on time, off time, ramp on or off, intensity (or goal)
  Specific treatment characteristics: with volitional contraction, against static
    resistance, or during ambulation
TENS Unit
  Name of unit for home use
  Parameter settings: frequency, pulse duration, modulation
  Electrode placement sites
  Type of electrodes utilized: self adhering brand name, carbon electrodes and
    gel with tape

A=Assessment   The assessment portion of the documentation deals with the patient's response to treatment. The tendency for the use of the phrase "Pt. tolerated treatment well" should be avoided, since the word "tolerated" gives little information regarding the response to treatment. To tolerate something means to bear up under or to endure without injurious effect; it offers no positive or specific negative comments regarding the preceding treatment approach.

P=Plan   The plan should involve a description of anticipated treatment sessions, based on the assessment of the current approach. It also includes information regarding potential discharge or new techniques or exercises for the next therapy session.

4. Why wouldn't it be more important to take however long a treatment session would take to apply every indicated modality for a given symptom than to conserve time?

5. What is the rationale for the statement that chronic conditions typically take longer to treat than acute problems? Is it a valid statement?

6. Of what importance is the medical stability of a patient, and how could it adversely affect the course of treatment?

7. Why was a section of the chapter devoted to availability of equipment? Shouldn't that be a nonissue with regard to treatment? If you need to utilize something with a given patient, then schedule a treatment time when it will be readily available for your use with that patient. How realistic is this scenario?

8. Objectivity of responses to therapeutic interventions is not always in synch with the patient's subjective complaints or responses; why would this occur? Discuss the influence of job-related injuries, lack of support of significant others, or full support of significant others, and the potential for secondary gain.

9. Identify positive functional outcomes that would be measurable. How would they be measured?

10. Documentation of treatment serves as a physical record of the course of events. Where would information regarding inappropriate responses to the treatment be documented and how should they be addressed within the progress note?

REFERENCES

1. Kloth, LC and Feedar, JA: Acceleration of wound healing with high voltage, monophasic, pulsed current. Phys Ther 68:503, 1988.

2. Griffin, JW, et al: Efficacy of high-voltage pulsed current for healing of pressure ulcers in patients with spinal cord injury. Phys Ther 71:433, 1991.

3. Gault, WR and Gatens, PF: Use of low intensity direct current in management of ischemic skin ulcers. Phys Ther 56:265, 1976.

4. Alon, G, Azariz, M, and Stein, H: Diabetic ulcer healing using high voltage TENS. Phys Ther 66:775, 1986.

5. Twist, DJ: Acrocyanosis in a spinal cord injured patient—effects of computer controlled neuromuscular electrical stimulation: A case report. Phys Ther 70: 45, 1990.

6. Griffin, JW, et al: Reduction of chronic posttraumatic hand edema: A comparison of high voltage pulsed current, intermittent pneumatic compression, and placebo treatments. Phys Ther 70:279, 1990.

7. Delitto A, et al: Electrically elicited co-contraction of thigh musculature after anterior cruciate ligament surgery. Phys Ther 68:45, 1988.

8. Delitto, A, et al: Electrical stimulation versus voluntary exercise in strengthening thigh musculature after anterior cruciate ligament surgery. Phys Ther 68:660, 1988.

9. Nitz, AJ and Dobner, JJ: High intensity eletrical stimulation effect on thigh musculature during immobilization for knee sprain. Phys Ther 67:219, 1987.

10.   Lentell, G, et al: The use of thermal agents to influence the effectiveness of a low-load prolonged stretch. J Orthop Sports Phys Ther 16:200, 1992.

11.   Lehmann, JF, et al: Effect of therapeutic temperatures on tendon extensibility. Arch Phys Med Rehabil 51:481, 1970.

12.   Warren, CG, Lehmann, JF, and Koblanski, JN: Heat and stretch procedures: An evaluation using rat tail tendon. Arch Phys Med Rehabil 57:122, 1976.

13.   Paris, DL, Baynes, F, and Gucker B: Effects of Neuroprobe in the treatment of second degree ankle inversion sprains. Phys Ther 63:35, 1983.

14.   Melzack, R, Vetere, P, and Finch, L: Transcutaneous electrical nerve stimulation for low back pain. Phys Ther 63:489, 1983.

15.   Brill, MM and Whiffen, JR: Application of 24-hour burst TENS in a back school. Phys Ther 65:1365, 1985.

16.   Longobardi, AG, et al: Effects of auricular transcutaneous electrical nerve stimulation on distal extremity pain: A pilot study. Phys Ther 69:10, 1989.

17.   Mannheimer, JS, and Lampe, GN: Pain and TENS in pain management. In Mannheimer JS and Lampe GN (eds): Clinical Transcutaneous Electrical Nerve Stimulation. FA Davis, Philadelphia, 1984, pp 7–10.

18.   Waddell, G, and Richardson J: Observation of overt pain behaviour by physicians during routine clinical examination of patients with low back pain. Psychosom Res 36:77, 1992.

19.   Vlaeyen, JWS, et al: Assessment of the components of observed chronic pain behavior: The checklist for interpersonal pain behavior (CHIP). Pain 43:337, 1990.

20.   Herrara-Lasso, I, et al: Comparative effectiveness of packages of treatment including ultrasound or transcutaneous electrical nerve stimulation in painful shoulder syndrome. Physiother Can 79:251, 1993.

21.   Soderberg, GL: Skeletal muscle function. In Currier, DP and Nelson, RM (eds): Dynamics of Human Biologic Tissues. FA Davis, Philadelphia, 1992, pp 92–93.

22.   Miller, CR and Webers, RL: The effects of ice massage on an individual's tolerance level to electrical stimulation. J Orthop Sports Phys Ther 12:105, 1990.

SUGGESTED READINGS

1.   Kettenbach, G: Writing SOAP Notes. FA Davis, Philadelphia, 1990.

2.   Daulong, MR and Nye, MF: Issues and trends in reimbursement. In Matthews J (ed): Practice Issues in Physical Therapy. Slack Inc., Thorofare, NJ, 1989.

3.   Palmer, JL and Toms, JE: Manual for Functional Training, ed 3. FA Davis, Philadelphia, 1992, pp 305–331.

4.   Stolov, WC, Cole, TM, and Tobis, JS: Evaluation of the patient; goniometry, muscle testing. In Krusen, FH, Kottke, FJ, and Elwood PM (eds): Handbook of Physical Medicine & Rehabilitation, ed 2. WB Saunders, Philadelphia, 1971, pp 17–87.

Index

An "f" following a page number indicates a figure; a "t" following a page number indicates a table.